T0123025

Artificial Hearts

Artificial Hearts

The Allure and Ambivalence of a Controversial Medical Technology

Shelley McKellar

Johns Hopkins University Press
Baltimore

Johns Hopkins University Press
2715 North Charles Street
Baltimore, Maryland 21218-4363
www.press.jhu.edu

Library of Congress Cataloging-in-Publication Data

Names: McKellar, Shelley, author.
Title: Artificial hearts : the allure and ambivalence of a controversial medical technology /
    Shelley McKellar.
Description: Baltimore, Maryland : Johns Hopkins University Press, 2017. | Includes
    bibliographical references and index.
Identifiers: LCCN 2017008834 | ISBN 9781421423555 (hardcover : alk. paper) |
    ISBN 9781421423562 (electronic) | ISBN 1421423553 (hardcover : alk. paper) |
    ISBN 1421423561 (electronic)
Subjects: | MESH: Heart, Artificial—history | History, 20th Century | History,
    21st Century | United States
Classification: LCC RD598.35.A78 | NLM WG 11 AA1 | DDC 617.4/120592—dc23
LC record available at https://lccn.loc.gov/2017008834

A catalog record for this book is available from the British Library.

*Special discounts are available for bulk purchases of this book. For more information, please
contact Special Sales at 410-516-6936 or specialsales@press.jhu.edu.*

Johns Hopkins University Press uses environmentally friendly book materials,
including recycled text paper that is composed of at least 30 percent post-consumer
waste, whenever possible.

CONTENTS

List of Illustrations and Tables   *vii*

Acknowledgments   *ix*

Introduction. Fighting Heart Disease with Machines and Devices   1

1 Multiple Approaches to Building Artificial Hearts: Technological Optimism and Political Support in the Early Years   29

2 Dispute and Disappointment: Heart Transplantation and Total Artificial Heart Implant Cases in the 1960s   60

3 Technology and Risk: Nuclear-Powered Artificial Hearts and Medical Device Regulation   95

4 Media Spotlight: The Utah Total Artificial Heart and the Charge of Bioethics   123

5 Clinical and Commercial Rewards: Ventricular Assist Devices   180

6 Securing a Place: Therapeutic Clout and Second-Generation VADs   211

7 Artificial Hearts for the Twenty-First Century   240

Abbreviations   *267*

Notes   *269*

Index   *339*

PLATES *Color illustrations follow page 130*

1. A woman's body with superimposed replaceable organs and tissues, 1965.
2. Six air-driven devices designed to replace or assist damaged hearts, under development during the early to mid 1960s.
3. Eight experimental total artificial hearts, dating from 1957 to 1981.
4. *Life* magazine cover featuring the feud between Houston surgeons Michael DeBakey and Denton Cooley, April 1970.
5. *Life* magazine cover displaying the Jarvik-7 total artificial heart, September 1981.
6. Willebrordus Meuffels, in the operating room, implanted with an Akutsu III total artificial heart, September 1981.
7. Dr. Tetsuzo Akutsu and the Akutsu III total artificial heart, September 1981.
8. *Newsweek* magazine cover showing the AbioCor total artificial heart, June 2001.

FIGURES

The placement of a total artificial heart in the body. 3
The placement of a left ventricular assist device in the body. 4
Drs. Willem Kolff and Tetsuzo Akutsu examine their experimental mechanical heart, 1957. 34
Dr. Michael DeBakey and President Lyndon B. Johnson, 1964. 44
Dr. Adrian Kantrowitz and his brother Arthur examine their "booster heart" device, 1966. 50
Dr. Michael DeBakey and pump implant patient Esperanza Del Valle Vasquez, 1966. 53
Drs. Christiaan Barnard, Michael DeBakey, and Adrian Kantrowitz discuss the challenges of heart transplantation, 1967. 70
The Liotta-Cooley artificial heart, 1969. 77
Drs. Denton Cooley and Domingo Liotta with artificial heart recipient Haskell Karp, 1969. 78
Dr. Denton Cooley at a press conference, 1969. 88
Dr. Norman Shumway speaks to journalists, 1968. 89
Drs. Willem Kolff and Denton Cooley admire the Liotta-Cooley artificial heart, about mid-1970s. 93
Schematic diagram of the Atomic Energy Commission nuclear-powered heart. 103
Illustration of a nuclear-powered heart-assist device, sponsored by the National Heart and Lung Institute, positioned in a calf. 104
Dr. Willem Kolff, standing next to a display of artificial hearts developed in his laboratory. 127

Drs. Don B. Olsen, Willem Kolff, and Robert Jarvik, posing with two Jarvik-7 artificial hearts.   131

Dr. William DeVries, holding a Jarvik-7 artificial heart next to a model of the human heart.   139

Artificial heart recipient Barney Clark with his wife Una Loy, December 1982.   142

William Schroeder's diseased heart is placed on a tray next to a sterilized Jarvik-7 artificial heart, November 25, 1984.   149

Artificial heart recipient William Schroeder visits his hometown of Jasper, Indiana, August 4, 1985.   150

Artificial heart recipient Michael Drummond with Dr. Jack Copeland and others at Tucson's University of Arizona Medical Center, 1985.   157

Dr. William S. Pierce, holding a paracorporeal ventricular assist device developed at the Pennsylvania State University College of Medicine.   186

Dr. Peer Portner talks to the press about the Novacor left ventricular assist system, 2001.   193

Former vice president Dick Cheney holds up the battery and control unit of his implanted HeartMate II left ventricular assist device, September 2011.   212

Drs. Richard Wampler and O. H. Frazier with Hemopump patient Herb Kranich, April 1988.   223

The HeartMate XVE Left Ventricular Assist System and the HeartMate II Left Ventricular Assist Device.   225

The Jarvik 2000 Ventricular Assist Device.   229

Dr. Gerson Rosenberg, holding the Penn State Electric Total Artificial Heart.   242

The AbioCor implantable replacement heart.   244

Artificial heart recipient Robert Tools with Dr. Robert Dowling, July 31, 2001.   247

Artificial heart recipient Tom Christerson with Drs. Laman Gray and Robert Dowling, March 12, 2002.   248

The SynCardia temporary Total Artificial Heart.   255

TABLES

5.1. Selected pulsatile VADs and FDA regulatory status.   196

6.1. Selected continuous-flow VADs and FDA regulatory status.   231

7.1. Selected total artificial hearts and FDA regulatory status.   254

This book reflects my interest in medical artifacts and exploring history through objects. The "things" of the past have always intrigued me. I like to wonder about and handle objects, speculating about their use and ownership, as an access point to better understand people and their practices in the past. Anyone privileged to visit the Smithsonian Institution's collection storage areas knows that there is no shortage of medical artifacts to inspire a research project. Artificial hearts, however, are a real showstopper. The mechanical hearts implanted in Haskell Karp (1969), Murray Haydon (1985), Michael Drummond (1985), and Robert Tools (2001) are among the more popular artifacts at the Smithsonian's National Museum of American History, which houses an impressive cardiac device collection. I, too, was drawn to these objects—enthralled with the design and construction of these devices, amazed that such technology might work, and a bit awestruck to be handling the actual artificial hearts once implanted in patients.

I was introduced to artificial hearts through Project Bionics, a collaborative history project of the American Society for Artificial Internal Organs, the National Library of Medicine at the National Institutes of Health, and the Smithsonian Institution's National Museum of American History, which was initiated in 2000 to document and preserve the rich history of the development of artificial organs. Formerly in real danger of becoming lost from the historical record, the papers, devices, and recollections of many artificial organ pioneers are now safeguarded in national repositories because of this project. I am indebted to Ramunas (Ray) Kondratas, Robert (Bob) Bartlett and Jean Kantrowitz for selecting a Canadian historian with a new PhD to participate in this project in its early years. I greatly enjoyed being part of this documentary history project; it was a wonderful opportunity to capture the history of artificial organs from the involved participants, researchers, and clinicians, and I came to appreciate and respect the commitment, ability, and compassion of many individuals working in the field. For the many personal conversations, lab visits, and project activities, I thank the Project Bionics Working Group (circa 2000–2005) of Bob Bartlett, Judy Chelnick, Arthur Ciarkowski, Walter Dembitsky, Brack Hattler, Jean Kantrowitz, Ray Kondratas, Mark Kurusz, Paul Malchesky, Don B. Olsen, George Pantalos, Steven Phillips, Peer Portner, W. Gerald Rainer, Wayne Richenbacher, Gerson Rosenberg, Paul Theerman, and John Watson. The energy and passion of Bob and Jean in leading this successful project cannot be overstated; both of you are truly remarkable and I learned much from each of you.

I also thank other members of the American Society for Artificial Internal Organs who kindly took time to speak with me at various scientific meetings. I shall never forget the meeting of the society at which I met artificial organs pioneer Willem Kolff, then in his 90s, who asked if I was "that lady interested in history." After I nodded, Dr. Kolff smiled and, with both hands, flung open his suit jacket to show me his most recent device prototype—a wearable artificial lung—and proceeded to tell me how it worked. One of the advantages of doing contemporary history is the privilege of such interactions, discussing past events directly with the historical participants, grasping the different personalities at play, and witnessing professional exchanges and research dissemination at such meetings. I am grateful for these experiences, both formal and informal, and applaud ongoing Project Bionics activities, such as the recent video interviews conducted by Steven Phillips and others, that serve to retain the device innovation stories and perspectives of the historical participants for posterity.

Over the years, I have benefited from the tremendous generosity and knowledge of curators, librarians, archivists, and others who have provided me with research materials. I have many people to thank for this kind of assistance. I thank Ray Kondratas and Judy Chelnick for providing me with access to the Smithsonian Institution's collections and imparting their knowledge about working with objects, interviewing historical participants, and conducting artifact research. Judy, I am enormously grateful to you for sharing your significant knowledge of the cardiac device collection and supporting my research with unwavering enthusiasm. From unending object questions to last-minute image requests to research trip accommodation, I am deeply indebted to you. The History of Medicine Division at the National Library of Medicine holds numerous manuscript collections that were central to my project, and I thank Paul Theerman (now at the New York Academy of Medicine), John Rees, Susan Speaker, and Steven Greenberg for making this material available to me, whether the records were fully processed or not. Thank you to numerous kind and knowledgeable individuals at various university and national repositories that I visited during this book project, notably Stan Larson, Louise Crouse, Sara Davis, Roy Webb, Krissy Giacoletto, and Julia Huddleston at the Special Collections, University of Utah; Kirk Baddley and Clint Bailey at the University of Utah Archives; Lois DeBakey at the Baylor College of Medicine; Philip Montgomery at the John P. McGovern Historical Collections and Research Center, Texas Medical Center Library; Fred Lautzenhesier at the archives of the Cleveland Clinic Foundation; Daniel Hartwig at the Special Collections and University Archives, Stanford University; Michael Kemezis at the Gordon Library, Worcester Polytechnic Institute; Meredith Weber at the Penn State University Archives; Jennifer Johnson at the Office of History and Heritage Resources at the US Department of Energy; and Marjorie Ciarlante at the National Archives and Records Administration. For anyone with an interest in this topic, who happens to be in Houston, I recommend visiting the DeBakey Library and Museum at the Baylor College of Medicine as well as the Wallace D. Wilson Museum at the Texas Heart Institute, which displays historical documents, photos, and objects referred to in this book.

I would like to thank several people for responding to specific research queries at key moments in the writing of the book. To Jodi Koste at the Special Collections and Archives at Virginia Commonwealth University, Michele Lyons at the Office of NIH History and Stetten Museum, Susan Speaker and John Rees at the National Library of Medicine, and Suzanne Junod and Tara Smith at the Food and Drug

Administration, thanks for sending me research material electronically and providing long-distance assistance! Geoffrey Stewart and Carlen Ng provided research assistance during the early stages of this project. At Western Libraries, Elizabeth Mantz never flinched at my "research help" questions and found ways to access material, for which I am truly grateful.

Thank you to everyone who provided me with historical images for these pages. Several of these individuals are listed above, but the following persons are included as well: Linden Emerson and Ken Hoge at the Public Affairs Office at the Texas Heart Institute; JoAnn Pospipil and Tiffany Monet Schreiber at the Baylor College of Medicine Archives; Margaret Harman and Alexis Percle at the Lyndon Baines Johnson Library and Museum; Mark Wilson and Susan Brailey at *Physics Today;* Katie Maass, Jeb Zirato, and Richard Smith at the University of Arizona Health Services; Janelle Drumwright at SynCardia Systems LLC; Barbara Mackovic and Jill Scoggins at the University of Louisville Health Science Center; Robert Jarvik at Jarvik Heart Inc.; Dana Gordon and Joelle Sedlmeyer at Getty Images; Matt Lutts at Associated Press; and St. Jude Medical Inc. I thank Charlotte Strode for granting me permission to publish the photos taken by her late father, William Strode. I thank Martha Saxton for granting me permission to publish the photos taken by her late husband, Enrico Ferorelli, which are now being processed as the Ferorelli Photographic Archive under Amy Bowman's direction at the Dolph Briscoe Center for American History at the University of Texas at Austin. I thank Kathilyn Allewell, Media Specialist at the University of Western Ontario, for her terrific digital skills in the preparation of images for this book.

Throughout this project, I greatly appreciated my conversations with clinicians, researchers, patients, historians, bioethicists, and other individuals interested in artificial hearts and the issues related to the development of this technology. Thank you all for your enthusiasm and engagement, and in particular those individuals who clarified medical or legal details, discussed thorny clinical issues, read draft chapters and book proposals, assisted with securing image use permissions, and donated historical material to appropriate collections. Thank you Bob Bartlett, Joanna Bourke, Gordon Campbell, Judy Chelnick, Renée Fox, Bruce Fye, Bert Hansen, Ray Kondratas, Rande Kostal, Barron Lerner, Francine McKenzie, David Nagpal, Stuart Smith, Jane Tucker, and Bill Turkel. A shout-out to two physicians, both experts in their fields, who gave me their time and wisdom at key points in the book's preparation: Bob Bartlett, a surgeon and the medical researcher who developed ECMO technology, read an early draft of the entire manuscript, correcting my errors in describing some surgical techniques and explaining how devices move from the research laboratory to the medical marketplace. Bruce Fye, a cardiologist and a historian, read a later draft of the entire manuscript, also with a sharp eye to medical details, and shared his vast knowledge of the history of cardiology and cardiac surgery. Thank you both for spending hours on the phone discussing my work, taking time away from your summer and Thanksgiving holidays!

I am sincerely grateful for financial support of this project from the Associated Medical Services (AMS), a key sponsor of medical history research and activities in Canada. The impact of AMS is significant and wide-reaching within the history of medicine community in this country. An early research grant-in-aid award from the AMS–Hannah Institute for the History of Medicine launched this artificial heart research project. I thank AMS for its support of the Hannah Chair in the History of Medicine at Schulich School of Medicine and Dentistry at the University of Western Ontario, which allows me to pursue my research. As well, I would like to acknowledge the assistance of the J. B. Smallman Publication Fund and the Faculty of Social Science, both of the University of Western Ontario, for publication and research support.

Portions of chapter 2 were previously published in my article "Clinical Firsts: Christiaan Barnard's Heart Transplant Operations," *New England Journal of Medicine.* Copyright © 2017 Massachusetts Medical Society. Reprinted with permission. An early version of chapter 3 appeared as my article "Negotiating Risk: The Failed Development of Atomic Hearts in America, 1967–1977," *Technology and Culture* 54, no. 1 (2013): 1–39, copyright © 2013 The Society for the History of Technology. It is used with permission of Johns Hopkins University Press. Portions of chapter 4 were previously published in my article "The Promissory Nature of Artificial Hearts," *The Lancet,* 2017. Reprinted with permission. Chapter 6 includes excerpts from my chapter "Disruptive Potential: The 'Landmark' REMATCH Trial, Left Ventricular Assist Device (LVAD) Technology and the Surgical Treatment of Heart Failure in the United States," in *Technological Change in Modern Surgery: Historical Perspectives on Innovation,* ed. Thomas Schlich and Christopher Crenner (Rochester, NY: University of Rochester Press, 2017), 129–55.

I enjoyed working with everyone at the Johns Hopkins University Press. Jackie Wehmueller was always encouraging to me. Thank you to Matt McAdam, Catherine Goldstead, Juliana McCarthy, and Kim Johnson for their editorial guidance and for looking after me so well. I sincerely thank the anonymous peer reviewer assigned by the Press who read through each chapter very closely and provided substantial, valuable comments to improve the manuscript. I am truly grateful to Lois Crum, a freelance copyeditor for Johns Hopkins, for polishing this manuscript with her word skill and reader-friendly suggestions. Thank you to Alexa Selph for creating the book index.

Not all the individuals whom I have acknowledged may agree with my conclusions, and they are certainly not to be held responsible for any of my interpretations, errors, or omissions.

I dedicate this book to Doug and Delaney. Thank you for your patience and love.

Artificial Hearts

Fighting Heart Disease with
Machines and Devices

It [artificial heart] is amazing. I haven't felt this good in years. . . . What you're hearing is the sound of life.

Kathleen Shores, total artificial heart recipient (2012)

Heart failure sufferer Kathleen Shores battled extreme fatigue, dizzy spells, heart palpitations, shortness of breath, and bouts of edema (fluid retention) that prevented her from driving, walking, and sometimes eating, before she had an artificial heart implant. In November 2012, Shores lay dying of heart failure in the intensive care unit at Froedtert Hospital in Milwaukee, Wisconsin. Refusing to surrender, she permitted her surgeon, Dr. Robert Love, to remove her diseased heart and replace it with an artificial heart. The mechanical device sustained Shores's life, and within weeks she was back home resuming daily activities with her family, tending to her teenage children, exercising, and shopping, while waiting for a donor heart.[1] Heart failure patient Troy Golden in Oklahoma City would also have died if not for the availability of an artificial heart, which kept him alive for an additional 15 months. Time had run out for Golden, but a strong desire to live trumped his anxieties about receiving an artificial heart. No longer at death's doorstep, Golden returned home after his device implant and resumed preaching at his church. According to Golden's surgeon, Dr. James Long, it was "almost like performing a resurrection . . . taking someone who was checking out and giving them life."[2] However, the technology was not a cure; it provided extra months for patients to spend more time with family or, for the lucky ones, to receive a donor heart. For Shores, the device served as a bridge, for one year, until she underwent a successful heart transplantation.[3] Golden died with his artificial heart, still waiting for a donor heart, from other disease complications.[4]

Artificial hearts are life-sustaining but imperfect devices with a controversial history but also ongoing relevance regarding the desirability and sustainability of expensive end-stage disease therapies. Their clinical use elicits questions of "success," costs, hopes, fears, and more in a high-technology medical world. Do these devices "save lives" (as a curative fix) or "buy time" (as an expensive, makeshift measure prolonging the inevitable) for end-stage heart failure patients? Are the two aims mutually exclusive? Is one intention less valid? For decades relegated to science fiction and outlandish notions of bionic people, artificial hearts faced seemingly insurmountable problems of device design, biomaterials, and power sources. Building mechanical hearts to replicate the human heart was a daunting bioengineering undertaking. By the twenty-first century, implantable mechanical hearts were a clinical reality, and for some individuals, like Shores and Golden, these devices extended their lives in a meaningful way. These patient experiences embodied the near-ideal scenario that had been envisioned by device researchers and hoped for by medical and public audiences for decades, and they can be situated on one end of the implant patient "success" spectrum.

It was clinical necessity that prompted researchers to build artificial hearts, as Americans battled an epidemic of heart disease in the twentieth century. For decades, the development of artificial hearts continued, sustained by dedicated and passionate investigators, crucial US federal government support, and key industry collaboration that converged during a period when Americans speculated about the potential of organ replacement in end-stage disease scenarios. The values and expectations that were articulated and mobilized by American medicine and society played an influential role in the negotiated development of this technology by stakeholders, advocates, and objectors who managed enthusiasm and disappointment over the devices to sustain or challenge mechanical heart research programs. The history of artificial hearts is fraught with controversy, and its clinical realization was never certain. In 2017, artificial hearts are part of the therapeutic armamentarium in specialized heart centers—alongside pacemakers, defibrillators, artificial valves, stents, and other devices—in the broader fight against cardiac disease. Smaller, more durable artificial hearts are under development, which, along with improved clinical management of heart failure patients, will almost certainly contribute to the greater use of these devices in the future. A historical perspective reveals that, after more than 60 years of development, many of the technological, socioeconomic, and bioethical issues that dog this imperfect technology have been ongoing and at times have come close to burying the technology. In the end, it was the promise of this technology that offset those issues, persisting during cyclical, spirited debates within medical circles and the public media.

This history of artificial hearts is about the allure and ambivalence that surrounded the technology, the interpretative flexibility of "success" that nourished the promise of these devices, and the persistent uncertainty regarding their efficacy and effectiveness that elicited scientific and public discussions. The promissory nature of the technology as a curative fix for heart failure aligned with the view of the body as an entity of replacement parts. Who would not want a life-saving, off-the-shelf device fix for a loved one dying of heart failure? Medical and public debate evolved from the desirability of artificial hearts to the feasibility and sustainability of such expensive end-stage disease therapies. The discussion of "could we do it" became one of "should we do it" as a greater number of stakeholders, including medical practitioners, politicians, bioethicists, patients, and the public, weighed in after often-sensational clinical cases.

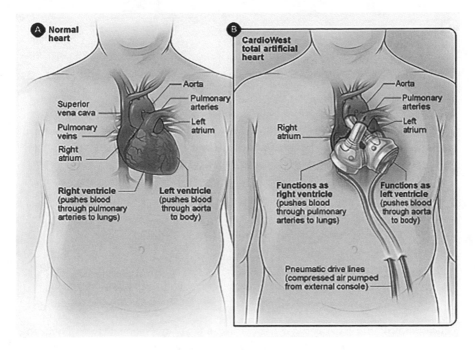

The placement of a total artificial heart in the body. National Heart, Lung, and Blood Institute, National Institutes of Health, US Department of Health and Human Services.

The term *artificial hearts* refers to a variety of mechanical devices that work to increase blood flow and to sustain life for the end-stage heart failure patient. The heart works like a pump—it moves blood entering the right side of the heart (the right atrium and ventricle) to the lungs to become oxygenated, and then through the left side (the left atrium and ventricle) and out into other parts of the body, from which it returns to the heart. The left ventricle works the hardest among the four chambers of the heart, as it propels blood out of the heart to nourish tissues and organs in the body with oxygen-rich blood (systemic circulation). In the cases of Shores and Golden, both sides of the heart were irreversibly damaged; they were experiencing biventricular failure. Each person's heart was removed and replaced with a SynCardia Total Artificial Heart. More common is left ventricular impairment, for which surgeons may recommend ventricular assist devices (VADs), or partial artificial hearts, that attach directly to the weakened ventricle to assist in pumping. In VAD cases, the diseased native heart is not removed.

Different heart failure patients require different cardiac devices, depending on their needs. Postoperative cardiac surgical patients may need temporary support until their repaired heart recovers, other cardiac patients may need longer-term support

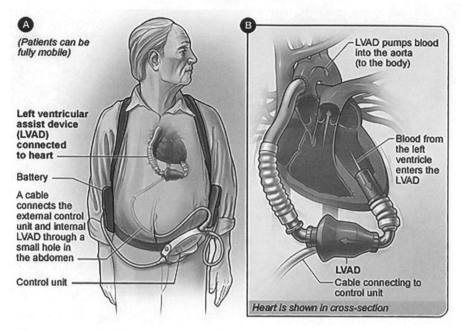

The placement of a left ventricular assist device in the body. National Heart, Lung, and Blood Institute, National Institutes of Health, US Department of Health and Human Services.

while waiting for a heart transplant, and still other patients, ineligible for a transplant, may need permanent replacement or support of their severely damaged heart to ward off death. The cardiac output (the amount of blood expelled) of a healthy adult heart is about 5 to 6 liters (less than 2 gallons) per minute while resting. When exercising, the heart needs to generate three to four times that cardiac output. When a patient's cardiac output lowers to about 2 liters per minute despite maximal medical therapy (cardiogenic shock), clinicians sometimes suggest mechanical support to keep patients alive and revive failing organs. In this situation, there is a spectrum of devices available to assist or take over blood circulation: smaller pumps restore cardiac output up to 5 liters per minute; stronger VADs pump 4 to 6 liters of blood per minute; and more robust total artificial hearts (TAHs) generate a cardiac output of 7 to 9 liters per minute.[5] The idea of pumping blood and restoring life with a mechanical device—connecting patients to machines situated outside, or sometimes inside, the body—may have initially seemed far-fetched. In the twentieth century, however, the allure of medical technology and the idea of the rebuilt body had taken hold in American society and medicine with the clinical use of artificial kidneys, artificial heart valves, synthetic grafts and tissue, cochlear implants, and other mechanical devices.

Spare Parts for People

The media played a notable role in promoting American fascination with medical devices and the prospect of a rebuilt body. In 1965 *Life* magazine heralded the time as an "era of rebuilt people" and published a two-page color spread of a woman's body superimposed with replaceable organs or tissues, including transplanted kidneys and livers, electronic bladder stimulators and blood pressure regulators, and more.[6] Similarly, in 1989 *National Geographic* editors published an article entitled "Rebuilding the Body from Nose to Toes," with photos illustrating how joints and bones may be replaced with titanium, plastic, and ceramic parts, while silicone rubber and Dacron may substitute for tendons, arteries, and cartilage.[7] In 2013 a Smithsonian Institution documentary presented Rich Walker and Matthew Godden's bionic man, an android of prosthetic human body parts and artificial organs donated by various scientific laboratories.[8] Several devices remained experimental, such as an implantable artificial kidney (that would make hospital dialysis treatments unnecessary), while other bionic body parts were more common clinically, such as prosthetic hips and cochlear implants. Is there anything about humans that bioengineers are not striving to mimic, replace, or alter? Such popular imaginings of rebuilt bodies tantalized the public about the possibility of replacement technology. In this setting, artificial hearts buoyed between investigational lab prototypes and clinically viable devices.

Throughout the history of this experimental technology, the media documented the varied experiences of artificial heart patients, shaping public understanding. Some of the more well-known heart failure patients who received mechanical pumps include former US vice president Dick Cheney, Robert Tools, Peter Houghton, Michael Drummond, Barney Clark, Haskell Karp, and Esperanza del Valle Vasquez. These individuals garnered a certain public profile because of their heart problems and their choices to be implanted with artificial hearts, but not all had positive experiences. In 2011, Cheney publicly demonstrated how his HeartMate II pump worked, sometimes disconnecting his pump from its power source and setting off alarms on the unit that flustered his interviewers, before reconnecting.[9] Journalists reported how Robert Tools, who received an AbioCor TAH in 2001, left the hospital on a day trip to White Castle to eat a hamburger. (The report was intended to demonstrate patient improvement, of course, but one certainly queries the food choice and spots the disconnect between therapeutic and prevention strategies in the battle against heart disease.) Photos of Tools, smiling and enjoying such daily pleasures with relatively free mobility, implied that a successful recovery was at hand.[10] In sharp contrast was the media's reporting of the bumpy medical course of Barney Clark, who survived 112 days with an implanted Utah artificial heart, connected by drivelines to an external 418-pound pneumatic drive unit, at the University of Utah Medical Center in Salt Lake City in 1982–83.[11]

These heart failure patients were the "sickest of the sick," those who had exhausted all conventional therapies and now faced imminent death. Significant morbidity and mortality accompanied early artificial heart implant cases, because of the compromised organs and additional medical problems incurred from the progression of heart failure in these very sick patients. The therapeutic goal of artificial hearts was to extend the life of a near-death heart failure patient by weeks or possibly months by mechanically restoring adequate blood circulation. The degree to which life was sustained, however, did not always match the quality of life that patients may have expected an artificial heart implant to provide. In 1981 Houston patient Willebrordus Meuffels was, at best, only semiconscious for the two days that he lived with an Akutsu III TAH in his chest, and he died a week after undergoing a heart transplant.[12] In 2002 James Quinn, after battling complications for weeks and never fully being discharged from hospital care, told Philadelphia reporters that he regretted his decision to undergo an AbioCor TAH implant.[13] Technological device challenges and patient postoperative care remained difficult despite reported success in thwarting death for these patients. The different groups and communities—stakeholders, supporters, and objectors—who weighed in on the use of artificial hearts held varying definitions of success, thus fueling debates about the continued development of the devices.

With the aid of medical technology, physicians are able to diagnose and treat many diseases. Diagnostic technologies such as x-ray, ultrasound, and magnetic resonance imaging machines permit physicians to see into the human body, while such therapeutic technologies as mechanical respirators, artificial kidney machines, and cardiac pacemakers replicate the function of damaged organs in the body. Medical practitioners work to identify diseased parts and to restore their functions, reflecting the conceptualization of the body as an entity made of organs, bones, and tissues with specific structural and functional roles. Fixing damaged body parts sometimes has meant replacement. As shown by medical historians Thomas Schlich, David Hamilton, Susan Lederer, and others, transplantation became "the technological fix of choice" for any number of medical issues tied to organ malfunction in the twentieth century.[14] Transplantation bolstered the idea that body parts were interchangeable. This concept of replaceable body organs supported the development of mechanical parts, which was boosted once again when it became apparent that the supply of human organs would never meet the demand.

The possibility that artificial organs could replace damaged human parts invigorated a surgical imaginary that did not necessarily reflect contemporary surgical reality. Still it encouraged an influential core group of surgical and bioengineering researchers to persist with their research when many scientists dismissed artificial hearts as fanciful and impractical.[15] As Lederer argues, blood transfusion and organ transplantation were radical treatment approaches for technical and sociocultural reasons. Replacing human blood or organs required invasive and dangerous surgical procedures and rattled some cultural, ethnic, and religious beliefs. Lederer's work shows that the American public's lack of reluctance to exchange body parts was partly due to the promissory science that framed these procedures as early as the beginning of the twentieth century.[16] This history of artificial hearts extends Lederer's work on public enthusiasm for replacement procedures along the themes of surgical imaginary and remaking the human body. By the mid-twentieth century, the visions of physician-researchers Michael DeBakey and Willem Kolff found support within the larger cultural context of understanding the body as composed of replaceable parts and within the growing technological imperative in medicine. At this time, American society accepted the use of medical technology as both diagnostic and therapeutic tools to fight disease, to alleviate pain, and to extend life.

Still, not all organs are considered equal in terms of their function or perceived value for individuals. An implicit hierarchy of organs, led by the brain and the heart in comparison to the spleen or the appendix, caused some individuals to pause before parting with some of their native bits. Are all parts of the body equally replaceable? Culturally influenced, traditional views of the heart as an organ of mystery, or the seat of the soul, or the holder of one's individual personhood and emotional core were not totally eclipsed by the new reductionist and mechanical view of this organ as a replaceable pump in Western medicine. As in discussions of brain death at the same time, which also addressed concepts of the body and personhood, there emerged some questioning within the medical community and the general public. Not all individuals reduced the heart to a simple pump, thus resisting this technological body concept.

The early clinical use of artificial hearts produced ambiguous results, raising strong concerns and vocal opposition in American society. Would the vision of replaceable parts match the reality? If an artificial heart could be built, would it work as well as the native one? The device needed to be biocompatible, interacting with the body and not fighting against it, moving blood at the right speed—not too slow, with the risk of clotting, nor too fast, risking blood damage— to nourish organs and tissue sufficiently. Mechanical failure of the device would almost certainly result in patient death. Questions of efficacy (did it work?) and effectiveness (did it help patients?) were debated within medical and related political communities, while bioethicists, social scientists, and others also questioned the expansion of mechanical organ replacement on socioeconomic and moral grounds. Practical concerns of cost and quality of life for implant patients added to rising doubts that medical science could actually build affordable, acceptable mechanical hearts. This debate exploded after the permanent TAH cases of the 1980s.

In 1988 a *New York Times* editorial labeled the artificial heart "The Dracula of Medical Technology," applauding the recent decision by NIH administrators to cancel funding for its development after "this Dracula of a program [had already] sucked $240 million out of the National Heart, Lung and Blood Institute."[17] This contemptuous moniker—The Dracula of Medical Technology—stuck with the device for many years. Despite the dramatic stories of surgeons rebuilding bodies and patients warding off death with an artificial heart, could a mechanical device truly replace the human heart? Various stakeholders in the development of artificial hearts remained steadfast in their commitment to develop this technology, supported by both public and private funding. The American public, facing increasing reports of an epidemic of heart disease in the country and strongly believing in American technological superiority and fixes, hoped that artificial hearts were possible. Politicians, bioethicists, academics, and industry people weighed in at different times on the issue, their views often amplified by journalists. Even within the medical profession, opinions about the clinical use of artificial hearts differed. Many medical practitioners and health policymakers asked, Where best should we direct our attention and resources—preventive measures or therapeutic options? There emerged the debate that there might be a limit—a technological, economical, or ethical limit—to what therapeutic devices could or should do in medicine. Expensive, high-technology fixes like artificial hearts allude to the failure of prevention but also to the expectation of curative, or at least life-sustaining, therapy to treat end-stage disease. American values and structures supported technological fixes and, in general, played to both therapeutic and preventive sides of disease management. In the case of artificial hearts, proposals of sidelining this technology in favor of greater support for preventive strategies were hotly debated, reflecting strong and vocal expectations of treatment as well as an awareness of the growing burden of chronic and degenerative disease.

Amid uncertainty and dispute, the development of artificial hearts openly confronted the role played by technology in our understanding of disease and its treatment. To what extent did the technological imperative in medicine promote the building and use of artificial hearts? How long and at what cost would medical researchers and the public persist with the artificial heart's development? Researchers pursued multiple lines of investigation simultaneously that led sometimes to incremental gains and other times to dead ends. Clinical achievements and setbacks were duly reported at professional medical meetings, while patient triumphs and disappointments made media headlines. Decades of witnessing the "hype" and "crashes" of these devices challenged the expectations of stakeholders and advocates and contributed to shifting definitions of success. Surely the cost and questionable benefits of the artificial heart, particularly in the case of early patients who experienced a debatable quality of life with the device, gave researchers and the public pause?

The "spare parts pragmatism" and rebuilding of people disturbed social scientists Renée Fox and Judith Swazey, who were appalled at the overzealous commitment of American medicine and society to fixing people through organ replacement, based on what they saw by 1992 as "the human suffering" and consequent "social, cultural, and spiritual harm" emerging thereafter. Granted access to the events as they unfolded, Fox and Swazey observed and interviewed medical team members related to the Jarvik-7 artificial heart implant cases of the 1980s. They argued that the use of artificial heart technology propagated an untenable concept of "limitless medical progress" and displayed an "escalating ardor about the life-saving goodness of repairing and remaking people."[18] I explore their proposed "courage to fail" ethos, the perseverance of individuals to act despite probability of failure, to see if more layers appear across a broader time period and additional locales. I suggest that a longer historical perspective, examining research activities well before and after the Jarvik-7 heart cases, and a broader study of individuals and centers beyond the University of Utah reveal a complicated and nuanced set of visions and expectations, affected by shifting political, economic, and social factors. A courage-to-fail spirit existed, yet it manifested itself differently among various individuals and clinical settings, tempered by the context of the period.

Artificial Hearts as a Case Study

This book is a case study of a controversial medical technology; its development sustained by its powerful allure in American medicine and society as a therapeutic possibility and characterized by persistent ambivalence concerning its realization and clinical use. The acceptance or rejection of a medical device is better understood within the political and sociocultural circumstances in which it is conceived, tested, and clinically used. Many medical researchers, patients, politicians, and industry partners shared the vision of replacing worn-out parts of the body with mechanical devices and thus supported the development of artificial hearts. But artificial hearts, with their seemingly endless problems, seemed to suggest that there was a limit to what devices would be worth living with and paying for. Objectors to the clinical use of artificial hearts reinforced this concept of a boundary based on technological challenges and, later, various bioethical issues associated with the device. In the case of artificial hearts, the promissory science of mechanical organs shaped questions of efficacy and effectiveness that consistently threatened to end their development. In part, this was due to the interpretative flexibility of "success" around which stakeholders and supporters could mobilize to neutralize the uncertainty that surrounded mechanical hearts and technological fixes.

The case study presented here elicits implications for medical technology more generally. When is medical technology not the answer, particularly when it only "sort of" works? When is it time to declare "No more!," and who gets to declare it? Levels of acceptable efficacy and effectiveness were malleable, clearly different among the various stakeholders in, advocates of, and objectors to this technology. Their positions were shaped and influenced by individual circumstances as well as broader political, economic, and social circumstances. For different but synergistic reasons, the "promises" of many new technologies may certainly have held more sway over the "pitfalls" for dying patients and their families, the device industry, and determined medical researchers. The characterization of artificial hearts as a "halfway success," as stated by one bioethicist in the 1980s, reflected the many economic, social, and moral problems associated with the technology.[19] It challenged the binary characterization of therapeutics as either successes or failures and acknowledged fears of unwanted near-success. Questions of device efficacy and effectiveness were manipulated by individuals and groups to substantiate often contrasting stances. In the end, it was groups or communities with shared visions related to the promissory nature of this technology who mobilized resources well enough to maintain its ongoing development throughout its rocky history. The allure and ambivalence of artificial hearts as a technological solution (or at least a treatment strategy) to heart failure, alongside variable characterizations of success, anchor this story of how and why this problematic technology continued to be developed.

The history of artificial hearts is predominantly an American story. It was, as cardiologist-historian Bruce Fye notes, a "tiny but awe-inspiring artificial heart universe" that was dominated by a handful of American researchers and clinicians in elite, specialized American medical centers.[20] Mechanical heart research programs existed elsewhere in the world, including Russia, Germany, Japan, Australia, and Canada, but it was the artificial heart program of the National Institutes of Health in the United States that was the largest, best funded, and ultimately most successful one in the twentieth century. Greater achievement by Americans can be attributed to this country's medical research structure, leading university researchers, industry involvement, and federal government financing, along with an American culture that supported technological fixes. Key individuals working in the United States animated the field, including Willem Kolff, Michael DeBakey, Adrian Kantrowitz, Denton Cooley, William S. Pierce, Robert Bartlett, Peer Portner, Robert Jarvik, Victor Poirier, John Watson, Jack Copeland, O. H. Frazier, Richard Wampler, Gerson Rosenberg, and others.

Taking a leadership role, American artificial heart researchers made alliances with surgeons and bioengineers worldwide to exchange ideas and test prototypes. Under the Nixon administration, an intergovernment agreement between the United States and the USSR, announcing an official collaboration championed by surgeon-researcher Michael DeBakey and Soviet artificial organ pioneer Valeriy I. Shumakov, stimulated joint conferences and visiting delegations between Houston and Moscow in the hopes of expediting the development of mechanical hearts.[21] Much of this collaboration was politics, of course. Cognizant of the political importance for their respective artificial heart programs, DeBakey and Shumakov supported many scientific working visits between their two countries, touting the "friendly and fruitful" environment in which their joint work took place.[22] A discernible political and technological momentum carried artificial hearts through and around potential limits to their development. The course was not a smooth, linear path but a multiple-pronged approach to a wide variety of scientific goals that edged forward, shifted sideways, even abandoned some lines of investigation, before eventually producing several acceptable, clinically viable devices for heart failure patients.

The history of artificial hearts is situated within the period after World War II during which American science and technology expanded, the federal government invested in medical research, heart failure became increasingly prevalent in American society, technological medicine came to the fore in Western health care, and the business aspects of health care became more prominent in the United States. The development path of artificial hearts faced innumerable barriers, and their commercial success was never certain. The realization of mechanical circulatory support systems by the end of the twentieth century represented decades of incremental medical and bioengineering gains, contested program directions, wavering research funding, capricious industry partnerships, and ever increasing device regulation. Their clinical use speaks to values and priorities of American medicine and society in the second half of the twentieth century. At midcentury, US public health officials were sounding off about a heart disease epidemic, stimulating serious research into both the prevention and the treatment of heart disease. Within this context, the development of artificial hearts began in earnest in response to the problem of heart failure.

Heart Disease: A Leading Cause of Death

In 1910 heart disease was the leading cause of death in the United States, bypassing tuberculosis and pneumonia as the top disease killer of Americans. By 1950, almost 40 percent of all deaths were due to heart disease, which claimed more lives than the next three leading causes of death combined.[23] The life expectancy of white men and white women had increased from ages 50 and 53 in 1910 to ages 66 and 71 in 1950, with heart disease gaining prevalence in the aging society.[24] With cardiovascular X-rays, electrocardiograms, and other tools, physicians diagnosed more cases of rheumatic heart disease, coronary artery disease, endocarditis, and other forms of heart disease among their patients. In 1948 the US Congress passed the National Heart Act, which established the National Heart Institute (later renamed the National Heart, Lung, and Blood Institute) to conduct research and training into the causes, prevention, diagnosis, and treatment of diseases of the heart and circulation. Although initial funding was modest—only $500,000, which was the same amount allocated to the eradication of a potato parasite in Long Island at the time—it nevertheless stimulated a variety of basic and applied research projects, most notably the Framingham Heart Study.[25] In Framingham, Massachusetts, a long-term, ongoing cardiovascular study of the city's residents identified several common factors or causes leading to heart disease. Data collected in this study established the concept of risk factors, specifically hypertension, high cholesterol, and cigarette smoking, as major contributors to the problem of heart disease in America.[26] In 1955 President Dwight D. Eisenhower suffered a heart attack, requiring a seven-week stay in the hospital for recovery, and the seriousness of heart disease was made ever more apparent. As Paul Dudley White, a leading cardiologist and one of Eisenhower's physicians, wrote in his classic textbook *Heart Disease,* "heart disease has become the chief public health problem of our day."[27]

Heart disease is a broad term, used to describe any number of conditions or symptoms of the heart, and cardiovascular problems or diseases of the blood vessels may also be included. The most common type of heart disease is coronary artery disease, caused by the accumulation of cholesterol and plaque in the arteries that provide blood to the heart muscle.[28] These arteries become hardened and narrowed, reducing blood flow to the heart and causing the possible formation of a blood clot, which result in chest pain (angina) or a heart attack (myocardial infarction). A heart attack results in the death of the part of the heart muscle that is deprived of oxygen-rich blood, and there is permanent heart damage. Other heart diseases include heart rhythm difficulties (arrhythmias), heart muscle troubles (cardiomyopathy), heart valve problems (stenosis, regurgitation, prolapse), heart infections, and congenital heart defects. Heart failure thus is not a specific heart disease, but rather a condition that develops as a result of cardiac damage from heart diseases such as these.[29]

Heart failure is a chronic, progressive condition that occurs when the heart muscle can no longer efficiently pump enough blood to the lungs (pulmonary circulation) or to the rest of the body (systemic circulation). Blood backs up in the venous system, blood pressure decreases, and the body's organs and tissues suffer from poor perfusion (or blood circulation). Heart failure is not a heart attack, nor does the patient's heart stop (which is a cardiac arrest, when there is no pulse). The heart of a patient in heart failure is simply not working or pumping blood as it should. The problem may be a case of left-sided heart failure (most common), right-sided heart failure, or both. To compensate, the heart and the body adjust in a variety of ways. Struggling to pump, a heart ventricle becomes enlarged, with thickened muscle but less contracting power to move blood through the body. In the body, blood vessels may narrow to maintain blood pressure and blood may be redirected from less important tissues and organs to the most vital organs (heart and brain).[30] When the body's organs and tissues do not receive enough nutrient-rich, oxygenated blood, they do not function properly. The heart failure patient may feel extreme fatigue, a shortness of breath, and possibly an increased heart rate, which will make everyday activities like walking and climbing stairs increasingly difficult. As the condition worsens, the patient experiences a buildup of fluid in the feet, ankles, and legs (edema), a congestion of blood in the lungs, and perhaps memory problems and even impaired thinking. Based on the severity of the symptoms, a patient's heart failure is typically classified according to the New York Heart Association's four-stage functional classification system, ranging from Class I (cardiac disease causing minimal limitations in physical activity) to Class IV (cardiac disease causing severe limitations and discomfort with any physical activity).[31] Heart failure is life threatening, with poor long-term prognosis; most heart failure patients die within five years after diagnosis from complications arising from poor blood flow (such as organ failure) or from contracting infections in their weakened condition (such as pneumonia).[32] There is no medical cure for heart failure. As one physician commented, "Heart failure is a lethal disease with a worse life expectancy than many types of cancer."[33]

In 2014 an estimated 26 million people were living with heart failure worldwide—including 5.8 million Americans—and the incidence and prevalence of this condition were on the rise.[34] With approximately 3 percent of the world's population affected by symptomatic heart failure, the condition is emerging as a global health and financial burden. In the United States, a greater proportion of the population suffers from heart failure each decade. The direct and indirect costs of caring for these patients, including hospitalization, medications, and so forth, is about $31 billion, and this number is expected to more than double by 2030.[35] More people are surviving heart attacks and other cardiac conditions, perhaps because of more successful therapies or better education about heart disease. As a result, people are living longer with damaged hearts and thus carry the risk of heart failure. (To be clear, mortality rates from coronary heart disease have been declining since the 1970s, yet it still remains the leading cause of death in most developed countries.)[36] Various medical and epidemiological studies report that heart failure in the United States is most common in older people (age 65 and older), African Americans, overweight individuals, and previous heart attack patients.[37] Slightly more men than women battle this condition, although roughly 47 percent of American heart failure patients are women.[38] Medical researchers point to coronary artery disease, high blood pressure, and diabetes as the common causes leading to heart failure.[39] Medical practitioners thus aim to treat these underlying causes in an attempt to relieve the symptoms and improve the quality of life of their heart failure patients.

In general, the public is aware of the rising incidence of heart failure and, to some extent, the various treatment options available. The state of our understanding and ability to treat heart failure is directly related to the initiatives of government, medical research, and patients to do more against a condition framed as something preventable, reparable, or at the very least amenable to improvement. Contributing to such initiatives has been the significant amount of information and statistics regarding heart disease in general and heart failure specifically amassed by public health agencies, disease advocate groups, and medical practitioners, among others, and presented in the medical literature and the public media. Throughout the twentieth century, the culture of biomedical medicine endorsed research efforts to identify the causes of heart disease, to better understand the resulting structural and functional alterations to the heart, and to provide innovative and beneficial therapies. As outlined in White's textbook, the standard treatment for heart failure at midcentury was rest, digitalis, and diuretic drugs to help relieve dyspnea (difficulty breathing) and edema (fluid buildup).[40] Yet mortality rates remained alarmingly high, motivating medical researchers and practitioners to push for greater understanding and better treatment of heart failure.

Surgical Fixes for Damaged Hearts

In the twentieth century, many new surgical procedures and technologies altered the care of patients with heart disease, as historians Bruce Fye, David Jones, Harris Shumacker, and others have shown.[41] Jones's history of coronary artery bypass surgery and coronary angioplasty is a useful case from which to draw potential similarities with artificial heart technology. All are expensive cardiac procedures that are often characterized as life-saving. Jones states that the "simple, intuitive logic" of bypass surgery and angioplasty, alongside a plumbing analogy, forged a seemingly inevitable case for their efficacy and effectiveness, despite a lack of consensus among physicians about the cause of heart attacks.[42] Medical and nonmedical groups held expectations of therapeutic benefit for bypass surgery and angioplasty, arguably in varying degrees, as did early clinician-researchers and patients for artificial hearts. As Jones argues, their reasons for support emerged out of medical uncertainty, inconclusive evidence, and competing theories that nevertheless were shaped by individual values and external interests. Similarly, there was an intuitive aspect to building mechanical hearts—basically a pump to move blood—that fostered belief in its feasibility and mobilized support for the development of artificial hearts as a therapeutic option for heart failure patients.

Famed aviator Charles Lindbergh, known for his 1927 transatlantic flight more than for any medical innovation, delved into the problem when he learned that his sister-in-law's heart condition could not be fixed because surgeons were unable to stop the heart for such reparative operations. During the 1930s, Lindbergh worked with Nobel Prize–winning scientist Alexis Carrel at the Rockefeller Institute for Medical Research in New York, exploring ways in which the heart might be artificially kept alive outside the body for improved study and observation by medical scientists. Carrel and Lindbergh produced a glass perfusion pump, which successfully kept small explanted organs of birds or cats alive by circulating a fluid of oxygen, salts, and nutrient through the blood vessels to these organs.[43] Carrel and Lindbergh published their work in *Science,* and afterward several *New York Times* stories announced the researchers' success in building an "artificial heart."[44] (It was not an artificial heart but a perfusion pump.) The *Times*'s science writer William Laurence described Lindbergh's "chamber of artificial life" as a combined mechanical heart and lungs, an artificial blood supply and even synthetic air that kept body parts alive for the first time outside the body.[45] Not long after, a photo of Lindbergh, Carrel, and the pump made the cover of *Time* magazine in 1938.[46] It made for spectacular reporting, feeding the imagination of society for such a device. But World War II and the declining novelty of the Lindbergh-Carrel pump pushed interest in artificial hearts to the sidelines. In the 1950s, investigation of a mechanical solution to the problem of heart failure resumed and became less fanciful when the introduction of several key technologies in cardiac surgery demonstrated its very real possibility.

With better control over patient pain, bleeding, and infection by the early twentieth century, surgeons increasingly intervened into the inner cavities of the body. By removing, repairing, and later replacing damaged body parts, surgeons offered cures by scalpel. They cut out cysts, patched up soft tissue wounds, repaired abdominal wall hernias, excised tumors, removed inflamed appendixes, fixed birth defects, and more. Twentieth-century views of the body as an entity made of parts supported surgical intervention as a curative solution to specific anatomical or structural problems. The twentieth century is often described by medical historians as the century of surgery, owing to the technological advances of the period as well as the public's general willingness to go under the knife. In 1933 Henry E. Sigerist wrote, "The American patient wants to be cured as quickly as possible. Faced with the choice between surgery and prolonged medical treatment, he will unhesitatingly choose surgery."[47] This mind-set reflected a shift from understanding the body as a functional whole to an assemblage of fixable parts.

Initially, the heart was considered off-limits to the surgeon's scalpel because of technical challenges. Only a few bold nineteenth-century surgeons sutured puncture wounds or drained the pericardium (the sac around the heart). In a few exceptional cases, foreign bodies lodged in the walls of the heart may have been removed. Patients rarely recovered from such injuries, though. Such outcomes discouraged most surgeons and supported the conventional wisdom of the medical profession that warned against operating on the heart. In the 1880s, Theodor Billroth of Vienna, one of the world's most prestigious surgeons, stated, "Any surgeon who would attempt an operation on the heart should lose the respect of his colleagues." In 1896 Sir Stephen Paget of London declared, "The heart alone of all viscera has reached the limits set by nature to surgery. No new method and no new technique can overcome the natural obstacles surrounding a wound of the heart."[48]

During the first half of the twentieth century, several new diagnostic technologies contributed much to the clinical knowledge of heart disease. The electrocardiograph, a machine that produces electrocardiograms, or ECGs, recorded the electrical action of the heart and allowed doctors to document irregular heartbeats of their patients. Catheterization (injection of a flexible tube into the arm, up a vein, and into the atrium of the heart) and angiocardiograms (X-rays of the blood vessels injected with a dye via a catheter) improved diagnosis of heart disease. Constricted arteries and swollen vessel walls (aneurysms) could be detected, and experimental surgical treatments emerged. As more knowledge about the heart was gained, surgeons like Robert E. Gross in Boston, Clarence Crafoord in Stockholm, and Alfred Blalock in Baltimore began devising surgical procedures to treat various malformations of the heart. The celebrated blue baby operations of the mid-1940s, in which surgeons operated on the great vessels of the heart (arteries leading away from the heart) to compensate for congenital heart defects, validated surgical endeavors to repair problems and improve heart function.

By the late 1940s and into the 1950s, there was no doubt that heart surgery was a new and exciting field. Undergoing rapid change, it moved through three distinct phases—extracardiac to closed-intracardiac (closed-heart) to open-heart surgery—in two generations. Alfred Blalock and Helen Taussig's blue baby operation of 1944 gave momentum to closed-heart surgery.[49] Surgeons and researchers studied and performed these early palliative heart procedures; they made improvements and devised new techniques; and before long corrective open-heart surgery rendered these operations obsolete. Leading surgeons daring to operate on the heart in this period included British surgeon Russell Brock; Swedish surgeon Clarence Crafoord;

Canadians Gordon Murray, Arthur Vineberg, Wilfred Bigelow, and William Mustard; and a longer list of Americans: Alfred Blalock, Robert E. Gross, Michael DeBakey, Charles P. Bailey, Dwight Harken, C. Walton Lillehei, Denton Cooley, and Norman Shumway.[50]

The public's feelings toward heart surgery changed with the sensational blue baby operations of the 1940s. The surgeons' success in saving the lives of cyanotic children soon led to more successful procedures for other congenital and acquired heart disease conditions. Misgiving gave way to confidence in the skills of the cardiac surgeon. Society was less inclined to imbue the heart with special cultural meanings as either the seat of the soul or the mysterious center of emotional identities. Romantic notions of the heart were being replaced with a mechanistic understanding of the heart as a pump that could be repaired.[51]

The Heart-Lung Machine: Setting the Stage

Technological innovations in the 1950s began to alter dramatically how surgeons operated on the heart. This was the beginning of open-heart surgery. As Bruce Fye states, about two dozen surgeons in North America and Europe were exploring methods by which they could open the chest and, under direct vision, perform longer, more complex cardiac operations on a quiet, bloodless heart.[52] Toronto surgeon Wilfred Bigelow introduced hypothermia, a surgical technique involving total body cooling, to a skeptical audience at the American Surgical Association in 1950. Bigelow's idea was to "cool the whole body, reduce the oxygen requirements, interrupt the circulation, and open the heart."[53] In 1952 in Minneapolis, John Lewis successfully operated on a 5-year-old girl who was suffering from atrial septal defect, using the open-heart hypothermia technique.[54] This technique allowed surgeons to temporarily cut off blood circulation to a beating heart, providing a bloodless field and direct vision to correct heart anomalies. But it could not be sustained for long periods of time. After about four minutes of no blood supply, irreversible brain damage occurs; using hypothermia to reduce the brain's oxygen demand offered the surgeon another minute or two before risking permanent brain damage. This limitation obviously restricted the surgeon to simple cardiac operations.[55]

To extend operating time, several investigators, notably Clarence Crafoord in Sweden, Jacob Jongbloed in Holland, and John Gibbon Jr. in the United States, built machines to assume the function of the patient's heart and lungs in maintaining blood circulation during surgery. As they offered several hours of support, these machines also provided the surgeon with a nonbeating, bloodless heart on which to conduct delicate repairs. Yet it was a steep technological challenge to remove the blood from the body, oxygenate it, and return it without damaging its properties.[56] Tubes were inserted in the inferior and superior vena cava, redirecting to the machine the oxygen-poor blood going into the heart. The machine then pumped the blood to an oxygenator, replicating the functions of the lungs by removing carbon dioxide and adding oxygen. The blood was then pumped through a filter to remove clots and bubbles before it was returned to the patient via a tube inserted in the aorta.[57]

Widely acknowledged as the inventor of the heart-lung machine, Gibbon began work on his machine in the 1930s, later collaborating with Thomas Watson, an engineer and chairman of International Business Machines, who provided financial and technical support. At Jefferson College of Medicine in Philadelphia, Gibbon was constantly modifying his machine, experimenting with different materials and configurations of mesh screens, and operating on bypassed dogs to assess its function. His first clinical success with the machine occurred in 1953, when he corrected an atrial septal defect in 18-year-old Cecilia Bavoleck, who was suffering from heart failure. It was a historic operation, and with the hole in her heart now closed, Bavoleck lived more than 40 years after the surgery.[58] Improvements to the pump still needed to be made, but Gibbon had shown that mechanical circulatory support—allowing a machine to do the work of the heart and lungs—was possible. It took several more years to refine the machine as well as to encourage other surgeons to use the pump.

Crafoord's, Jongbloed's, and Gibbon's heart-lung machines all worked on the same operating principle but had different oxygenators that were later refined and improved upon. John Kirklin at the Mayo Clinic modified the Gibbon machine, and the inexpensive, easily assembled DeWall bubble oxygenator (or Lillehei pump-oxygenator) became available after that.[59] By the late 1950s, heart surgeons had the potential to perform cardiac bypass, combining hypothermia with extracorporeal (outside the body) circulation. With such technologies, they could cool and bypass the heart, stopping it for up to an hour and then starting it again without inflicting any damage to the organ. Heart operations became more numerous and complex, and cardiac patients were being supported by bypass for longer periods of time under the watchful eye of trained medical technicians called perfusionists. By the late 1960s, several cardiovascular surgeons were performing previously unthinkable coronary bypass and cardiac transplant operations. In Houston, Texas, superstar cardiovascular surgeons Michael DeBakey and Denton Cooley performed more operations in one week than most other medical centers scheduled in one month. The Baylor College of Medicine and the Texas Heart Institute became the best known cardiovascular surgical centers in the world, serving, in the words of one journalist, as "the Lourdes to heart-diseased pilgrims from everywhere."[60]

The importance of the heart-lung machine cannot be overstated, for it made greater reparative and replacement cardiac surgery possible. It dramatically ushered in a new era in heart surgery. With the heart-lung machine, surgeons could open the chest and, under direct vision, perform complex, reparative cardiac operations on a quiet, bloodless heart. However, cardio-bypass procedures had high rates of operative mortality in the 1950s and 1960s, as well as high rates of complications for survivors. After four cases, out of which only one patient survived, John Gibbon refused to perform any more operations using the heart-lung machine.[61] Many other surgeons did continue to use the heart-lung machine, though, envisioning its potential to allow them to remedy complex cardiac abnormalities and structural damage to the heart in patients with congenital and acquired heart disease. Coronary artery bypass grafts, aortic and mitral valve replacements, septal defect closures, and aneurysm repair operations became successful surgical treatments. A handful of pioneering surgeons began transplanting hearts in the 1960s, but with disastrous results until the introduction of immunosuppressant drugs in the 1980s allowed them to counteract the problem of organ rejection.

A momentous technological feat, the heart-lung machine established the feasibility of mechanical circulatory support. The pump-oxygenator served as an acceptable substitute for the patient's heart and lungs, but the technology was not without problems. The heart-lung machine could only be used temporarily; it was not a cure for the failing heart. Patients are kept on bypass only for the length of their operation, ideally not longer than six hours, to avoid risks of blood clotting, blood damage (hemolysis), air embolism, or postperfusion syndrome (neurocognitive damage). When coming off bypass, some patients went into severe cardiopulmonary failure and died. There was a need for prolonged extracorporeal circulation to allow weakened hearts and lungs extra time to recover. Prompted by surgeon Robert E. Gross to investigate this matter further, surgeon-researcher Robert Bartlett developed membrane lungs, or extracorporeal membrane oxygenation technology, in the 1970s, which provided days, not hours, of support for failing hearts and lungs to recover.[62] The importance of the heart-lung machine was as a means for greater corrective cardiac surgery rather than as a therapeutic solution for the failing heart. It provided proof-of-concept that mechanical support and replacement was feasible, stimulating development of other technologies. When diseased heart structures could not be repaired, open-heart surgeons implanted mechanical replacement devices to restore function and prevent further damage to the heart. Two key replacement devices—the artificial heart valve and the artificial pacemaker—contributed to the growth of mechanical replacement parts in this period.

Artificial Valves and Artificial Pacemakers

Heart valve disease impairs the function of one of the four heart valves that control blood flow through and out of the heart. With each heartbeat, the flaps of each valve open and close to regulate the forward motion of blood as it circulates into and out of the heart. A congenital heart disease, coronary artery disease, high blood pressure, heart attack, or cardiomyopathy may cause a valve to thicken, stiffen, open or close improperly, or become leaky or plugged, interfering with adequate blood flow and making the heart work harder.[63] If valve repair is not possible, then surgeons advise valve replacement with either a tissue valve (pig, cow, or human) or an artificial valve. Mechanical valves are made of titanium, carbon, and other durable, biocompatible materials. Finding the right materials, which would be tolerated in the body and specifically compatible with the blood, produced important research transferable to the development of other implantable devices. Different designs of artificial valves emerged, highlighting the multipath development course of this device and the advantages of surgeon-engineer collaboration.

In 1952 Georgetown University cardiac surgeon Charles Hufnagel implanted his caged-ball artificial valve into the descending thoracic aorta of a woman with a leaky aortic valve. The new procedure worked to alleviate the patient's symptoms of chest pain and fatigue, but, since Hufnagel was operating without bypass (it was before the open-heart surgery era), the artificial valve did not actually replace the faulty human valve, which was left in place. Still, the significance of the Hufnagel valve lies in its success in demonstrating the feasibility of artificial valves to regulate blood flow in the human body. In 1960 surgeon Albert Starr and engineer Lowell Edwards at the University of Oregon developed the smaller Starr-Edwards ball valve, which was inserted directly into the hearts of patients on bypass. In this case, cardiac surgeons removed the patient's diseased valve and implanted the Starr-Edwards valve in its place. Other surgeon-engineer partners also tinkered with the design and materials of the ball valve, removing struts, changing the silicone ball material, covering the ring with Dacron, and so forth. During the 1960s, a new overall design change was put forward by Walt Lillehei and Anatolio Cruz, by Viking Bjork and Donald Shiley, and by other teams who proposed tilting and nontilting disc valves, which they argued caused less damage to the blood. Many of the early disc valves battled strut fractures, however, requiring better design and biomaterials to withstand the mechanical pressure, and improved versions were built. Other teams experimented with different valve designs. Surgeon Vincent Gott and mechanical engineer Ronald Daggett devised a flexible bileaflet valve, which emulated the human heart valve by allowing blood to flow directly through the center. The Gott-Daggett valve, the St. Jude Medical bileaflet valve, and other bileaflet valves began to be used clinically. But some physicians commented on a blood backflow problem in their patients, prompting more device modifications. In the end, no one design dominated, and a variety of valves became available on the market; all valves held advantages and drawbacks, leaving patients and their surgeons to choose which artificial valve best fit the cardiac condition of the patient and the implant preference of the surgeon.[64]

Like artificial valves, the development of the artificial pacemaker also contributed to this trend of building mechanical replacement parts for the heart. A pacemaker is a device that sends electrical impulses to the heart to stimulate the heart muscle, replacing the patient's natural electrical signal when it is slowed or disrupted.[65] Like the development of artificial valves, building a pacemaker required surgeon-engineer collaboration, but it faced different technological challenges, notably the task of making the device small enough to be implanted inside the body. In 1952 Boston cardiologist Paul Zoll kept a patient alive through numerous episodes of cardiac standstill using his external pacemaker, a bedside machine with a strap to hold two chest electrodes in place on either side of the patient's heart.[66] It was a closed-chest treatment meant as an emergency action to revive patients by stimu-lating contraction of the ventricles (bottom of the heart). A certain voltage was necessary to stimulate the heart, which patients found too painful for extended use. Nevertheless, Zoll's pacemaker gained a place in hospitals. Cardiac specialists found the machine easy to set up, to use, and to interpret the results, and while the treat-ment was not pain-free for patients, it did seem to keep them alive for short periods. But Zoll's machine had only limited clinical use.[67]

The introduction of transistor circuitry significantly changed the development and acceptance of pacemakers. With this new technology, the pacemaker evolved from large, external machines to smaller, implantable devices. Engineer and business-man Earl Bakken, whose company Medtronic Inc. later grew to dominate the pace-maker market, developed the first wearable (but external) transistorized pacemakers in the late 1950s. The first fully implantable pacemaker operation took place in 1958 at the Karolinska Institute in Stockholm, Sweden, by heart surgeon Åke Senning. Designed by Rune Elmquist (of the Elema Company, now owned by St. Jude Medical), the pacemaker was about the size of a hockey puck, and it failed after six hours, necessitating its replacement with a second, identical pacemaker that worked for six weeks.[68]

Pacemakers needed to last longer and function better, and so engineers searched for better power sources and control systems. Mercury batteries, which were typi-cally used, caused these pacemakers to fail within 18 months of implantation. In the 1970s, nuclear-powered pacemakers emerged but had limited clinical use owing to the social and political anxiety at this time surrounding the use of plutonium in the body and all things nuclear.[69] By the end of the decade, lithium-battery pacemakers supplanted nuclear power as the better power source. Lithium (and later lithium-ion) batteries contributed to smaller, more sophisticated, and longer-lasting pacemakers. But would the device still function appropriately as the individual aged? The intro-duction of integrated circuits and microprocessors significantly improved the func-tionality of pacemakers, allowing for adjustable and programmable features, thus better meeting individual patients' needs.[70] A pacemaker's computer would record the heart's electrical activity and heart rhythm as well as blood temperature, breath-ing, and other information that could be relayed to physicians. At first, pacemakers seemed limited as "emergency" machines intended to resuscitate patients from heart stoppage, but they evolved into complex devices with "on demand" pacing to pro-vide reliable heart rhythm regulation. With the new implantable cardiac defibrilla-tor, artificial pacemakers emerged as a technological solution to society's anxieties concerning sudden cardiac arrest as well as heart failure caused by a prolonged ir-regular heartbeat.[71]

Paget's 1896 pronouncement of surgical limits surrounding the heart was clearly out of date. By the mid-1960s, the clinical use of artificial valves and the artificial pacemaker exemplified the willingness of medical practitioners and their patients to intrude upon the boundaries once set around the heart. Artificial valve researchers wrestled with valve design and suitable biocompatible materials, while engineers and surgeons developing artificial pacemakers sorted out power challenges and reliability issues. Surgeons began treating heart valve disease and problems of arrhythmia with these new devices. More broadly, the clinical success of artificial valves and pacemakers depicted a trend of using artificial means to replace damaged human parts. How far-fetched was the possibility of an artificial heart as a treatment for heart failure? A small number of artificial heart researchers deemed it worthwhile to investigate, joining a large and growing group of individuals choosing to fight disease with machines and devices.

Artificial Hearts: A Seductive Technology

Artificial hearts are a seductive technology in that the promise of this technology induced groups and communities to "buy in" and to consolidate their support based on their hope for the technology and its future role. Stakeholders' and supporters' shared expectations influenced their activities, provided structure and legitimation, attracted interest, and secured investment. Conversely, objectors mobilized around the pitfalls of the technology and their fear of it and its future. Promissory science involves managed and negotiated possibility, with constructed "regimes of hope," to navigate uncertainty and varying levels of expectations.[72] Expectations and visions connect variable groups, often bridging or mediating across different boundaries. As sociologist Nik Brown and others point out, society's expectations are not historically constant, and they can "change over time in response and adaptation to new conditions or emergent problems."[73] Highlighting the ways in which expectations and visions are articulated and reconstituted deepens this history of artificial hearts from a descriptive narrative of devices and people navigating disease and technology challenges, so that it also reveals American values and priorities in medical research, therapeutic trends, and the concept of rebuilt bodies.

Concerned about the problem of heart failure, the American public vacillated between hoping artificial hearts would be a technological fix and fearing that the devices might make patients worse off. Without a doubt, the allure of artificial hearts played a powerful and constant role, dulling pangs of uncertainty, throughout the controversial development of this technology. Divergent characterizations of success are key to understanding how and why this problematic technology continued to be developed, countering recurrent uncertainty over the appeal of mechanical hearts. The desire and potential to replace worn-out parts of the body galvanized medical researchers, government agencies, device companies, and patient groups to support artificial heart development. From its earliest stages, shared expectations and visions among both supporters and objectors aligned groups, consolidated infrastructure, and built momentum, as these groups responded to the highs and lows that played out during the development of artificial hearts. Additional matters addressed in this study include the technological complexity of building replacement organs, the contested and negotiated process of medical research, and the constructed drama of "clinical firsts." A clear tension emerged regarding the place of government regulation of medical devices—did it serve to protect the public or simply hinder innovation and development? What role did the media play in shaping expectations as well as bridging medical and nonmedical communities on the complexities of this technology?

In addressing these questions, I aim to tell an engaging story of cardiac specialists, researchers, and patients battling heart failure by the use of an experimental and controversial technology, with all the conflict and uncertainty that it entailed. Building artificial hearts was a significant technological challenge; thus it is necessary to delve into the technical specifics of these devices—to remove the "black box" and describe the inner workings of the devices—illuminating how the task both reflected and challenged contemporary understanding of heart function and the feasibility of its mechanical replication. I include images of devices and their clinical use alongside sometimes dense technical information. During my research, I handled many of these artificial hearts and spoke with device investigators to learn how the technology worked. In the process I was able to explore the necessary collaborations, connections, and tensions between engineers and heart specialists, industry and academic researchers, surgeons and patients, hospitals and the media, medical and nonmedical communities. I discovered that the influence and authority of American medical and societal views were less fixed and more nuanced when situated within a decades-long development course. Intended neither as a triumphant nor a negative history of artificial hearts, this book presents a thoughtful account of events and expectations, drawing attention to the vigorous debates over device success and mechanical organ replacement approaches. It was the imperfect nature of the technology that led to an unmistakable ambivalence throughout its development and clinical use.

This book traces the history of artificial heart development during the second half of the twentieth century and into the twenty-first century, with chapters presented more or less chronologically. Each chapter roughly focuses on the development of a specific device or group of devices to highlight distinct themes and events. Organizing the book in this way allows for stand-alone chapters but at the cost of repeating some material and understating the simultaneous nature of device development. The first chapter explores the early years of building artificial hearts and the daunting technological complexity of designing mechanical circulatory support systems. During the 1950s and early 1960s, a foundation for artificial heart research solidified, owing to the work of three important researchers—Willem Kolff, Michael DeBakey, and Adrian Kantrowitz—who developed three different devices independently but who, together, nurtured a nascent artificial organs research community and secured political support for the development of mechanical hearts. Their device research and lobbying efforts contributed to the establishment of the Artificial Heart Program at the National Institutes of Health, which provided crucial government funding and a national structure for this multidisciplinary undertaking.

I argue that two significant outcomes emerged in this period as a result of these three researchers. First, Kolff, DeBakey, and Kantrowitz demonstrated the value of supporting different approaches and building multiple devices. Their work corroborated the policy of the Artificial Heart Program to support development of a "family" of mechanical circulatory devices; there would not be one artificial heart but many artificial hearts to support patients with different types of heart failure. This policy reflected the uncertainty of the period regarding the best device option when it came to the technological challenge of building artificial hearts. The research community agreed that the spectrum of possibilities was wide; as Kantrowitz later stated, "When hundreds of thousands of these [artificial hearts] are used . . . then it'll be clear which one is a little bit better."[74] Second, Kolff, DeBakey, and Kantrowitz emphasized the engineering challenges of building mechanical hearts, which framed and biased assessments of device success to the question of efficacy (does it work?) over effectiveness (does it help the patient?) for decades. Having seen the desperate clinical need for mechanical hearts at first hand, cardiac surgeons DeBakey and Kantrowitz may very well have dismissed efficacy-versus-effectiveness discussions as absurd. In those early days, these researchers were confident in their belief that artificial hearts, if engineering challenges were overcome, would contribute to improved treatment of heart failure. The context is important to remember. It was a period of great scientific and technological optimism in America, a time when the Congress endorsed many grand projects, including landing a man on the moon. Convinced of the scientific community's ability to replicate heart function mechanically, National Heart Institute director Ralph Knutti predicted the availability of artificial hearts for clinical use by Valentine's Day 1970. When DeBakey reported that his use of a partial artificial heart had worked well enough to bridge a surgical patient to recovery in 1966, it seemed that public confidence in artificial heart research had not been misplaced. But significant technical and physiological problems existed, which researchers nevertheless maintained would be surmountable with more time and money for research.

The second chapter examines the impact of heart transplantation on the development of artificial hearts and the medical debate over whether human hearts or mechanical pumps were the better replacement therapy for heart failure. Dramatic transplant and implant cases seized headlines during the 1960s, forging medical allegiances to one approach or the other, both of which tantalized the American public about the possibilities that seemed within reach. The development of artificial hearts and the marvel of heart transplantation surgery soon became intertwined in several ways. At the time, it was not evident which procedure would emerge as the better treatment or whether both therapies should be abandoned. In Cape Town, South Africa, Christiaan Barnard performed the first heart transplantation in 1967, and 16 months later, Denton Cooley performed the first TAH implant in Houston, Texas. Both patients died within a matter of days. Neither case immediately ushered in a new era of life-saving surgery, nor was the field certain of which approach to pursue.

I argue that over the next several decades, the challenges and uncertainties experienced in heart transplant surgery augmented the standing and perceived value of artificial heart implantation as a complementary, not competing, cardiac replacement treatment. Within the medical community, debates ensued over which was the better treatment—human or mechanical parts—with neither treatment offering satisfactory outcomes at this time.

The 1960s media coverage of heart transplantation and device implantation surgery bolstered the allure of replacement therapy and also exposed professional conflicts and transgressions. Notably, the 1969 TAH implant surgery incited a well-publicized feud between Houston cardiac surgeons Michael DeBakey and Denton Cooley over an accusation of device theft and lack of authorization to perform the procedure. The allegation raised significant issues of innovation credit and institutional reputations. Who can claim device ownership? And does ownership confer license to decide when the time is right to perform an experimental procedure on a human? Was it not premature of Cooley to implant this device in a patient? The 1969 implant case appeared to be about testing an experimental device in a human as much as it was about "doing everything possible" to save the life of a moribund patient. The characterizations of success by Cooley and his team reflected and supported the framing and biased assessments of artificial hearts in terms of efficacy rather than effectiveness. Chapter 2 explores the high-profile transplant and implant cases of the 1960s, highlighting the medical disputes, the treatment disappointments, the role of the media, and the subsequent reverberating effects on artificial heart research programs.

Technology and risk is the theme of chapter 3. Between 1967 and 1977, medical researchers and engineers in two separate federally funded programs tackled the technological complexity of designing a radioisotope-powered mechanical heart, one in which the primary power source was heat generated by radioactive decay. One atomic heart was developed by the Atomic Energy Commission, which subcontracted work on the pump's design and biomaterial fabrication to Willem Kolff and his research team at the University of Utah. The National Heart and Lung Institute sponsored a different nuclear-powered device, which was a partial artificial heart system designed and tested by surgeon-researcher John C. Norman to temporarily sustain the failing heart. Between 1972 and 1974, Norman implanted early versions of his cardiac-assist device, powered by plutonium-238, in 15 calves in the research laboratories at Harvard University's School of Medicine and at Texas Heart Institute in Houston, but with poor results. In both devices, a plutonium-powered engine operated the blood pump, but the use of plutonium presented problems of continuous radiation exposure, heat dissipation problems and hence tissue damage in the body, and other limitations. At the time, a radioisotope-powered approach was a promising option since biological fuel cells were decades away from being practical and battery systems, which tended to overheat, had only a two-year life span and required daily recharging. Plutonium-powered pacemakers were being implanted clinically, so why not a plutonium-powered artificial heart? The development of nuclear-powered artificial hearts highlights the technological optimism of scientists and engineers, the intersection of science and government, and the broader context of public debates about risk and uncertainty during this period. Medical researchers and engineers claimed that atomic hearts were feasible and practical and that the technological complexities of these devices were surmountable. However, political and social concerns arising in the context of a heightened sense of risk awareness in the 1970s ultimately ended these atomic heart programs, as strong public support for increased government control of both atomic energy and medical devices overrode scientific assertions that further development could produce a safe and practical atomic heart. American society simply perceived nuclear-powered artificial hearts as too dangerous to support.

Chapter 4 focuses on the Utah TAH, its sensational clinical use, and the public debate that it incited during the 1980s. Developed by Willem Kolff, Robert Jarvik, Don B. Olsen, William DeVries, and others at the University of Utah, the Utah heart, more than any other TAH device, raised the profile of artificial hearts as a viable option for individuals with heart failure. Also referred to as the Jarvik-7 heart, this mechanical heart is one of the best known medical devices of the twentieth century, because of its extensive 1980s media coverage, which reported a dramatic story of medical technology triumph, devoted researchers, bold surgeons, and brave patients that captivated American society. The media took their cue from the steadfast characterization of the artificial heart as a success by Utah stakeholders and the apparent "resurrectionist capacity" of this device that extended the lives of near-death patients such as Barney Clark and William Schroeder. Artificial heart researchers gained valuable information from the 1980s clinical cases, and some implant patients reached levels of improved health that allowed them to attend family weddings or to undergo heart transplant operations. Yet the overall clinical experiences were more unsettling than not, exposing a flawed technology.

Politicians, medical professionals, bioethicists, academics, and industry people weighed in, leading to increasing public disillusionment and vociferous debate over artificial heart technology. Most outspoken against the clinical use of artificial hearts, bioethicists contested issues of informed consent and patient autonomy, access and cost, quality of life and patient self-determination, and the overall criteria for success. A discernible shift in medical and lay discussions was evident; once focused predominantly on the feasibility of developing artificial hearts, they now extended to the desirability of such a clinically acceptable device (perfected or otherwise). Chapter 4 examines the perspectives of artificial heart researchers, clinicians, patients, bioethicists, and the media, comparing public to clinical narratives of these events and identifying the tensions, discrepancies, and divergent interests therein. The chapter also draws attention to the regulatory and business path of the artificial heart, which contributed to both the rise and the fall of the Utah device in this period. In the end, I argue that a clear lack of consensus regarding the success and meaning of these 1980s clinical cases emerged, creating an ambiguous and difficult environment for the development of TAHs thereafter.

Chapters 5 and 6 examine the research and clinical gains made by investigators and clinicians in the design, manufacture, and testing of VADs. Since the 1960s, research on VADs had continued alongside that on TAHs, with knowledge gained from one technology transferred to the other. Not surprisingly, device projects overlapped in laboratories and even among investigators. At the University of Utah, Willem Kolff's laboratory experimented with both TAHs and VADs; Robert Jarvik lent his name to both a TAH, the Jarvik-7 heart, and later an assist pump, the Jarvik 2000 FlowMaker. Yet VAD researchers moved their devices through clinical testing and product positioning in the marketplace more successfully than TAH investigators. One key characteristic of VAD development was that academic researchers worked more collaboratively with experienced medical device companies like Baxter Healthcare Corporation and Thoratec Laboratories Corporation to develop their technology. Not all devices transitioned from research prototypes to viable commercial products, however, and some companies spun off, sold off, or took over competing device product lines for a variety of reasons.

Chapter 5 argues that VADs, not TAHs, made the greater gains toward clinical acceptance because of their less complex nature, both technologically and conceptually, and also because pivotal industry collaboration helped to shepherd these devices through regulation, clinical trials, and commercialization. Intuitively, it seemed to all stakeholders more doable and less drastic to develop a viable device that would not require removal of the native heart. A VAD would not need to compensate completely for the native heart; it would leave the patient's organ in place as a somewhat reassuring back-up. Implanting a VAD—at a time when artificial heart valves and cardiac pacemakers were considered standard treatments—seemed much less radical than a TAH. In the 1970s and 1980s, VAD researchers addressed many of the technical bioengineering and patient care issues that had beset TAHs, and they developed smaller, assist devices that worked more reliably and had better patient outcomes. Key research funding for VAD development and testing on biocompatible blood materials, power sources, percutaneous (through the skin) or transcutaneous (across the skin) energy transmission mechanisms, and integrated systems readiness trials flowed through the NIH's artificial heart program as well as other academic and federal granting agencies. Investment by industry, such as by Thermo Cardiosystems Inc. and Thoratec Laboratories Corporation, significantly contributed to the marshaling of several VADs through product development, testing, and launching, positioning them within a marketplace already prepared for cardiovascular devices. In comparison to TAHs, more VAD prototypes were under development by industry groups in this period. Chapter 5 foregrounds the science and business that shaped VAD technology as the more rewarding mechanical heart technologically, conceptually, and commercially.

Chapter 6 explores how second-generation VADs secured therapeutic clout and greater clinical acceptance in the 1990s and the first decade of the 2000s. Former US vice president Dick Cheney directly benefited from this second-generation VAD technology. He lived with an implanted HeartMate II LVAD for 20 months before undergoing a heart transplant operation in 2012, and he credited the device for saving his life. Two key turning points that preceded the clinical availability of the device implanted in Cheney were the favorable results of a first-generation left ventricular assist device (LVAD) clinical trial and the development of second-generation, continuous-flow assist pumps. First, the Randomized Evaluation of Mechanical Assistance for the Treatment of Congestive Heart Failure (REMATCH) study provided convincing, high-quality data supporting first-generation VAD device safety and clinical effectiveness over conventional medical treatment for end-stage heart failure patients. This data compelled heart specialists and their patients to consider mechanical pumps more seriously and secured Food and Drug Administration (FDA) approval and third-party payer reimbursement for clinical use. Second, a key change in technology platforms shifted the design of VADs from volume displacement, pulsatile devices to continuous-flow, nonpulsatile pumps, resulting in second-generation assist devices, such as the HeartMate II LVAD. These devices were smaller, quieter, safer, and more effective than the clunky first-generation VADs. The new, continuous-flow VADs significantly reduced the problems of thromboembolism, infection, patient mobility, and device breakdowns. Greater clinical use of VADs, not TAHs, was seen in this period owing to the improved technology, better patient outcomes, and proficient commercialization of these devices. Among device stakeholders, the medical community, and society, a shared definition of success coalesced around the aim of returning the implant patient to a near-normal life, with the medical, social, and economic factors that that entailed. This purpose fed into the promise of artificial hearts (in this case VADs) as a viable and acceptable treatment option for end-stage heart failure. The rising number of VAD implants emerged out of the convergence of interests held by researchers, cardiac specialists, industry, the government, and patients, all of whom wanted these devices to work well for various synergistic reasons.

Chapter 7 shifts back to TAH devices and describes events in the clinical testing of two different mechanical hearts—the AbioCor TAH and the SynCardia TAH. *Time* magazine proclaimed the experimental AbioCor TAH to be one of the best inventions of 2001, but persistent technical difficulties and disappointing clinical trial data ultimately prevented the commercial fruition of this device. By the end of the decade, the SynCardia TAH attained FDA, Health Canada, and Conformité Européene approval as a bridge-to-transplantation device for end-stage biventricular (both sides) heart failure. This success has prompted some practitioners to advocate for its use as a permanent treatment for non-transplant-eligible patients. With the increasing number of TAH cases, there is a sizable cohort of implant patients whose experiences of living with these devices can now be documented, contributing to better understanding of this technology's implications for patients and caregivers. Nevertheless, the ideal mechanical heart has yet to be built. Current investigations with continuous-flow TAHs represent one line of research under development, among other possibilities. American medicine's and society's technological optimism remains, fueled by the success of some devices for some patients, thus sustaining the allure of mechanical hearts. In 2011, given the rising prevalence of heart failure and acute donor organ shortages, cardiac surgeon Jack Copeland asserted that artificial hearts might displace cardiac transplantation as the dominant treatment for end-stage heart failure in the future.[75]

The history of artificial hearts is an important story of scientists, clinicians, and patients choosing to fight heart failure with complex, imperfect devices. It is a case of persistence and resiliency in the face of uncertainty and dispute. A formidable group of stakeholders have battled incessant technical problems and public criticism, forcing them to shift, adapt, even abandon some lines of research. Ardent researchers, maverick surgeons, brave "guinea pig" patients, discordant bioethicists, and others have played various roles in the development of artificial hearts, at times in spectacular ways. This history is about the promissory nature of medical technology, the desire for curative fixes, and the expectation of meaningful life-sustaining treatments. The potential, the promise, and the "what if" have held a powerful allure that has shaped the development of this controversial medical technology. In turn, it has influenced how success has been characterized and by whom, demonstrating an interpretative flexibility of success when it comes to device assessment.

A discernible level of confidence and optimism, varying in its professional and public intensity over the decades, has sustained the pursuit of artificial hearts for more than 60 years. It has been a daunting task from the outset, and as early investigators in the field—including Selwyn McCabe, Bert Kusserow, Frank W. Hastings, Willem Kolff, Michael DeBakey, Adrian Kantrowitz, and others—embraced the challenge, they truly underestimated the complexity of the undertaking. In the 1950s, the possibility of mechanical hearts was legitimate and its clinical need was compelling for this small but innovative group of researchers. Getting on with the actual building of artificial hearts was now the job at hand.

CHAPTER ONE

Multiple Approaches to Building Artificial Hearts

Technological Optimism and Political Support in the Early Years

I believe that the symbol of life, the site of love, and the habitat of the soul, the human heart, will be replaced by a mechanical pump.

Dr. Willem Kolff, artificial organs researcher, 1966

The human heart is characterized as possessing so many loaded emotional, spiritual, and functional attributes that it seems ludicrous to think that it could be replaced with a mechanical one. Medicine and society sidestepped the conundrum by emphasizing the physiology and function of organs when discussing replacement, grouping the heart alongside the kidney, the liver, and other internal organs. In so doing, researchers positioned the task of building artificial hearts as an engineering problem, using technology to the practical end of treating heart failure, which capitalized on American technological optimism and enticed political backing. This approach to the heart shaped the type of researchers attracted to the project, the setting in which it was pursued, and the structure through which it secured support. Reducing the function of the heart to that of a blood pump—leaving discussions of love and the soul to those outside of medical science—made the pursuit of building artificial hearts appear doable and desirable at a time when medicine and society exuded hope and confidence about science and technology projects.

Motivated by the success of heart-lung machines, a handful of medical researchers pursued the idea of building artificial hearts in the late 1950s, focused on pushing the boundaries in mechanical circulatory support systems (MCSSs). If the heart-lung machine could sustain cardiac function temporarily, why not build a device that could support circulation for longer periods, to support cardiac recovery after surgery or, more spectacularly, to replace incurable, diseased hearts? According to one cardiac surgeon, the heart-lung machine shifted the attitude and imagination of many in the field, which, until then, had been generally dismissive of such fanciful ideas.[1] The heart-lung machine demonstrated that heart function could be mechanically replicated, at least for several hours, and that some patients benefited from mechanical cardiac support in their recovery after surgery. This success inspired numerous medical men to develop bold, new cardiac devices—artificial hearts—that would assist, even replace, failing diseased hearts.

In these early years of building artificial hearts, three medical men—Dutch-American physician and researcher Willem Kolff, Texas surgical titan Michael DeBakey, and cardiothoracic surgeon-investigator Adrian Kantrowitz—developed different mechanical devices for different patient needs, reflecting the nascent state of the field and the experimental nature of the endeavor. All three researchers were motivated by the clinical need for extended mechanical circulatory support. Kolff, credited with the invention of the artificial kidney, had built that machine during World War II and now wanted to create mechanical replacement devices for other failing body parts, including the heart. DeBakey and Kantrowitz, in their surgical practices, saw many cases in which a mechanical heart might extend the life of a patient. Each investigator recognized the tremendous physiological and technological challenges of building an artificial heart, yet they tackled it anyway. None of them were engineers, but engineers were key members of their research teams. As clinician-researchers, Kolff, DeBakey, and Kantrowitz shared a similar vision of mechanical circulatory support—or mechanical replacement of the blood pumping function of the heart—but each approached the task differently in terms of device design, placement, and clinical application. Was one approach better than another? Who would be first in delivering a viable device, and would firstness ultimately decide the better research direction to pursue?

In this period, the most promising mechanical hearts under development were Kolff's total artificial heart, DeBakey's bypass-type ventricular assist device, and Kantrowitz's serial-type VAD. In Cleveland, Kolff pursued the development of a TAH as a permanent mechanical replacement for a removed, failing human heart. He transferred the knowledge of and experience with blood flow, gained from his artificial kidney work, to build his implantable mechanical heart. This was the most ambitious, arguably fanciful aim for such a device at this early stage. (Kolff's team later experimented in a more limited way with assist devices.) In Houston, DeBakey also came to the endeavor with experience building mechanical or artificial devices that interacted with the blood; he had invented the roller pump used in John Gibbon's heart-lung machine and was investigating the viability of artificial arteries for vascular bypass procedures. His initial approach to a feasible artificial heart focused on developing ventricular assist pumps for temporary assistance as a bridge to surgical recovery. This was a more realistic aim, driven from the operating room and aimed at clinical utility for extended mechanical support beyond the heart-lung machine. (DeBakey also experimented with longer-term biventricular mechanical support and TAH replacement during this period, but he discouraged its clinical use.) In Brooklyn, Kantrowitz applied his theory of diastolic augmentation (or synchronized arterial counterpulsation) in the development of several cardiac assist devices or "booster hearts" intended for permanent support. Like DeBakey, Kantrowitz had seen the usefulness of such a device in his surgical practice. But in contrast to DeBakey's bypass-type pumps, which pumped independently of the heart and reduced blood flow by the natural heart, Kantrowitz's serial-type devices worked in tandem with the heart and augmented the natural heart's blood flow. These three devices differed in size, shape, how they worked, and intended clinical use. Collectively, these multiple approaches helped to sort out best biomaterials, device mechanics, implant tolerance in the body, and other issues.

This chapter argues that the foundation for artificial heart research that solidified in the 1960s was due to the work of these three important researchers—Kolff, DeBakey, and Kantrowitz—as well as the establishment of the Artificial Heart Program, which provided key research funding and a national structure to this multidisciplinary undertaking. Kolff, DeBakey, and Kantrowitz demonstrated the value of supporting different approaches and emphasized the engineering challenges associated with building artificial hearts; in these ways they contributed to consolidating confidence, interest, and funding for the development of artificial hearts but also to biasing assessments of success toward efficacy (does it work?) over effectiveness (does it help the patient?). In this early period, assumptions that efficacy would translate into effectiveness overlooked issues of patient expectations, suffering, and quality of life; such issues were not immediately discussed, but they soon would be, within medical and lay communities.

Artificial hearts depicted as an engineering problem shaped the early scientific and political framing of their development at a time of technological optimism and endorsement of science and technology fixes in American medicine and society. The daunting device challenges of designing satisfactory blood interface materials, power sources, control drives, and pumping mechanisms did not discourage artificial heart researchers like Kolff, DeBakey, and Kantrowitz. They embraced the challenges to solidifying collaboration and endorsement. In speaking to federal agencies, they narrowed the solution down to securing proper funding and expertise from industry and universities. Lobbying for support, they were selling the American capability to achieve this grand undertaking. The requirements and needs of building artificial hearts were really unknown, producing a wide-open game board that permitted different research paths. DeBakey's savvy in Washington and with journalists produced a narrative of potential, promise, and "what if"—in words and photos—that circulated among political and public audiences. However, the less confident National Institutes of Health director, James Shannon, questioned whether the basic science existed, accurately foreseeing the development of artificial hearts as a much longer-term undertaking and foreshadowing a battle of priorities for research dollars in the fight against heart disease. Shaky political support threatened research funding and a fragile momentum that was being nurtured by Kolff, DeBakey, and Kantrowitz.

From Kidneys to Hearts: Willem Kolff

At the early meetings of the American Society for Artificial Internal Organs (ASAIO), a scientific forum attended by "disciplined scientists and free-spirited, gadgeteer-geniuses," members discussed the future development of the artificial kidney and the heart-lung machine, the two artificial organs of primary interest in the 1950s.[2] Originally physician centered, the society welcomed engineers, biologists, and representatives of industry to its annual meetings to discuss the creation of new devices that would serve medical goals. There was a palpable excitement and energy at these meetings as attendees openly shared their experimental work and suggested new research directions.[3] In 1957 ASAIO president Peter Salisbury challenged members to think beyond the short-term use of the artificial kidney or heart-lung machine.[4] What about treating chronic renal failure? How about a pumping device to assist failing human hearts? Could a mechanical heart machine be developed for use beyond the operating table? At the time, the heart-lung machine demonstrated the feasibility of mechanical circulatory support, specifically, replicating a patient's heart and lung function by pumping and reoxygenating blood outside the body. However, the machine caused blood trauma in the form of blood cell damage and bleeding, and therefore it was limited to short-term use for surgical procedures. Could a machine be developed to overcome these problems, possibly for long-term use?[5]

These expressions of device possibilities reflected a shared "scientific imaginary," an interpretative concept that considers the effects of science upon the imagination and, similarly, how imagination affects science.[6] Anthropologist Lesley Sharp points to the "what if" promissory qualities of experimental innovation in medicine, arguing that "the scientific imaginary simultaneously shoulders themes of longing, hope, promise and desire in contexts where the endpoint (or endpoints) remain(s) unknown."[7] Indeed Salisbury's words exude wonder, excitement, and conviction, which clinicians, families, politicians, and others seeking to alleviate patient suffering would find appealing. Scientific research requires imagination and confidence to tackle seemingly insurmountable obstacles or to pursue ideas "outside the box." But was the "what if" of artificial hearts really that far away in 1957? Salisbury raised the possibility of developing a prosthetic heart after the cardiac surgeon and physiologist Selwyn McCabe demonstrated his experimental implantable blood pump at the meeting.[8]

After accepting a research position in 1950 at the Cleveland Clinic Foundation, Kolff attended this 1957 ASAIO meeting to present his work on experimental blood oxygenator devices. Up to this time, Kolff's research had focused on treating acute and chronic kidney failure, a condition that occurs when the kidneys are no longer able to filter and remove waste and extra fluid from the body. He had invented an artificial kidney machine in 1943, and after World War II he worked to refine it, sharing his designs with others, hoping for broader clinical use.[9] The Cleveland Clinic hired Kolff to help it offer one of the first hospital-based dialysis programs in the United States, supporting his research and providing clinical access to improve mechanical device treatments for renal failure patients. Kolff wanted his experimental work never to be completely divorced from clinical work, and so this close cooperation with Cleveland Clinic colleagues and related specialties was ideal for him. As Kolff stated many times, his ultimate goal was "the well-being and happiness of the patient," and so he was a good fit for the Cleveland Clinic, which, while supporting research, was equally interested in timely clinical application.[10] (Later, the Cleveland Clinic Foundation's decision to remove the clinical part of Kolff's program "so that he himself could devote his entire full schedule to research and development" was a contributing reason to Kolff's departure in 1967.)[11] Kolff's strong advocacy for dialysis inspired him to investigate other mechanical means of assisting or replacing sick organs. In his early years at the Cleveland Clinic, Kolff transferred his knowledge of and experience with blood flow from the artificial kidney machine to blood oxygenator devices. Salisbury's line of inquiry at the ASAIO meeting struck a chord with Kolff, and he returned to his lab eager to begin work on an artificial heart.[12] Shortly thereafter, in January 1958, Kolff became head of the new Department of Artificial Organs at the Cleveland Clinic, an institutional recognition of the expansion of Kolff's research from kidneys to hearts.[13]

Kolff sought to build an implantable artificial heart to replace the human heart, which, being either diseased or damaged, would be removed from the body. He envisioned the natural heart as a double pump that pushed blood through the lungs and into the body. Could Kolff build a mechanical double pump small enough to fit in the exact position of the human heart, one that the hostile environment of the body would accept?[14] Working with Japanese medical researcher Tetsuzo Akutsu, Kolff first experimented with the plastic replacement of aortic and mitral valves in the hearts of dogs. (Akutsu traveled to the United States in the 1950s, and over the next several decades, he worked in Kolff's Cleveland laboratory, Kantrowitz's New York laboratory, and the Cullen Cardiovascular Surgical Research Laboratory at the Texas Heart Institute before he returned to Japan in 1982 to lead Japan's national artificial heart program.)[15]

In Cleveland, Kolff and Akutsu completed 27 experiments of implanting plastic valves in the hearts of dogs before they boldly jumped ahead to build an entire plastic heart, composed of two polyvinyl chloride pumps. It was a pneumatically driven device, built from a plastic cast impression of the heart of a 60-pound dog. The heart was connected to an air compressor by plastic tubes. This air-driven heart was tested first in mock circulation on the bench (to ensure mechanical function), then implanted into a dead dog (to study surgical procedure and fit), and finally placed into a living dog in December 1957. The dog lived for 90 minutes with the implanted heart before device complications terminated the experiment.[16]

Kolff and Akutsu promptly reported their experimental animal case to the professional community, eager to claim it as the first successful TAH implant in an animal in the Western world.[17] In their opinion, the experiment was a success because their device had functioned in vivo (in animals), keeping the dog alive for 90 minutes, and it was forever cited as such in medical textbooks thereafter.[18] For them, it was proof of concept. While it might have demonstrated the feasibility of mechanically maintaining circulation for a limited time, Kolff and Akutsu's device was certainly not successful enough to be implanted in humans. The efficacy of the device was questionable, given that the dog had hardly moved from the operating

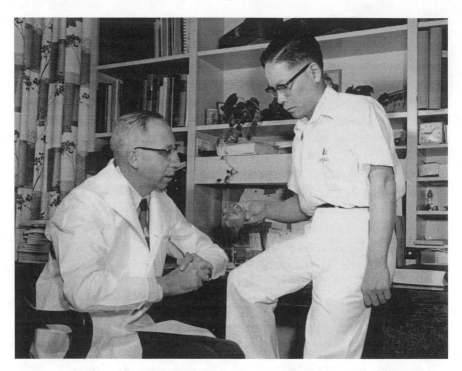

Artificial heart researchers Willem Kolff and Tetsuzo Akutsu (holding device) examine their experimental mechanical heart, implanted in a dog in 1957 at the Cleveland Clinic. Reprinted with permission, Cleveland Clinic Center for Medical Art & Photography © 2016. All Rights Reserved.

table. Obvious technological limitations were that the device was pneumatically driven, necessitating connection to an outside air compressor to power it, and that it had malfunctioned after 90 minutes. Equally problematic was the surgical procedure, which needed refinement. Heart removal was difficult and painstaking, and implanting the device required the tedious and time-consuming surgical connection of the mechanical heart to the major blood vessels. This was due to the design of this early device, which was modeled on the natural heart and the complexity of blood vessels surrounding it. Researchers questioned the suitability of the human heart as the ideal form for a mechanical heart model. During the next several years, the Cleveland group developed different artificial heart devices, varying in form and method of operation. Medical researchers worked closely with engineers to come up with the best biocompatible materials and reliable components, the best source of energy, the best driving mechanism, and the best regulating controls. In the end, all of the early artificial heart devices of the 1950s were abandoned because of technical complexity, poor durability, biomaterial problems, and their large size.

Two examples of the flawed but interesting designs that Kolff pursued in this period were the solenoid artificial heart and the pendulum artificial heart. The solenoid-driven artificial heart involved a magnet-driven pump. This heart was a six-sided flat box, about 2 inches high and 4 inches across, and weighed only 3.5 pounds. Five coordinated electromagnets, arranged in a rosette, were activated by electric current, which entered through two wires, creating mechanical energy. The electromagnets (or solenoids) pushed disks inward, compressing hydraulic fluid that squeezed two collapsible plastic ventricles, situated on either side of the rosette, simulating diastole (filling phase) and systole (emptying phase) of the heart.[19] The pendulum artificial heart was an electromotor-driven pump based on the pendulum principle. It contained a motor, suspended by pivots, which swung back and forth within a rigid housing. The device compressed each ventricle alternately. The pendulum heart was implanted in a dog and maintained circulation for more than five hours; Kolff reported that the animal breathed spontaneously and retained reflexes.[20] Both the solenoid and the pendulum hearts were electrically driven, but their battery power lasted only a few hours before needing to be recharged in an electric converter plugged into a wall socket. As Kolff acknowledged, the solenoid-driven heart was inefficient and produced heat at a level intolerable to the body, while the pendulum heart was too bulky and heavy within the body and the energy derived from the driving power was limited.[21]

Engineers from the National Aeronautics and Space Administration (NASA) persuaded the Cleveland researchers to return to pneumatically driven devices. Air power was plentiful and simpler and resulted in less heat production in comparison to electrically driven hearts, which generated too much heat for the body to tolerate. Pulsating air pressure, generated outside the body, could be easily channeled through small flexible tubing to any device in the chest. At first Kolff recoiled at the thought of returning to air-driven hearts. He stated, "This idea would commit us to a system in which the power supply would have to be outside the body. I had visions of the possessor of an artificial heart walking around with something like a garden hose sticking out of his chest!"[22] Kolff's reaction reflected his orientation as a physician, not an engineer.

When it came to building artificial hearts, engineers and physicians viewed the technology and the body differently. Engineers are mechanical experts, focused on design possibilities and parameters, who draw from their training in structural design, electrical engineering, fluid mechanics, aviation, and so on, and work in laboratories. In their task of building mechanical pumps, which one engineer described as "essentially sophisticated fluid propulsion devices," engineers fixated on such things as materials, rotors, tubes, writing systems, power sources, and battery packs.[23] In comparison, the training of physicians is oriented around people, for whom maintaining health, treating disease, and alleviating pain mandates a clinical focus. As such, clinician-researchers respond to the patient issues associated with artificial hearts, which also make socioeconomic and bioethical matters relevant. At times equally caught up in the technical difficulties associated with these devices, physicians nonetheless want mechanical pumps to be effective and to improve the condition of the heart failure patient. Engineers are biased by their focus on perfecting device design—designing, testing, reconfiguring, testing, redesigning, and so forth—according to anthropologist Lesley Sharp, who also states that patient suffering is an abstract to many engineers in the field. Describing the human body as prone to "failure" and "breakdowns," engineers concentrated on device performance, not patient experiences with the technology.[24] (Biomedical engineering, or bioengineering, with its application of engineering principles to biological systems, is a relatively new field, emerging only in the late 1960s and 1970s as a recognizable, science-based discipline.) What made the collaboration of engineers and physicians work in these early years was their shared development commitment and belief in the therapeutic purpose of artificial hearts.

Wanting NASA design assistance, Kolff eventually agreed that efforts should be concentrated on building a reliable heart pump mechanism that was air-driven, and later the team explored alternative power sources. NASA engineer Kirby W. Hiller, who devised controls for nuclear-powered rockets, worked with Kolff for a short time during the mid-1960s, designing a more flexible self-regulating control mechanism and adapting it to a variety of Kolff's pump designs.[25] Soon thereafter, Kolff, Akutsu, and engineer S. Harry Norton devised a sac-type artificial heart, a flexible plastic ventricle fitted into a slightly larger rigid housing.[26] Air pressure directed into the space between the ventricle and the housing resulted in the compression and release of the sac-type ventricle, moving the blood in and out of the device.

This project was not just an engineering problem; the greater challenge was getting a foreign device, such as a mechanical heart, to work compatibly with the human body. After bench testing and animal implants, Kolff reported the sac-type heart as reliable, small, light, and easy to fit into the chest cavity. Dogs survived up to 20 hours with this device. However, technical difficulties arose when the device interfaced with body fluids and functions. Kolff documented the common occurrence of thrombosis and emboli as a result of blood clotting on the plastic components of the device. In dogs who survived more than 12 hours, emboli dislodged, causing strokes and other conditions.[27] The Cleveland group immediately enlisted the help of chemists to help them find a more biocompatible plastic. Research then continued into alternative designs, new biomaterials, and different power sources, giving rise to a larger, but necessary, multidisciplinary team.[28]

Kolff was not alone in the development of artificial hearts during the late 1950s and early 1960s.[29] In 1957 Bert Kusserow of Yale University implanted a small blood pump into the abdomen of a dog to take over the function of the right side of the animal's heart.[30] Following up on this work, Kusserow reported a similar replacement pump for the left side of the heart in 1959.[31] Both of his pumps destroyed red blood cells (hemolysis), however, so his lab worked to revise pump design as well as to investigate new power sources, surgical implant procedures, and anticoagulant therapy to control blood clotting. At Miners Memorial Hospital in Harlan, Kentucky, Frank W. Hastings, William H. Potter, and John W. Holter developed a mechanical heart device driven by a reciprocating fluid column. It was a two-chambered diaphragm pump with an electric motor and a hydraulic pump that, when implanted in dogs, failed to maintain blood pressure and led to organ failure.[32] Problems with pump motors, valves, blood flow, and more kept William S. Pierce's research team at the University of Pennsylvania from keeping any dogs alive for more than a few hours.[33] At the University of Cordoba in Argentina, Domingo Liotta and his colleagues began implanting artificial hearts in dogs in 1959, experimenting with various types of pumps and materials. He recorded dogs surviving up to 13 hours, although none regained consciousness.[34] Liotta remarked, "From a mechanical point of view, the ventricular function of the heart-pump is not difficult to replace; the problem is to preserve the functional integrity of the rest of the circulatory system."[35] Testing these devices in vivo in dogs amplified problems that had seemed less an issue with mock circulation and in vitro (bench) testing. Only a handful of researchers pursued artificial heart research, and all reported dismal results at this early stage. These precarious beginnings soon gave way to a clearer course when Michael DeBakey took the stage.

Assist Pumps for Surgical Recovery: Michael DeBakey

In the 1960s, DeBakey emerged as a top authority in the field of heart disease as a result of his busy and innovative surgical practice at Houston's Methodist Hospital, his robust research program at Baylor College of Medicine, and his advocacy for a national heart disease research and treatment policy. DeBakey was visible and active; he served on national committees that would influence medical research and public health policies. Well-known celebrities and public figures, such as Marlene Dietrich, the Duke of Windsor, the Shah of Iran, and others, traveled to Houston and DeBakey's operating table for corrective surgery. Plentiful media coverage, press conferences, and photos of such high-profile visits augmented DeBakey's public profile. DeBakey was the presumptive leader in the field of bold, innovative cardiovascular procedures, repairing arteries with Dacron grafts or replacing damaged heart valves with plastic ones. He was also engaged in the development of artificial hearts, telling Congress in 1964 that mechanical pumps were "not a panacea" but "a definitely feasible program" with promising benefit for the pressing problem of heart failure.[36] For the development of artificial hearts, DeBakey's engagement as a clinical researcher and a medical statesman incited momentum, altered the research dynamics, and shaped the expectations of this technology.

DeBakey moved fluidly between the operating room and the laboratory. He investigated and performed numerous innovative vascular and cardiac procedures, such as carotid endarterectomy, heart valve replacements, and aneurysm surgery. His research ranged from the development of artificial Dacron arteries that bypassed damaged blood vessels to MCSSs that assisted or replaced failing hearts. From the outset, DeBakey acknowledged the complexity of designing a TAH. Initially his multidisciplinary team pursued experimental work similar to that of Kolff's lab, specifically focusing on a TAH as a permanent cardiac replacement device. But what was clinically needed more, according to DeBakey, was an assist device to prolong mechanical support for the heart beyond what was possible with the heart-lung machine. Alongside TAH research, DeBakey focused his attention on building both implantable and extracorporeal (outside the body) VADs for short-term cardiac assistance.[37]

In the early 1960s, DeBakey persuaded C. William Hall and Domingo Liotta, two cardiac surgeons already pursuing research on heart devices, to join his Baylor research team. Hall was working on aortic valves at the University of Kansas, and DeBakey lured him to Baylor College of Medicine to become his artificial heart program director.[38] Liotta, visiting from his native Argentina, spent several months as an observer in Kolff's laboratory in Cleveland, after which DeBakey offered him a surgical fellowship and a research position at Baylor.[39] Hall worked with DeBakey on mechanical design ideas and challenges, while Liotta implanted the experimental devices into animals in the surgical research laboratories.[40] Other technicians and assistants, "perhaps as many as 40 people," working in the machine and plastics shops in DeBakey's lab, also contributed to the building of early devices, according to one machinist-technician, attesting to the integrative nature of the technical knowledge and skills required in this research.[41]

One of the earliest assist pumps to emerge out DeBakey's research program was a small implantable tube of double-lumen silicon elastomer (rubber) that propelled blood from the weakened left side of the heart into the descending aorta and into the body. This intracorporeal tube-type pump consisted of a rigid outer tube with an inner, more flexible tube that collapsed by pressurized air entering the housing. This collapse pushed the blood in a unidirectional flow, with ball valves at either end of the outer tube. Pneumatically driven, the device required external lines penetrating the chest to connect to an external power source. Over many months, the research team, which included Liotta, Hall, and DeBakey, put the experimental pump in 51 dogs to refine the surgical implant procedure and to assess the performance of the device. Throughout the research, they published encouraging reports: this device took a portion of blood from the left atrium and pumped it into the descending aorta, off-loading or relieving the left ventricle from pumping all of the blood into the aorta.[42] The feasibility of assisting cardiac circulation by mechanical means had been demonstrated, at least on the healthy hearts of dogs.

The pump's first clinical use took place on July 19, 1963, when a 42-year-old man in congestive heart failure received this intracorporeal tube-type pump.[43] The patient had a severely damaged heart. He suffered pulmonary edema (buildup of fluid) caused by left ventricular failure, which had developed after he underwent an aortic valve replacement surgery, and then a heart attack that had necessitated a second operation to perform open-chest massage to restart the heart. The problem now was that the patient's left ventricle, severely weakened from long-standing heart disease, could not pump enough blood to maintain circulation. Arguably, this was the first patient to be implanted with any artificial pump, and it was an unplanned, last resort treatment that became the patient's third operation in less than a week. For three and a half days, the experimental device functioned adequately, as an assist device that rerouted some oxygenated blood out of the heart and into the descending aorta. Still the patient died, from widespread damage to other organs, but "not from failure of the pump," according to DeBakey, who successfully spun the outcome from a failure (patient death) to an endorsement for continued device research.[44]

At a meeting of the American Heart Association, DeBakey told colleagues that the pump had worked well enough, off-loading the damaged heart, and the patient's blood pressure and pulse rate had improved. To journalists, DeBakey emphasized the patient's improvement as a proof of concept for mechanical pumps, which some reporters embellished. *Time* magazine praised the device as a success, "a rest cure," and identified the problem as being the patient, who was described as a "doomed" man owing to his "old" and "hopelessly damaged" heart and "irreversible damage to his liver, lungs and kidneys."[45] Reporters described the pump as a device of promising potential against the backdrop of rising heart failure prevalence and mortality. The reality was that device problems existed that would take years to resolve. In examining the pump at autopsy, DeBakey's team identified fibrinous, clotted material inside the device that obviously had interfered with blood flow and needed to be fixed. Over the next three years, they worked on improving the device before attempting another clinical case.

Purposely, DeBakey searched for a better blood interface or contact surface to reduce the detrimental changes in the blood when it flowed from its normal habitat within the heart and blood vessels to the artificial environment of the mechanical pump. Fibrinous masses or blood clots formed, anchored in various locations in the device, which led to embolism (blockage of an artery), a life-threatening condition. DeBakey's previous experience with artificial arteries contributed to the team's development of a surface similar to the natural lining of arteries.[46] He proposed Dacron velour, which allowed the fibrinous material deposited by the blood to enmesh in the loops of the velour surface to create a new blood-compatible surface. For several days or weeks of device use, the Dacron velour proved satisfactory as a blood interface, producing minimal and tolerable damage to the blood. For longer periods, however, DeBakey warned that the fibrinous material continued to build up and ultimately impeded blood flow and pump performance. Thus, better blood interface materials remained a critical problem in the development of longer-term artificial hearts.[47]

Recognizing the scale and diversity of the problems at hand, DeBakey invited physical scientists and engineers from Rice University to collaborate with his Baylor team on pump design, pump control and power systems, and device materials research, for which he secured substantial National Heart Institute funding, approximately

$750,000 annually.[48] Together, the Rice engineering teams led by William O'Bannon and William Akers and the Baylor medical group directed by DeBakey, Hall, and Liotta experimented with different pump sizes, shapes, output, valves, and attachments to combat the problems of blood damage caused by device turbulence and blood clotting owing to blood stagnation and interfacing with foreign material. The teams devised different methods of automation to power and to regulate the pump, and they tested the strength, elasticity, and flexibility of the valves, diaphragms, pump housing, and connectors used in the fabrication of these devices.[49]

Over the next several years, the Baylor-Rice team developed several types of assist pumps that underscored, rather than resolved, the technological and biological complexities of building an artificial heart device.[50] For example, the Baylor-Rice team developed a sac-type assist device made of two layers of Dacron-reinforced Silastic (a silicone-plastic substance that was rubberlike and biologically inert). An external pneumatic pump forced air into the device, expanding and collapsing the inner layer to expel the blood into the circulation system. With some success, De-Bakey implanted this device in animals as both a left and a right VAD, suggesting that leaving the natural heart as a reservoir might be better functionally than excising the organ. He described the device as "the most promising," but adverse physical properties of the materials used in it caused blood problems and poor host acceptance.[51] A device of contrasting design and approach was an intraventricular pumping device, which consisted of a Silastic sleeve and was placed into the ventricles. Also pneumatically driven, this one required air transmission tubes from the device to penetrate the atrium wall and the chest of the patient and connect to the external source. But the problems of poor materials and interaction with the body plagued this device too.

DeBakey's team grappled with various power sources, including electrical and skeletal muscle power, for their devices. They explored electromagnetic induction by means of a primary coil outside the body to energize an implanted secondary coil, eliminating the need for penetrating wires. They examined the use of skeletal muscle (the latissimus dorsi muscle) to drive air bellows, which were connected to the devices by air transmission tubes. Neither proved realistic at this time.[52] What is significant about these diverse device designs and power source investigations is DeBakey's support of multidisciplinary, collaborative research, illustrating his recognition of the complexity of artificial hearts and the number of remaining ill-defined problems with MCSSs.

In addition to traditional medical and professional venues, DeBakey talked to journalists about his research work; the resulting publicity raised his public profile as a surgeon and researcher and encouraged public support for the development of artificial hearts. DeBakey did not shun press attention, and he intended to control the narrative. He believed in the need for communication—from researcher to researcher, from researcher to clinicians, and to the public—but with purpose. He recognized the public relations aspect of informing society about the impact of publicly funded programs, the value of research, and the possibilities of new disease treatments. To members of Congress, he stated, "We must communicate to the public what the potentialities of research may be," letting the people know that the value of research was its promise of knowledge and clinical application to address heart disease problems more effectively.[53] He recognized that good public relations would contribute to his status as an authority in the field, would help to secure public and private funding for heart disease research, and would promote the value of research centers (with Baylor College of Medicine situated as an obvious cardiovascular research center).

During the 1960s there was considerable publicity surrounding DeBakey's research work and surgical practice. He spoke regularly to journalists at news conferences and other media appearances, always in surgical garb, talking to the press despite traditional medical convention to avert lay publicity. In 1963 DeBakey performed a heart valve replacement surgery before a live television audience—the first such broadcast—drawing criticism from some of his peers for what they saw as courting the media and inviting personal attention.[54] "Only a few years ago, the publicity received today by physicians and scientists would have curled the hair of most ethics committees," stated Irvine H. Page, physician and director of research at the Cleveland Clinic Foundation.[55] But this was DeBakey crafting and publicizing an image of himself and Baylor College of Medicine, creating a narrative that focused on research possibilities, new surgical procedures, and patient benefits in which he fully believed; yet others labeled his actions medical propaganda. According to journalist Thomas Thompson, "DeBakey welcomed cameras and notebooks into his cloistered world. . . . [DeBakey] acted, he said, to inform the public about the progress made with federal funds—the *people's* money . . . and if Michael DeBakey became, coincidentally, the most famous surgeon in America, then it was a by-product over which he had no control."[56] DeBakey was a powerful organizer and promoter, and his critics panned his efforts as self-aggrandizement.[57] The publicity most certainly fed DeBakey's ego as well as drawing national and international recognition for his cardiovascular practice.

In 1965 DeBakey appeared on the cover of *Time* magazine, and the accompanying story recounted, and contributed to, the ongoing drive to develop an artificial heart. The cover story had been building; DeBakey had been the topic of three previous *Time* stories printed in the previous 19 months, reporting on his mechanical pump research, his findings as chair of the President's Commission on Heart Disease, Cancer, and Stroke, and his aortic aneurysm repair for His Royal Highness, the Duke of Windsor.[58] Entitled "Toward an Artificial Heart," the 1965 cover story told of DeBakey's many surgical accomplishments and his "confident prediction" of an artificial heart, his self-imposed, backbreaking schedule of operations, his robust research program, and his "drive for perfection." The six-page article ended on a note that DeBakey had most certainly orchestrated: it said the hold-up on the delivery of an artificial heart was the need for well-funded, collaborative research of scientists, clinicians, and industry to solve the problems of materials and power supply.[59] The article made a case that the development of artificial hearts was possible with DeBakey at the helm, showcasing the man and his work. It illustrated how savvy De-Bakey was in his relations with journalists and public relations, for it was not coincidental that during this period, after years of lobbying by DeBakey and others, the new federally funded Artificial Heart Program was established.

The Establishment of the Artificial Heart Program

Key to launching the fledgling field of mechanical circulatory support was the National Heart Institute (NHI). In 1964, after much lobbying by DeBakey, the Congress announced the artificial heart as a development priority and established the Artificial Heart Program at the NHI, part of the National Institutes of Health in Bethesda, Maryland.[60] The NHI, created 14 years earlier under President Harry Truman, supported research and training into the causes, prevention, diagnosis, and treatment of diseases of the heart and circulation.[61] Within the NHI, the newly created Artificial Heart Program constituted a federally sponsored, large-scale research and development program and contributed substantially to the advancement of MCSSs as it lured both academic and industry investigators into this line of work. Federal funding legitimated the research and framed how development would proceed. The Artificial Heart Program was the NHI's first targeted, extramural development program that adopted a systems development approach, as did many US space and defense science and technology projects, to plan, manage, and produce key deliverables toward the goal of building an artificial heart.

During the late 1950s and early 1960s, Kolff, DeBakey, Kantrowitz, and other investigators received some research funding for their artificial heart work from the NHI, but they wanted more. DeBakey's funding of $750,000 annually was unusual; the typical grant was far less. For example, in the years leading up to 1964, Kolff received roughly $340,000, Kantrowitz totaled about $200,000, Peter Salisbury collected approximately $50,000, and Bert Kusserow received about $56,000 in total NHI research grants for work related to the artificial heart.[62] In the postwar period, with a booming economy and popular backing for science and technology projects, congressional support for ambitious, new medical research programs was ripe for the picking. So, in an uneasy alliance with NHI administrators, artificial heart researchers pushed for the creation of a large-scale, government-sponsored development program.[63]

Well known in Congress for his prior testimony advocating greater federal research support, DeBakey first pitched the idea of funding artificial heart development before the Senate Subcommittee on Appropriations in 1963, stating, "Experimentally, it is possible to replace the heart with an artificial heart, and animals have been known to survive as long as 36 hours. This idea, I am sure, could reach full fruition if we had more funds to support more work, particularly in the bioengineering area."[64] NIH (National Institutes of Health) director James Shannon, a nephrologist by training, with a PhD in physiology, also testified in support of more funding for heart programs, but he was not as passionate as DeBakey for targeted artificial heart research. Still, it seemed that the NIH "was on notice to do something," according to cardiologist Thomas Preston, and the potential of artificial hearts captured more supporters.[65]

Several months later, the National Advisory Heart Council, a policy advisory body to the NHI made up of predominantly heart research and clinical specialists, endorsed the proposed artificial heart program "as one of high priority," enticed by its promise of making valuable contributions.[66] In early 1964, the NHI convened the Ad Hoc Advisory Group on the Mechanical Heart, which consisted of several leading artificial heart investigators including Kolff and DeBakey, who, not surprisingly, agreed with the National Advisory Heart Council and made recommendations regarding the next steps for implementation of a large-scale NHI program.[67] DeBakey was increasingly involved in securing federal support for heart disease research, capitalizing on President Lyndon B. Johnson's expectation to do something about the problem of heart disease.[68] In March 1964, Johnson asked DeBakey to chair the President's Commission on Heart Disease, Cancer, and Stroke.[69] Johnson's personal history of heart disease, dating back to his 1955 heart attack, intensified his commitment to increasing funding for cardiovascular research and treatment.[70] DeBakey became a prominent medical statesman and had increasing political clout with the Johnson administration. The White House viewed DeBakey as "the unquestioned leading vascular surgeon in the world," and DeBakey received numerous invitations to White House dinners, health events, committee participation, and bill signings during Johnson's presidency. Johnson thanked DeBakey for his "selfless service," declared his "warm admiration" for his work and how he valued his and DeBakey's "long friendship."[71] The pervasiveness of heart disease meant that many members of Congress or their family members also suffered cardiovascular problems, thus stimulating action and support. For example, Senator Lister Hill, who was the son of a surgeon, and Congressman John Fogarty, who suffered heart disease, were strong supporters of medical research related to heart problems, and they worked tirelessly to win broader congressional backing. Following suit, Congress members approved the program, convinced of its merit and its anticipated short-term development, and recommended that it be pursued "with a sense of urgency."[72]

In mid-1964 the NHI officially launched the Artificial Heart Program with the mission "to reduce death and disability from heart disease through the development and use of a variety of therapeutically effective, safe, and reliable cardiac assist and total replacement systems."[73] Frank W. Hastings, a surgeon and a researcher in the field of MCSS, became the first director of the Artificial Heart Program and played an influential guiding role in the program. From the outset, program administrators stressed a philosophy of rehabilitation rather than the mere prolongation of life, emphasizing the goal of developing a family of cardiac devices. NHI funded six contracts for system analysis studies, which would include an assessment of the entire

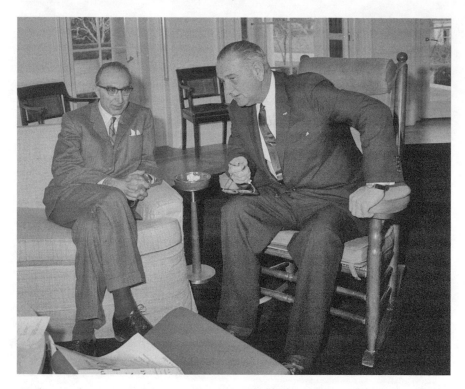

Cardiovascular surgeon and researcher Michael DeBakey (*left*) and President Lyndon B. Johnson in the Oval Office, White House, Washington, DC, March 20, 1964. LBJ Library Photo by Cecil Stoughton.

field of mechanical circulatory support and how best to proceed.[74] Their reports confirmed Hastings's position that, while some important work had been carried out by individual investigations under NIH grants, a systematic, goal-oriented, contract-supported approach to the total problem of building artificial hearts would be more effective.[75] In 1965 the Artificial Heart Program adopted this directed approach, funding contracts to academic, medical, and industrial organizations on the various subsystems (such as materials, energy, blood pumps, and physiology). Hastings intended "to speed the day when safe and effective devices could reach the bedside," and to do this, he mobilized resources and skills not fully utilized under the grant system.[76] By focusing on targeted device components, mostly engineering in nature, the NHI hoped to be more effective in developing better artificial hearts sooner.

Initially, the Artificial Heart Program received from Congress a fairly small budget of $1.1 million, or less than 1 percent of the NHI's total budget for research contracts and grants.[77] It was not enough, according to DeBakey, who returned to testify before congressional appropriations committees over the next several years to impress upon them the need for more funding for the program. "What we need is money," insisted DeBakey. "If we have the money, we can put the right kind of people to work on it."[78] Nobel Laureate and geneticist Joshua Lederberg wrote a letter to the Appropriations Committee stating, "We are spending millions and millions and millions of dollars in space and trying to get a man on the moon and on foreign aid. Here we are losing a million people who are dying every year because of some form of heart disease, and we quibble at trying to get a few million dollars to get going on this project."[79] In the end, federal funding for the program increased considerably, in large part because of the active lobbying of DeBakey and others. By the late 1960s the Artificial Heart Program annual budget was roughly $8 million, and it was supporting approximately 100 contracts.[80] The funding was a noticeable increase in just five years for this new program, but still a fraction of the total NHI annual budget of roughly $165 million at the time.[81] Artificial heart investigators welcomed the new funding, from which DeBakey, Kantrowitz, and Kolff received hundreds of thousands of dollars for their research programs over the next three decades.[82] DeBakey's optimism for the program was clear, if not overexaggerated, as he stated, "Because of the [recent] intensified effort, we are now . . . way ahead of schedule."[83] It did seem that the development of a practical artificial heart was in sight, the path forged by key, high-profile researchers with federal funding, and this confidence permeated throughout cardiovascular communities.[84]

The Artificial Heart Program was the first NHI targeted-research program, signaling a departure from the traditional funding structure of small grants and basic research. Its modified systems approach, a development model applied to many science and technology projects, including the space and military programs, stipulated research goals and set tight production schedules. In this approach, researchers worked in competing parallel programs, exploring similar and alternative systems to be adopted or discarded based on their contribution to targeted-research goals. It was a structured program intended to solve problems and achieve set objectives. Industry and academic researchers vied for contract or grant funding for independent development of valves, biomaterials, blood interface studies, control mechanisms, or power systems, which, at a later date, the program intended to integrate into a workable device. It supported basic research in universities and also incorporated the expertise of industry, such as electronics corporations, engineering firms, and chemical companies.[85] But the contract mechanism was not as complementary as NHI administrators had hoped, and they struggled with industry rivalries and collaboration difficulties despite NHI-facilitated contractor conferences. Nevertheless, in mid-1965, another Ad Hoc Advisory Group of medical scientists, engineers, physical scientists, and individuals experienced in systems analysis and development endorsed the modified systems approach for the development of artificial hearts.[86]

Profuse optimism beyond simply the enthusiasm of artificial heart researchers characterized these early program years. Bolstered by advances in the space program, Lederberg confidently stated that the building of the artificial heart was not as difficult as constructing a communications satellite or a lunar-probe vehicle.[87] NHI director

Ralph Knutti announced an ambitious four-phase development plan, predicting the availability of artificial hearts for widespread clinical use by 1970.[88] Administrators and scientists confidently presented a straightforward but flawed vision of its development. As argued by historian Barton Bernstein, "this strategy rested upon the optimistic but unfounded assumption that the problems of building an artificial heart were those of engineering, and that the basic scientific knowledge was available and had only to be harnessed. In short, it was assumed that the skills that had launched Americans into space could quickly build an artificial heart."[89]

The artificial heart was not just an engineering problem but also a biological problem as well as a foreseeable socioeconomic problem. The artificial heart had to function in a human body, an inhospitable environment for foreign objects of metal and plastic, which would require it to adjust spontaneously, such as speeding up or slowing down, to the body's needs and activities. The socioeconomic problems associated with complex devices like artificial hearts included costs, access, treatment support, patient quality of life, and autonomy in the patient's relationship with the technology. The artificial heart represented a failure of prevention; because it supported end-stage disease therapies, issues of health care priorities and cost containment in medicine would be debated. Most of these issues were not addressed at this time. Still, identifying the building of artificial hearts as an engineering problem was useful. It made the endeavor appear doable and desirable to nonmedical groups and communities at a time when medicine and society talked about rebuilding people and replacing parts. It positioned artificial hearts as a deliverable product at a time when the federal government was supporting applied research projects. As a result, the engineering emphasis contributed to, or shaped, the understanding of success that placed device efficacy as the first objective and device effectiveness as second. But assumptions of efficacy translating into effectiveness overlooked issues of patient expectations, suffering, and quality of life; these were issues with which many individuals in medicine and society would soon engage.

Broadly encompassing, the Artificial Heart Program proposed the development of a range of MCSSs that included both assistive and total replacement devices for short-term and long-term use, different devices to be used in different clinical situations to battle heart failure in America. While advocating mechanical support systems, DeBakey, Lederberg, and other researchers did not oppose basic research studies on the cause and prevention of cardiac disease. In the booming economy of the period, government largesse could certainly support a diverse assault on heart disease. However, DeBakey took issue with NIH director James Shannon's redirection of some artificial heart funding to support research on acute heart attacks, interpreting this as a lack of confidence in mechanical devices. Publicly Shannon supported artificial heart development to increase budget allocations from Congress, but privately he had serious doubts. In a memo to the surgeon general and secretary of the Department of Health, Education, and Welfare, the NIH director stated his opinion that "total cardiac replacement is not a feasible program objective at the present time" and that funding should be channeled to alternative strategies in the fight against heart failure.[90] Shannon argued that the scientific foundation necessary for the development of artificial hearts did not yet exist.[91] Specifically, the major obstacles included inadequate biomaterials to prevent blood clotting and the lack of an implantable power source, both of which required basic research rather than the industry contract support system of the Artificial Heart Program.

In 1966 Shannon established the Myocardial Infarction Branch as a sister program to the Artificial Heart Program, diverting more than half of the annual artificial heart budget to supporting this new branch of related cardiac research. The activities of this sister program would provide an essential base of medical knowledge relevant to the continued development and evaluation of mechanical circulatory support devices.[92] Shannon did have a bias toward basic over clinical research, and, as NIH director, he imposed what he felt was a better research balance in response to Congress's lavish funding of clinical research in the push to conquer disease. Based almost entirely on mortality rates, Congress targeted cancer, heart disease, and other leading disease threats of the period.[93] The research priorities within these areas were then directed by Shannon, who resisted any personal research agendas, as health research activist and philanthropist Mary Lasker found out when she challenged the priorities of cancer research.[94] Bernstein described Shannon's actions as "a deft bureaucratic strategy to whittle away at the artificial heart project," a strategy that, with the support of the Department of Health, Education and Welfare and the Bureau of the Budget, politically trumped DeBakey and his allies.[95]

Shannon did not favor the Artificial Heart Program, and neither, apparently, did the next NIH director, given the leveling off of the program budget. Annual requests for huge budget increases for the program were repeatedly refused by Shannon during his tenure. In 1966 the program budget was a paltry $4 million, but for 1967, NHI director Robert Grant requested a significantly higher program budget of $17 million, with annual increases to $44 million by 1972, for artificial heart development. Shannon did not approve the requests. Instead, for 1967 the program received an annual budget of $8 million, where it more or less remained for the next ten years.[96] In 1968 Shannon stepped down as NIH director. It is hard to fault Shannon and his immediate successors for their conservative funding of the Artificial Heart Program; their training as basic scientists contributed to a certain inertia to respond hastily to new, applied research projects, especially when they believed the fundamentals to be missing. Shannon was unequivocal in his views that judgments concerning allocations of resources required the competence of biomedical scientists and were simply beyond the capabilities of social and political scientists or nonscientific administrators in government. Shannon believed that NIH needed to stick with basic investigations into the nature and causes of diseases until enough knowledge was gained to allow for practical clinical application.[97] He recognized that the initial promises of artificial heart development had been set very high, in a context that included public pressure to arrest rising heart disease statistics and the convictions of a small group of artificial heart researchers. Not unrelated, a "novel technology" strategy to secure development support contributed to stimulating "agenda-setting processes" (both technical and political) and building "protected spaces."[98] The establishment of the Artificial Heart Program supported and protected the development of this technology in this way. Expectations had been set, but the hype was in jeopardy of turning into disappointment if DeBakey, Kantrowitz, and other device researchers could not demonstrate positive clinical use of the technology.

"Boosting" Patient Survival: Adrian Kantrowitz

In 1966 DeBakey and Kantrowitz independently reported clinical successes with their respective mechanical pumps and thus contributed to the maintaining of stakeholder expectations and device development. In Houston, DeBakey implanted in a series of patients his improved left ventricular assist pump, with mixed results. This pump was most likely the sixth DeBakey model, counting the pump used in his 1963 case as the first one.[99] Unlike the earlier pump, DeBakey's newest device rested outside the body (paracorporeal), with two connecting tubes (for blood flow) penetrating the patient's chest to attach to the left atrium and a systemic artery. The hemispherical, pneumatically driven pump was made of Dacron-reinforced Silastic with a molded diaphragm separating the gas chamber from the blood chamber. Pressurized air pulsed into the gas chamber, which collapsed the blood chamber and pumped the blood into the systemic artery for circulation into the body.[100] DeBakey viewed this device as temporary, to be used for only a matter of days or weeks, so placing the pump outside the body permitted easier surgical implantation and removal.

In April 1966 DeBakey implanted the pump in 65-year-old former coal miner Marcel DeRudder, who required the device to assist his severely diseased heart after an aortic valve repair operation. The mechanical pump assumed the workload of roughly 50 to 80 percent of the natural heart, allowing the weakened organ to heal before resuming full function. DeBakey could only guess how long DeRudder would need the pump.[101] DeRudder spent most of the next five days in a coma before he died from a collapsed lung (a result of complications unrelated to the device.) According to DeBakey, autopsy results provided evidence of cardiac healing that was due to the assist pump, and he told reporters that he would not hesitate to use the device again.[102] DeBakey continued to court the media, inviting a *Life* magazine photographer and journalist into the operating room to document DeRudder's operation. DeBakey's operating room was also well equipped with in-house cameras to film the operation for purposes of teaching and analysis, a practice that came to be followed in many teaching institutions. Despite the poor outcome for the patient, DeBakey was celebrated for his innovative device. The nine-page color spread of the operation in *Life* established DeBakey as a leader in artificial heart research beyond just the medical community.[103]

Less than a month later, DeBakey implanted an identical pump in 61-year-old Walter McCans, a retired navy petty officer who had undergone aortic valve replacement surgery. After a day, DeBakey removed the pump to address surgically the accumulation of fluid (probably blood) in the patient's chest, which ultimately caused McCans's death several days later. Despite the outcome, DeBakey reported that the short use of the pump contributed to cardiac healing, and unlike DeRudder, McCans had been conscious for much of this period.[104] While DeBakey considered the use of the pump in these cases to be successful, both of his patients had died. DeBakey's characterization of success was based on the efficacy of the device; it worked to pump blood with fair tolerance by the human body. But the effectiveness of the device could hardly be deemed a success, since its use did not produce the desired result of meaningful patient improvement.

While the media praised DeBakey for this daring procedure, many medical colleagues did not. Their disapproval arose from the lay publicity that reported the details of the clinical cases, often with inflated and emotion-laden statements. Many in the medical community viewed DeBakey's media coverage in this period as too much, reeking of self-promotion and infringing on patients' privacy. In a letter to DeBakey, surgeon-innovator Eugene M. Bricker described the DeRudder case as "a public spectacle" that he and many colleagues found "distasteful and embarrassing."[105] In a six-page editorial in *Modern Medicine,* Irvine Page stated that over-exuberant medical reporting of this "highly experimental procedure" had misled the public; he called for "caution and skepticism." It was a "shabby excuse," argued Page, to defend such dramatic reporting as necessary to promote and consolidate support for continued artificial heart research. He warned, "This blow-by-blow exhibit under klieg lights may be stimulating, melodramatic, and celebrity-building, but it will, in my opinion, spell disaster if adopted as a way of conducting research."[106] To *Medical World News* publisher Maxwell Geffen, DeBakey wrote a 10-page response to Page's comments, stating, "I believe it [Page's editorial] can do much harm to the support of the entire program, not only our own but those of other investigators at a time when much momentum for this program has been developed. . . . The whole tone of the editorial reflects resentment, embitterment, and hostility and is not only not objective but highly distorted."[107] In September 1966, the Harris County Medical Society censured DeBakey for using his name in the media in connection with the care of his patients.[108]

Echoing DeBakey's interpretation of success but with less publicity, Kantrowitz announced similar results with the mechanical auxiliary ventricle, or "booster heart," that he had designed with his brother, physicist Arthur Kantrowitz, who was a founding director of Avco Everett Research Labs in Everett, Massachusetts.[109] Kantrowitz's device was smaller than DeBakey's pump and had no valves; it was intended for permanent use, operated continuously or intermittently, and was placed inside rather than outside the body. Kantrowitz's mechanical auxiliary ventricle was a sausage-shaped

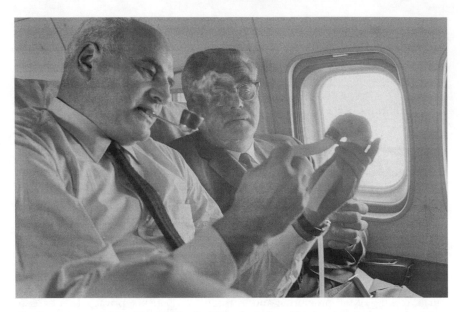

Cardiac surgeon Adrian Kantrowitz (holding device) and his brother Arthur, a physicist, examine their experimental, U-shaped auxiliary ventricle, or "booster heart," in June 1966. Used with permission from Getty Images.

double tube—a flexible silicone-rubber inner chamber encased in rigid fiberglass housing—with woven Dacron cuffs that connected surgically to the ascending and descending aorta. Its surgical position along the aortic arch formed the device into a U shape, and its proximity to the heart contributed to its greater effectiveness. The pneumatically driven device connected to an external control unit that admitted gas to the space between the outer housing and the inner chamber. Termed a "booster heart," the device worked in tandem with the natural heart and augmented blood flow by the natural heart. The inner tube filled with blood during the systole phase (contraction) of the natural heart. Compressed air then entered between the tubes, expelling blood from the inner tube into the circulatory system during the diastole phase (relaxation) of the natural heart.[110] This act reduced aortic pressure, decreasing the resistance against which the ventricle must eject blood, and thus reduced left ventricular work. In this way counterpulsation reduced the workload of the heart without reducing the blood supply.

Kantrowitz tested his mechanical auxiliary ventricle on 74 dogs over a period of several years to perfect the device, in the process attracting numerous researchers, including Japanese surgeons Tetsuzo Akutsu and Yukihiko Nosé, to join his team to study the counterpulsation approach in MCSSs.[111] In February and May 1966, Kantrowitz implanted his "booster heart" in two patients at Maimonides Hospital in New York.[112] The first patient was a 33-year-old man with chronic left ventricular failure caused by cardiomyopathy (heart muscle disease), who died less than 24 hours after implantation of the device.[113] Two months later, Kantrowitz implanted the same device into Louise Ceraso, a 63-year-old woman in congestive heart failure (impaired heart function) who survived 12 days.[114] The mechanical auxiliary ventricle operated intermittently—on for two hours, off for one hour—but longer if warranted. Although Kantrowitz intended the device to be permanent, he wanted to increase the patient's tolerance to unassisted circulation and not create full dependence on the mechanical device. According to Kantrowitz, the patient did relatively well; "she sat up, ate her meals, and visited with her family."[115] However, she died from a cerebral vascular event (stroke), which upon postmortem examination proved to be the result of a thrombus (clot) originating at the site where the device connected to the aorta. Despite the final outcome, Kantrowitz reported that his mechanical auxiliary ventricle worked (though arguably not well enough, given the patient's death) in assisting the circulation of patients dying of heart failure. He encouraged the use of such devices in more clinical cases, returning to the laboratory to improve his device before he proceeded.[116] Years later in an interview with Dr. Allen Weisse, Kantrowitz reflected, "[DeBakey] was smarter than I was; he realized that [these devices] could only be used as a temporary device and not a permanent one because of the clotting problem."[117]

Both DeBakey and Kantrowitz characterized the clinical use of their pumps as successes for a variety of reasons. Their device endorsement reflected their alliance with other artificial heart researchers, their shared belief in a clinical role for these devices, and their desire to maintain federal research funding for continued device development. For the researcher, success may be understood as incremental to address the various technical and biological problems associated with these devices and as reiterative to refine design form and function. For the surgeon, success tends to emphasize the curative or reparative nature of the treatment, with the patient experience and outcome playing a larger role in the assessment. As surgeon-researchers, DeBakey and Kantrowitz were sensitive to both device efficacy and effectiveness, and of course they wanted to prolong the lives of their desperately ill patients. But in these 1966 implant cases, both men described their cases as successes in a narrow way that focused on device performance. At some level, they no doubt believed that these cases were not failures despite patient death, because what was learned could be applied to the next case with an improved pump. They also were savvy enough to recognize that continued research funding and political support rested on the demonstration of knowledge gained toward meeting the larger goal. The interpretative flexibility of success used to assess these early 1966 device cases worked to retain the promissory nature, rather than concede disappointment or disillusionment over this technology. Arguably, "success" was required to maintain individual motivation and confidence in this grand pursuit as well as to maintain the investment, structure, and legitimacy that had been built within the young field of artificial heart research. Overused, and at times misused, the word *success* was used often and purposefully when describing early implant cases to both medical and nonmedical audiences. It sustained momentum and expectations that the realization of clinically acceptable mechanical hearts would be forthcoming.

For the first time, DeBakey sustained a patient's life with the use of his experimental ventricular assist pump in August 1966. He implanted the external, bypass pump in 37-year-old Esperanza Del Valle Vasquez, whose weakened heart had failed to resume function after aortic and mitral valve replacement surgery. After 10 days, DeBakey assessed the patient's heart to be strong enough to pump on its own, and he removed the device. The patient made a full recovery and was discharged from the hospital one month after her valve surgery.[118] Thereafter DeBakey reported more clinical cases, in which other patients also benefited from short-term pump assistance after heart surgery. For example, in 1967 a 16-year-old girl recovered from mitral valve replacement surgery after using DeBakey's ventricular assist pump for four days.[119] But despite patient success, DeBakey ruled out wide clinical application of this pump based on its prohibitive cost, the major surgical intervention required, and imperfect blood interface materials. Collaborating with Statham Instruments, a producer of aerospace and biomedical instrumentation, the Baylor-Rice research returned to the laboratory to review pump designs, to explore better biocompatible materials, and to evaluate the pump's performance based on bench tests and recent clinical use.[120] DeBakey firmly stated that, in its present stage of development, the use of cardiac assist devices must remain an investigative procedure.[121]

Challenging this assessment, Kantrowitz designed and fabricated an intraaortic balloon pump, a second counterpulsating assist device, different from his "booster heart." He tested it first on animals and later on patients with clinical success, and he witnessed its transition from an investigational device to a commercial one by the early 1970s.[122] The intraaortic balloon pump was a long tube with a polyurethane pumping chamber, covered in flexible woven copper tubing, about 1 cm in length and 0.4 cm in diameter that expanded to 14.8 cm in length and about 1.8 cm in diameter. Inserted through the left femoral artery and into the aorta, the balloon pump inflated and deflated to assist blood flow from the heart into the body.[123] The pump attached to an electronic control unit and helium source outside the body. The idea of the intraaortic balloon pump was not new, as acknowledged by Kantrowitz.[124] It had originated in Kolff's laboratory, where Spyridon Moulopoulos and others tested the device on dogs but never used it clinically.[125] Kantrowitz revisited their work in the attempt to develop a practical system to offer temporary cardiac assist to patients in cardiogenic shock. He reconfigured the balloon to reduce occlusion (blockage) and used helium instead of carbon dioxide as the driving gas. After three successful cases (from a total of five) in 1967, Kantrowitz claimed that the intraaortic balloon pump constituted a simpler and more effective means of providing temporary mechanical circulatory support than DeBakey's left ventricular bypass system.[126] Over the next three and a half years, Kantrowitz and his associates implanted the balloon in a total of 30 cases, reporting more positive than

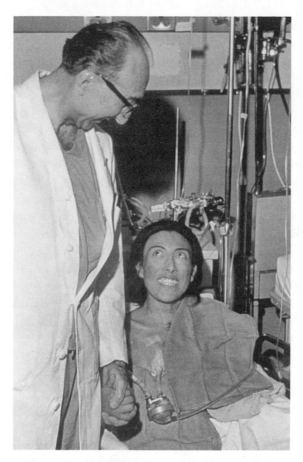

Cardiovascular surgeon Michael DeBakey with patient Esperanza Del Valle Vasquez, recovering from heart surgery with the support of an external cardiac assist pump, August 1966. Courtesy of the Baylor College of Medicine Archives.

negative patient outcomes. As a result, a larger, cooperative study of the intraaortic balloon pump was initiated at nine other medical centers.[127]

Stimulated by his success with this temporary pump, Kantrowitz continued research on a permanent left ventricular assist device, redesigning the U-shaped auxiliary ventricle, or "booster heart," into the "dynamic aortic patch." The patch consisted of a cigar-shaped silicone rubber pumping chamber, with a connecting air tube, that Kantrowitz sutured into the wall of the aorta in essentially the same location as the temporary intraaortic balloon pump. He reported preliminary experimental results obtained with the patch that paralleled those achieved with the temporary balloon pump. After a long-term dog study, in which one animal lived 22 months with the patch, Kantrowitz implanted the device in three patients in the early 1970s.[128] The longest surviving case was Haskell Shanks, a 63-year-old man in chronic congestive heart failure who had been bedridden for several years. He recovered from the operation, became ambulatory, and was discharged from hospital, returning home with different drive systems, including a portable battery unit.[129] He died three months after his implant from an infection at the site of the drive tube that connected his implanted device to the external power unit.[130] Whereas the acute heart failure patients had benefited from the balloon pump, Kantrowitz optimistically reported that the patch offered benefits to patients in severe, chronic left ventricular heart failure but that severe infectious complications thwarted its adoption.[131]

While Kantrowitz continued his research on a left ventricular device for permanent implantation, DeBakey returned his attention to the development of a TAH. From 1966 to 1968, the Baylor-Rice team explored designs for a biventricular, artificial heart utilizing the materials, control mechanisms, and power sources of the assist pumps. Unlike the earlier TAH designed in 1962–64 that left the natural heart in position, this new device required the removal of the natural heart before implantation. The newer DeBakey model consisted of two separate units—a right and a left ventricle—fabricated of Dacron-reinforced Silastic that were later bound together with Dacron. In the pneumatically driven device, air forced the diaphragm to collapse the blood chamber in each unit, thus pumping blood from the right and left ventricles into the pulmonary artery and the aorta, respectively. Surgical implantation of this device was not easy, requiring the removal of the ventricles of the biological heart and suturing the artificial heart to the remaining atria (top of the heart) and the patient's great blood vessels. Animal experiments in the first three months of 1969 demonstrated this surgical difficulty, as the first four calves died on the operating table owing to surgical and technical problems. The next three calves survived the surgery, but the device did not sustain life beyond a few hours. Dissatisfied with improper valves, weak arterial pressure levels, and unknown blood interface performance, DeBakey concluded that significant technical and physiological problems prevented this device from clinical use anytime soon.[132]

Foundations Laid: Uncertainty Remains

By the late 1960s, a research structure and greater clarity surrounding the requirements and needs for building artificial hearts had emerged as a result of the research of Kolff, DeBakey, and Kantrowitz and the establishment of the Artificial Heart Program. Each of these researchers benefited from the new federal funding of the Artificial Heart Program, and all continued to lead robust research programs for decades thereafter. Kolff, DeBakey, and Kantrowitz attracted a large number of younger researchers who were eager to study innovative new approaches in mechanical circulatory support. American surgeons and specialists Denton Cooley, Steven J. Phillips, Robert Jarvik, and William DeVries, as well as international researchers Tetsuzo Akutsu, Yukihiko Nosé, Domingo Liotta, and others, moved fluidly between these leading laboratories, contributing to a network of mobile researchers and cross-fertilization of ideas and approaches in the challenges of building artificial hearts.

Certainly Kolff, DeBakey, and Kantrowitz presented their results at professional conferences, such as the meetings of the American Society for Artificial Internal Organs, disseminating their views on the challenges and incremental research gains in MCSSs.

These three researchers were united in their commitment to the feasibility and desirability of artificial hearts, but they proposed three different devices. Was the approach of one researcher better than another? In contrast to Kolff's TAH research, DeBakey's and Kantrowitz's assist devices emerged as the more prudent development path in terms of feasibility, cost, and clinical (but still experimental) use. Of these two assist devices, which one was better—a device that worked independently to take over for a compromised heart (such as DeBakey's pump), or an implant that worked in tandem with the natural heart (such as Kantrowitz's serial-type device)? It depended on the patient case: clinical indication (such as the severity of the heart failure and functional heart limitations) would lend itself to one approach over the other, if these devices moved beyond experimental treatments. Other factors, such as cost, intended short-term or long-term use, and level of the surgeon's training and experience with a particular device, would also influence device choice. But at this point, none of the three proposed devices were ready for widespread clinical use.

Broader questions to ask include: When is there value in diversity of approaches? When is it sensible to converge on one approach to a problem? In general, multiple approaches are often taken as a way to gain confidence in the validity of research findings and data. It is useful to support various lines of inquiry when a field is young, when there is not one obvious research pathway, and when there are different constituents, with different backgrounds, identifying different needs to be fulfilled. Changing technology can also contribute to destabilizing set research approaches, and a level of flexibility afforded with multiple approaches may help to address such a situation. Multiple approaches to a problem can also signify a tension or lack of cohesion in a community grappling with uncertainty. What was the best approach to arrest rising morbidity and mortality rates of heart disease? Prevention or treatment strategies? American research communities support both, although there is debate about the level of research and funding priorities attached to each strategy. Within the treatment arena, an engineering approach to fixing medical problems contributes to high-technology diagnostic and curative ventures, drawing away from the ideal of preventing disease. Convergence on a single approach to a problem typically occurs when field experts reach consensus to do so, with expectations of producing a standard of care amenable to the context (such as evidence-based medicine) in which it will be provided.

In the case of artificial heart development, the three different approaches examined in this chapter reflect the beginnings of a specialized and multidisciplinary field, the uncertainty surrounding the state of engineering and biological sciences required to build artificial hearts, and the varied scope and clinical indications for these devices. A young field, such as MCSSs, often supports multiple device approaches, drawing in diverse constituents with different lines of inquiry, as a way to provide more information about device biomaterials, mechanics, implant tolerance in the body, and other factors. Producing new knowledge about heart failure, device-body interactions, technological limitations, device biomaterials, and power challenges contributed to what little was known, and it stimulated research interest and activity. Supporting a range of devices at this early stage allowed for a wide net to be cast, and no one knew which research teams, medical centers, and lines of inquiry would be most productive and what information would be learned. It allowed for a motley group of researchers—from disciplined scientists to free-spirited, gadgeteer geniuses—to connect as a community, fledgling as it certainly was in those early days. Artificial Heart Program administrators supported multiple approaches, and in adopting a systems development management strategy, they issued competing contracts to develop various components, intending that key points of convergence would occur, leading to technical consolidation and eventual device integration. Scheduled NIH reviews and reported research findings would bolster some lines of device development (such as pulsatile cardiac assist devices) and end others (such as the nuclear-powered heart). It made sense to support multiple approaches at this early stage of device development for the basic and applied knowledge that they generated at a time when federal coffers were willing to supply the funding to do so. It made sense to converge on one device approach to heart failure when evidence of efficacy was being matched with evidence of effectiveness. At that point, administrators hoped that the research and development process would be more fully in the hands of industry. The medical marketplace, with all the socioeconomic parameters and debates involved therein, also came to influence clinical acceptance. Only a few mechanical pumps reached this stage. In the case of artificial heart development, the multiple approach experience did not remove the uncertainty surrounding the feasibility of these devices, but it contributed a sense of legitimacy and momentum for the young field.

The growing research empires of Kolff and DeBakey placed them as the favorites in the quest to develop a clinically viable mechanical heart. With no less resolve, Kantrowitz conducted his research more modestly, initially at Maimonides Hospital in Brooklyn and later at Sinai Hospital of Detroit, where he moved in 1970; eventually he set up L-VAD Technologies, a bioelectronics development company devoted to cardiac assistive devices, with his wife Jean. All three researchers reported varying levels of success with their respective experimental devices, but none of these were ready for wider clinical adoption. Early patient cases of device "success"—an assessment arguably manipulated to serve political purposes that focused on incremental technical advances in this period—maintained program momentum and funding, fueling the hopes and promises of mechanical circulatory support devices. Whether astutely or unknowingly, the research community focused on the heart's mechanistic functions, foregrounding the feasibility of building an artificial heart that would sustain a patient's life. No discussion emerged regarding whether a mechanical replacement would be fully satisfying to the public in terms of how it altered the human body or how it traversed the cultural meanings of love and the soul associated with the human heart.

The role of the Artificial Heart Program was significant in providing the essential development funding and for buttressing academic-industry collaborations. It implemented a contracts-based, goal-targeted funding program as a result of effective lobbying by the artificial heart research community, most notably by DeBakey. Already involved in heart disease commissions on Capitol Hill, DeBakey had the ear of key decision makers to press for artificial heart development. Based on his petition for more research money and industry expertise, the decision of NIH to initiate an artificial heart development program that employed a contract-supported, components development approach made sense. It seemed a good fit for this program. It would support multiple approaches, multiple collaborations, responsible monitoring, and timely review and would also involve experts and provide opportunity for decision making on when or whether researchers should converge on one approach to the problem. By the early 1970s, greater support for the development of cardiac assist devices had accrued, in large part influenced by the work of Kolff, DeBakey, and Kantrowitz.

But there were two major drawbacks to the systems development approach for the Artificial Heart Program. First, it assumed that the basic science existed to support this applied research. As an engineering problem, the task of building artificial hearts privileged energy sources and pump construction, its feasibility as a workable device predominantly demonstrated through bench testing. It was also a biological problem in which questions about issues such as device implant and body tolerance, blood interface materials, and blood damage needed answers. Shannon had been correct in recognizing that more basic science research was needed and in encouraging work to be done in these related areas. In his view, extensive "hardware" building was premature, but this view was not well received by artificial heart researchers. It did not matter, given Shannon's position as NIH director, and he felt fully justified in siphoning money away from the Artificial Heart Program to related cardiac research projects during the 1960s.

Second, the contractors' meetings, arranged by program administrators to foster open exchange of device development work among all investigators for greater research gain and to assist with rigid timelines, produced mixed results. Administrators assumed that industry investigators would be as forthcoming with their research findings as academic researchers. They were not. Thomas Preston argues, "Instead of the usual academic process of prompt publications of results and full interchange of information, the parceling of contracts to competitive private companies put a premium on secrecy that undoubtedly impeded the program."[133] Industry was reluctant to share its work, professing that it was proprietary knowledge. Still, in the small world of artificial heart research, investigators navigated this line. Secrecy was not a major impediment to the program; the walls were not absolute, and there was professional exchange, owing to the scope of technical difficulties and the involvement of NIH administrators who insisted on it. Researchers talked among themselves, in a growing multidisciplinary network, presenting and publishing their findings to colleagues through their professional meetings and specialty journals. NIH administrators recognized industry concerns, and in the end, the two stakeholders found a workable middle ground of protected, limited disclosure. Given the lengthy, expensive research-and-development cycle of mechanical hearts, a cooperative relationship was necessary for a successful hand-off from federally funded research to industry funded commercial development.

The establishment of the Artificial Heart Program, as argued by physician and health policy consultant Michael J. Strauss, provided artificial heart research with a degree of autonomy and momentum that was both scientific and political.[134] This NHI targeted-research program exemplified the technological optimism and political support of the period. Artificial heart investigators in other countries, including Japan, Germany, and even Canada, worked in more modest federally funded research programs. As a result of political (and corresponding financial) support in the United States, Kolff, DeBakey, and Kantrowitz continued active artificial heart research programs that attracted and trained researchers from throughout the United States and abroad for decades thereafter. Periodic review of the Artificial Heart Program renewed political support for artificial heart research. Politicians were well aware of the potential of such cardiac devices for many Americans, and they hesitated to question the scientific authority of artificial heart researchers.

Building artificial hearts required decades of investigation, demonstrating the difficulty of mechanically replicating heart function and, more importantly, the biological adoption of artificial hearts. During these early years of building artificial hearts, serious research challenges emerged in the programs of all investigators, including those of Kolff, DeBakey, and Kantrowitz. Attempting to mechanically replicate the human heart was a daunting task for any researcher. Once investigators designed an artificial heart that actually worked, they struggled to refine their devices in four ways toward making its widespread clinical use realistic. First, and most obviously, the ideal artificial heart had to be small enough to fit into the chest and strong enough to match the power of the natural heart. Second, the power source for the device had to be safe and suitable for long-term use. Third, the mechanical heart had to adjust to the patient's physical and emotional responses, supporting the body's changing needs. Fourth, an artificial heart had to be composed of durable material to stand up to severe and constant pounding, and it had to overcome any problems of blood-prosthesis interface (to avoid causing thrombi, or clots). Early artificial heart research of the 1950s and 1960s contributed to identifying these parameters, with Kantrowitz most succinctly outlining these device requirements.[135]

Most researchers, if not all, were confident that these problems were surmountable and that devices could be constructed within these parameters. The clinical cases of Esperanza Del Valle Vasquez, Haskell Shanks, and others encouraged investigators to carry on. Were they not close to perfecting a family of cardiac devices, as envisioned by the Artificial Heart Program? Early artificial heart research of the 1950s and 1960s supported the development of many cardiac devices to treat the different clinical scenarios of heart failure patients. There would not be one artificial heart but many artificial hearts. Device improvements through more bench and animal research continued, with Kolff, DeBakey, and Kantrowitz shaping the field of MCSSs for decades. Their preeminence did not, however, preclude the involvement of other investigators, who, although less well known for their device research, also aspired to develop clinically useful mechanical hearts. The first case of a TAH implanted in a human occurred not by Kolff, DeBakey, or Kantrowitz but by an ambitious colleague—Denton Cooley—and it provoked drama, ethical questions, and an unanticipated impact on the development of artificial hearts thereafter.

CHAPTER TWO

Dispute and Disappointment

Heart Transplantation and Total Artificial Heart Implant Cases in the 1960s

Heart transplants should only be a stepping stone to the development of a mechanical heart. . . . these two lines of research should go on together.

Statement of leading American cardiac surgeons and cardiologists,
American Heart Association Press Conference (1968)

During the 1960s, few, if any, surgeons came close to matching the volume of cardiovascular surgery performed by American surgeons Michael DeBakey and Denton Cooley. Thousands of patients, suffering a range of acute and chronic cardiovascular disease problems, made their pilgrimage to Houston, Texas, hoping to benefit from the surgical skill of one of these men.[1] Remarkably, DeBakey and Cooley performed countless innovative and complicated procedures, from heart valve replacements to aneurysm surgery, that saved hundreds of lives and established Houston as a leading cardiovascular center. Both surgeons dared to operate when many others would not, and they introduced new surgical solutions arising out of their research programs, such as DeBakey's ventricular assist devices during the mid-1960s. But it was the bold, new surgery of heart transplantation, not mechanical devices, that captured greater public attention in this decade.

In 1967, in Cape Town, South Africa, cardiac surgeon Christiaan Barnard performed the first transplantation of a human heart into a patient. A tumultuous era in cardiac transplant surgery followed, with Cooley performing the greatest number of heart transplant operations in the United States in the early years of this procedure. In the 15 months between December 1967 and April 1969, Cooley and DeBakey performed 19 and 10 heart transplant operations, respectively. However, both surgeons reported staggeringly high mortality rates; most heart transplant patients died within weeks of the surgery owing to organ rejection or infection.[2] In early 1968 DeBakey identified the limitations of heart transplantation—namely, organ rejection and the availability of donor hearts—and urged further development of an artificial heart as a means, temporary or otherwise, to maintain the lives of transplant candidates and recipients in organ rejection.[3] Cooley apparently did not disagree, stunning DeBakey and other cardiac surgeons when he implanted a mechanical heart in 47-year-old Haskell Karp in April 1969.

Haskell Karp lived his life with three different hearts. In 1969 Cooley removed Karp's diseased native heart and implanted an experimental total artificial heart, which kept him alive for 64 hours; at that time he received a transplanted donor heart. But Karp lived only 32 hours with his third heart before succumbing to pneumonia and kidney failure. At this time, there was significant debate concerning the best cardiac replacement therapy—human or mechanical parts—to offer heart failure patients; neither produced satisfactory outcomes. The artificial heart operation stirred tremendous controversy within the medical community and society because of its experimental nature. It also severed the professional relationship of DeBakey and Cooley owing to allegations of device theft and lack of authorization to perform the implant procedure.

The sensational and sustained media attention on heart transplantation carried over to the daring artificial heart operation and the dispute between DeBakey and Cooley. Up to this point, the majority of media coverage on artificial heart research had been limited to DeBakey and his work, such as the multipage color *Life* magazine story on his assist pump operation in 1966.[4] The intense media interest and commentary that accompanied heart transplantation spilled over into artificial heart work, because of the overlapping cast of characters and the drama of both cardiac replacement therapies. Perceived by some journalists as companion fields, heart transplantation and the implantation of artificial hearts were daring medical acts, with surgeon-celebrity personas and inspirational patient stories, which were easily embedded in the medical and technological optimism of the period.[5] Sustained media coverage played a role in shaping public understanding of organ replacement therapy, highlighting the hopefulness of spare parts surgery as well as the medical and ethical complexities of cardiac replacement.

In the late 1960s, these two cardiac replacement procedures—heart transplantation and the implantation of artificial hearts—became intertwined, benefiting the development of artificial hearts. This chapter argues that the challenges and uncertainties experienced in heart transplant surgery augmented the standing and perceived value of artificial heart implantation as a complementary, not competing, cardiac replacement treatment. In this period, the research pursuit of artificial hearts gained greater stabilization in two specific ways as a result of overlapping events and debates with cardiac transplant surgery. First, the introduction and later success of heart transplantation expanded the role for artificial hearts. They no longer served only as promising bridges to recovery or as assist devices for postoperative cardiac patients, as demonstrated by DeBakey earlier in the decade; they now became also potential bridge-to-transplantation devices for heart failure patients when Cooley used one in this way in April 1969. Second, the initial favorable reception, then disillusionment, and later adoption of heart transplant surgery by medical communities and the public contributed to the overall legitimacy of organ replacement therapy. Allied with the heart transplant community, artificial heart researchers sustained funding, expectations, and a broader medical base by reinforcing the imagining and promise of heart replacement. In specialized cardiac centers, a relatively small number of surgeons explored both high-risk, experimental procedures, driven by the increasing number of their end-stage heart disease patients, that nonetheless led to professional and public expressions of concerns and misgivings. In addition, De-Bakey and Cooley's well-publicized rift over the April 1969 implant case highlighted issues relating to device authority and its clinical use that reverberated for years to come in the development of artificial hearts.

A Tale of Two Surgeons: Michael DeBakey and Denton Cooley

In 1948 Michael DeBakey accepted the challenge to bolster the surgical department at the Baylor College of Medicine, which had recently relocated from Dallas to Houston, Texas. DeBakey was a slight, dark-haired man, the son of a Lebanese merchant. He had spent more than a decade at the School of Medicine at Tulane University in New Orleans and had recently provided distinguished service in wartime medical operations, most notably the establishment of mobile surgical hospitals. From the outset of his career, it was clear that DeBakey was an innovative surgeon, who was hard-working and demanding of himself and, by extension, his staff. He was driven to strengthen Baylor's struggling surgical program, and he was determined to excel in his own surgical practice. He accomplished both goals. Within a few short years, De-Bakey established Houston as the center for aneurysm bypass surgery and cardiovascular repair. In the 1950s he argued that addressing the cause or even prevention of blocked arteries and veins was not necessary; as a surgeon, he could simply bypass such obstructions. DeBakey devised grafts—first human grafts from cadavers and later plastic grafts made of Dacron—to redirect the blood around obstacles in arteries that might otherwise rupture or cut off blood circulation. With his innovative Dacron graft, DeBakey repaired aortic and abdominal aneurysms and performed hundreds of these operations at a time when most surgeons refused to attempt such difficult procedures.[6]

DeBakey's reputation for taking on desperate cases grew, and he received referrals from across the country and the world. During the 1950s, DeBakey practiced volume surgery at Methodist Hospital, performing more aneurysm and vessel surgery in one month than most surgeons did in a year. Whereas the Mayo Clinic had long been recognized for its large number of common surgical procedures, such as removal of gall bladders, DeBakey forged a reputation as performing the greatest number of complex vascular procedures with success. He was an excellent surgeon, a perfectionist who was intolerant of mistakes, and a hard taskmaster. It was not unusual for him to spend 18 or 20 hours a day at the hospital. DeBakey kept a self-imposed, grueling schedule of operations. To a magazine journalist who was shadowing him for the day, he grumbled, "Too much to do and not enough time. Gotta get other people to move."[7] As a result of DeBakey's large caseload, the Methodist Hospital underwent four major additions; from its original 301-bed capacity in the early 1950s, it grew to become a 1,000-bed facility by 1970.[8]

DeBakey's research program bolstered his surgical practice and his international reputation. Like Willem Kolff and Adrian Kantrowitz, DeBakey experimented with mechanical cardiac devices to assist and replace the damaged human heart. Collaborating with researchers at Rice University, DeBakey's team developed several types of cardiac assist pumps and a TAH that underscored, rather than resolved, the technological and biological complexities of building an artificial heart device.[9] Nevertheless, DeBakey reported some positive results with his temporary assist pumps, notably the 1966 case of Esperanza del Valle Vasquez, who after 10 days attached to the pump made a full recovery.[10] Research on a total replacement artificial heart, however, presented more difficulties. Dissatisfied with improper valves, weak arterial pressure levels, and unknown blood interface performance, DeBakey concluded that significant technical and physiological problems prevented this device—the TAH—from clinical use anytime soon.[11]

At this time, DeBakey was also busy as a medical statesman for medical education and cardiovascular research; he served by invitation on numerous federal commissions and National Institutes of Health study groups. Politicians and senior health administrators in Washington solicited DeBakey's opinion on health matters ranging from medical research to training initiatives, awarding DeBakey political clout that he leveraged for greater government support of research on mechanical circulatory support systems. His reputation as a cardiovascular surgical innovator and authority extended beyond the medical community to political and public circles.[12] DeBakey garnered more and more support and a higher profile for cardiovascular surgery, and not surprisingly, the best and brightest surgeons sought to work with him, including Denton Cooley.

In 1951 Cooley accepted a surgical position at the Baylor College of Medicine, after completing medical school at Johns Hopkins University, where he trained under Alfred Blalock, the cardiac surgeon who introduced corrective "blue baby" operations, and one year of postgraduate training under the leading British chest and heart surgeon, Lord Russell Brock, in London. Being in the right place at the right time, Cooley participated in several early, investigational operations while in England. Open-heart surgery was still in its infancy at this time, with experimental bubble oxygenators and other heart-lung machines that made it possible for surgeons to reroute blood for oxygenation away from the heart temporarily, allowing them to stop the heart and complete repairs in a bloodless field. Technology promised to expand the field of heart surgery tremendously, and Cooley sought to be at the center of it. The position at Baylor College of Medicine offered Cooley the opportunity to work with DeBakey, who was attracting a larger number of cardiovascular patients than almost any other surgeon in the United States. Moreover, shifting to Houston was a homecoming for Cooley.[13]

Twelve years younger than DeBakey, Cooley was a tall, blond, and affable native Texan, who was born into a family of wealth and social prestige. Already a talented surgeon, Cooley joined DeBakey's team eager to do more. He assisted DeBakey during the early surgical years of aneurysm bypass and vascular repairs, keeping the demanding pace set by the tireless DeBakey for himself and his staff. Soon Cooley was performing countless cardiac operations, improving and refining his surgical techniques. Most of the heart operations performed by Cooley and DeBakey in the early 1950s were tricky "closed heart" or reparative procedures done on a beating heart; surgeons were not afforded the luxury of working on a still, bloodless heart until the introduction of open heart surgery a few years later. The type of "closed heart" and extracardiac operations attempted by surgeons included mitral commissurotomy (with a finger, opening a mitral valve that had been hardened by disease) and repairing congenital defects such as patent ductus arteriosus (blood vessel opening), coarctation of the aorta (blood vessel narrowing), pulmonary valve stenosis (blocked valve), and tetralogy of Fallot (abnormal heart structure). Cooley performed two to four closed-heart operations daily, an exceptional number for that period, when few surgeons attempted these intricate and lengthy procedures.[14]

After 1955, the more widespread use of hypothermia and heart bypass machines in cardiothoracic medical centers marked the beginning of open-heart surgery. By combining hypothermia with extracorporeal blood circulation, surgeons succeeded in cooling and bypassing the heart, stopping it for up to an hour or more, and then starting it again without inflicting any damage to the organ. Heart operations became more numerous, complex, and successful. In 1956 Cooley performed an astounding 95 open-heart operations, reflecting his energy and drive to push the new field of open-heart surgery further.[15] Cooley's great manual dexterity allowed him to perform delicate cardiac operations with encouraging results.[16]

During the 1950s, the surgical team of DeBakey and Cooley pioneered many cardiovascular operations at Baylor College of Medicine and Methodist Hospital. They reported impressive results in repairing cardiac aneurysms (vascular bulge), mitral and aortic stenosis (valve narrowing), septal defects (holes), and other abnormalities that weakened the heart.[17] Savvy with journalists and public relations, DeBakey cultivated the publicity surrounding his innovative bypass procedures, his mechanical assist devices, and his treatment of international leaders and celebrities, including the Duke of Windsor and Marlene Dietrich.[18] Cooley's name was not as well known to the public. Yet in the medical world, the names of DeBakey and Cooley were linked. DeBakey and Cooley worked independently and together in the operating room, and they coauthored many medical papers reporting their various surgical procedures. But what was once a polite and professional relationship had become detached and unfriendly by 1960.[19]

Constantly battling to book enough operating-room space for his cases, Cooley began to feel the constraint of working in DeBakey's house of surgery.[20] He quietly began doing pediatric heart operations at the Texas Children's Hospital, while continuing to perform cardiac surgery under DeBakey's service at Methodist Hospital. Then in 1960, Cooley officially left Methodist Hospital to set up his own surgical practice at nearby St. Luke's Hospital, and two years later, he founded the privately funded Texas Heart Institute (THI). Affiliated with St. Luke's Episcopal and Texas Children's hospitals, THI was dedicated to the study and treatment of cardiovascular disease. The institute had no patient beds, but its research and education programs transferred into improved patient care at their affiliated hospitals.[21] Over the next 10 years, St. Luke's Hospital grew to include a 27-story tower addition, and THI occupied seven full floors of it, as a direct result of Cooley's drive to build an internationally renowned cardiac center.[22] Cooley retained his clinical professorship at Baylor College of Medicine, but after he shifted his practice to St. Luke's and Texas Children's hospitals, he rarely spent time in a Baylor lab, skeptical that experimental work on dogs taught him anything useful about human physiology. Instead, Cooley refined and improved operations by doing, and his caseload continued to increase. According to journalist Thomas Thompson, there was never a dramatic break in the relationship between Cooley and DeBakey that led to his departure in 1960, only a gradual moving away. The dominant opinion was that the two surgeons had simply become "temperamentally incompatible"; after working with DeBakey for years, Cooley had had enough of being in DeBakey's shadow, and the two egos clashed.[23]

Thereafter, DeBakey and Cooley fell into an undeclared rivalry, according to colleagues.[24] Both were leaders in the growing field of cardiovascular surgery. With Cooley at the helm, THI quickly became one of the foremost specialized cardiac care facilities in the world. Cooley built an international reputation, maintaining a busy and successful surgical practice. He was a charismatic, talented, and highly praised surgeon in Texas who was confident and ambitious to do more operations, in less time, than any other practitioner. Many surgeons asserted that Cooley was a more technically gifted surgeon than DeBakey.[25] Cooley was certainly confident in his surgical abilities, never one to shy away from difficult operations, including the most daring and controversial procedure of this period—cardiac transplantation.

Heart Transplantation: From Celebration to Disillusionment

Heart transplantation captured tremendous public attention in the United States and around the world, beginning in 1967.[26] For the medical profession, the daring procedure of heart transplantation pushed organ replacement therapy beyond corneas (1905), sex glands (1920s), kidneys (1954), the pancreas (1966), and the liver (1967) toward a new surgical possibility in the quest to treat heart failure. As medical historian Susan Lederer argues, medical and public curiosity about organ transplantation, or the "surgical imaginary" of replacing worn-out body parts with new ones, began well before the organ transplants of the 1960s. Lederer challenges the historical assumption that Americans were reluctant to cut up the body, even exchange body parts. Beginning early in the twentieth century, news stories applauded patients for "going under the knife," and family members often donated or procured blood, tissue, and organs for possible surgical use. Fueling this ethos of "spare parts surgery" was the work of medical researchers at universities and medical centers across America, who, for decades, had been exploring organ transplantation on various levels, exchanging organs and tissue in hamsters and mice, and later dogs and calves.[27]

In the United States, cardiac surgeons Norman Shumway and Richard Lower led the research pack in heart transplantation. Beginning in 1959 at Stanford University, surgeon-researcher Shumway and surgical resident Lower started transplanting hearts in dogs and began publishing academic papers on the transplant procedure in these experimental animals and on their immunological aftercare. In 1960 Shumway and Lower reported the first successful heart transplant in dogs, which established the surgical technique for cardiac transplantation used by surgeons in both animals and humans for decades thereafter.[28] In addition to the surgical technique, the Stanford team contributed knowledge about how a transplanted heart functioned and about the body's immune response, knowledge gained through hundreds of animal experiments. By the mid-1960s, the Stanford team reported an 85 percent survival rate in dogs and proposed the possibility of human cases in the not-too-distant future.[29] Shumway and Lower's research gave them credibility and authority within the transplant field. However, neither of them performed the first human transplant cases.

In January 1964, at the University of Mississippi Medical Center, surgeon James Hardy implanted a chimpanzee heart into a 68-year-old white man who suffered severe coronary atherosclerosis, using the technique developed by the Stanford team. The patient, Boyd Rush, survived only a few hours, owing to the small size of the animal heart and its inability to maintain adequate circulation. The transplant team had planned to use a human donor heart, but an organ was not available, so instead they transplanted a chimpanzee heart that had been readied as a back-up.[30] Hardy's decision to implant an animal organ certainly raised a few eyebrows, but Hardy's many years of animal transplant research (which was arguably more on lung than heart transplantation) cushioned him from any deluge of harsh criticism from colleagues. The medical community assessed the operation as a desperate effort to save a man's life, and little else. Hardy's first clinical operation contributed little to the field and raised minimal media attention, and Hardy never repeated the procedure.[31] No flood of transplant operations with animal hearts occurred as a result of this case; the procedure of transplanting animal hearts into humans (xenotransplantation) remained contentious if not far-fetched.[32]

Three years after Hardy's failed chimpanzee heart transplant, the first human heart transplant case took place outside of the United States, much to the surprise of the American medical community. Everyone in the field assumed that the first clinical case would be done by Shumway, who had laid the research foundations for this procedure.[33] In November 1967, Shumway announced to the medical community, "The way is clear" to perform a human heart transplant. Moreover, his team was ready to proceed once a suitable donor and recipient were found.[34] The difficult decision regarding exactly when the experimental procedure should transit from bench to bedside had been made, arguably by the world's leading transplant research team.

According to Shumway, "Although animal work should and will continue, we are nonetheless at the threshold of clinical application."[35] The dog model had allowed Shumway to work out the surgical technique of transplantation, but it was limited in its use to nail down key indicators of cardiac rejection and corresponding dose schedules for immunosuppressive drug delivery. Shumway insisted that proper patient selection and close postoperative care would be crucial, from which early clinical cases would offer much needed information on managing organ rejection.[36] What was holding him up at this point was the arrival of an ideal donor and recipient at the same time. Shumway stated, "Thus far, the two requirements have not coincided."[37] In reality, Shumway was wrangling with academic neurosurgeons, who, upon the withdrawal of life support of their brain-dead patients, allowed for cardiac death (heart no longer beating), which then damaged the viability of the organ for transplantation purposes.[38]

South African cardiac surgeon Christiaan Barnard beat Shumway into the operating room, and overnight the lesser-known Barnard, not Shumway, became world renowned for performing the first human heart transplant operation. Barnard's South African hospital setting and his American training enabled him to take this bold clinical step. Affiliated with the University of Cape Town's medical school, the Groote Schuur Hospital offered a large and innovative cardiac clinic, which was cofounded by cardiologists Velva Schrire and Maurice Nellen in 1951.[39] Hospital colleagues collaborated with Barnard, supported his clinical research, and facilitated patient referrals. Barnard's formal training in the United States dated back to 1956, when he spent two years at the University of Minnesota learning from surgical pioneers Owen Wangensteen and Walt Lillehei. While in Minneapolis, Barnard met Shumway, who was completing his cardiac surgical residency under Lillehei.[40] (According to South African writer Donald McRae, the two men were contrasting personalities. "Shumway was as self-effacing as Barnard was self-absorbed; and they had never liked each other.")[41] In 1958 Barnard returned to Groote Schuur Hospital with a heart-lung machine, courtesy of Wangensteen, to launch an open-heart surgery program in South Africa. With Schrire and others, Barnard spent his time improving surgical techniques and devices, such as aortic and valve prostheses, moving toward introducing these procedures clinically.[42]

In 1966 Barnard returned to the United States to learn more about transplanting organs and controlling rejection. He and several South African colleagues had been conducting renal transplant experiments on dogs and had recently published their techniques for improved kidney storage.[43] From August to November 1966, Barnard studied under David Hume, a leading renal transplant surgeon at the Medical College of Virginia (MCV).[44] Barnard assisted in kidney transplant operations and learned how to manage transplant patients postoperatively, in preparation for launching a kidney transplant program in Cape Town. Hume assigned Barnard research work with rats and dogs to study organ rejection and its control with various immunosuppressive drugs.[45] Barnard also spent two weeks in Denver, Colorado, with Thomas Starzl, who had conducted the first liver transplant, to learn from his experiences with organ transplantation. Barnard learned about transplanting the heart through another leader in the field, Richard Lower, whom Hume had recruited from Shumway's program in 1965 to develop a transplant program at MCV. With great interest, Barnard watched Lower transplant hearts into dogs. It was clear to many that Barnard's attention had shifted from kidney to heart transplants, and some MCV researchers predicted that Barnard would not hesitate to attempt the experimental procedure "without delay" back in South Africa.[46] Indeed, Barnard "transplanted" operational techniques and patient management protocols from Hume's program in Richmond, Virginia, to Cape Town's Groote Schuur Hospital. He organized hospital treatment rooms, specialized equipment, required medications, a system of donor organ procurement, criteria for transplant eligibility, and an efficient transplant team. In October 1967 he performed a successful kidney transplant operation, which he dubbed his "run-through" surgery for his grander ambition of clinically transplanting a heart.[47]

On December 3, 1967, Barnard performed the world's first human heart transplant operation. He replaced the failing heart of 55-year-old Louis Washkansky, who suffered from coronary occlusive disease, with the healthy heart of Denise Darvall, a 25-year-old woman who had suffered extensive brain damage in an automobile accident. The donor heart began pumping in Washkansky's chest, and initial organ rejection subsided after drug treatment. However, on the 18th day after the operation, Washkansky died from a pulmonary (lung) infection that was misdiagnosed as a rejection problem and treated incorrectly.[48] Barnard's next transplant case, performed on January 2, 1968, produced better results. Philip Blaiberg, a 58-year-old patient suffering from congestive heart failure caused by coronary artery disease, received the heart of Clive Haupt, a 24-year-old who had died of a cerebral hemorrhage. Blaiberg lived more than 19 months with his transplanted heart, setting a long-term survival record that other cases aimed to match.[49] This case energized the surgical world, attesting to the possibility that lives could be extended beyond a few days.[50]

Barnard's transplant work garnered widespread and sustained media coverage nationally and internationally for months. As historian Ayesha Nathoo argues, the historic first transplant operation by Barnard was both a medical and a media phenomenon constructed by journalists in their "breakthrough" narratives that made international celebrities of the surgeon and the patient, causing thousands of eager readers and viewers to follow the outcome and consequences of such an experimental procedure.[51] Moreover, Nathoo explains that both Barnard and Washkansky were willing participants in the sustained media attention, a stark divergence from longstanding principles of the medical profession that physicians resist self-promotion and maintain patient confidentiality. In particular, Barnard drew much professional criticism as he traveled to Europe, England, and the United States, embracing his newfound fame in the early months of 1968.[52] Shumway later commented that Barnard became "consumed" by celebrity status. Shumway stated that since no one had anticipated the deluge of media attention, it was a "blessing" that Barnard went first, allowing him (Shumway) to continue his work away from the public spotlight.[53] What is significant about Barnard's cases for the development of the artificial heart is that they demonstrated the clinical feasibility of cardiac replacement and instigated a frenzy of cardiac transplant operations in the United States and worldwide thereafter. As certain political, social, and ethical issues arose surrounding heart transplants, such as interracial transplants and organ donor shortages, mechanical hearts were presented (incorrectly) as a less problematic alternative.

Unaware of Barnard's plans, American surgeons Adrian Kantrowitz and Norman Shumway prepared independently to go forward with their own human heart transplant cases after years of animal experiments.[54] Shumway must have felt cheated, if not bitter, that he had not performed the first clinical case. Upon hearing the news of Barnard's transplant case, Kantrowitz stated, "I was stunned. I would not have been surprised to hear that Shumway or Lower had done the operation, but I had never seen any heart transplantation studies published by Barnard."[55] No one expected that the first clinical case would take place outside of the United States, given the substantial American investment and expertise in heart transplantation research. As Lederer argues, Barnard benefited from NIH-sponsored work and resources, emanating from American research programs, that made his Cape Town operation possible.[56] In comparison to Shumway, Barnard was a relative newcomer to the transplant community, with a modest research program in South Africa. Barnard's limited animal research, in stark contrast to Shumway and Lower's lab work of nearly a decade, drew professional criticism that he was ill prepared to do this procedure clinically. Based on Shumway and Lower's work, Barnard proceeded, taking away what should have been their opportunity to introduce clinically what they had labored over in the lab for so long. Barnard was an aggressive surgeon, viewed by many in the medical community as a usurper; although not naive, he had less transplant research experience and training for a procedure for which other, more qualified colleagues advised caution in moving forward.[57] It reeked of professional insolence and a desire to secure notoriety for "being the first" by taking advantage of someone else's careful and systematic research. Of course, Barnard did not see it this way; he argued that he should not be criticized for reading the published research and then implementing these experimental procedures clinically.[58] The event speaks to American scientific research culture: of the value of basic research, of animal and bench testing, of paying one's dues, of acknowledging the work of others, and of shared professional courtesies in a community that shares research findings without fear of poaching. Barnard appeared oblivious to his indiscretion.[59]

Three days after Barnard's sensational first operation, Kantrowitz performed the world's second human heart transplant, in Brooklyn on December 6, 1967. Hardly rushing into a copycat operation, Kantrowitz had been stimulated by Shumway's surgical success in dogs and had experimented with Shumway's surgical technique

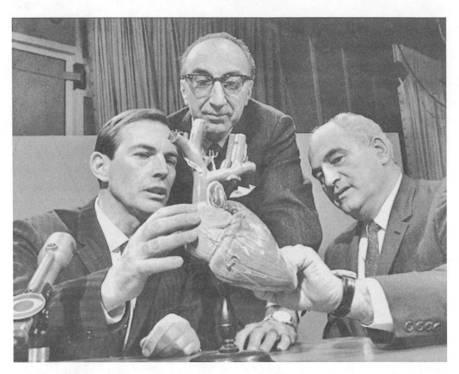

Cardiac surgeons Christiaan Barnard (*left*), Michael DeBakey (*center*), and Adrian Kantrowitz discuss the challenges of heart transplantation in Washington, DC, on the CBS television program *Face the Nation*, December 24, 1967. (AP-PHOTO/FILE)

in his own lab, beginning in 1961.[60] What made Kantrowitz's operation different was his decision to perform the surgery in an infant, not an adult: he transplanted the heart of an anencephalic infant (baby born without a brain) into an 18-day-old infant born with tricuspid atresia (baby born with an abnormal heart valve). Although the grafting of the new heart into the baby was completed technically without incident in the operating room, the child died 6.5 hours after the surgery owing to respiratory problems.[61] One month later, Kantrowitz performed another heart transplant, this time on a 57-year-old man with coronary artery disease who received the healthy heart of a 29-year-old woman with a fatal brain tumor. But the donor heart was unable to support the patient's circulation, and the patient died 10.5 hours after the operation. Having witnessed two failed cases, Kantrowitz chose not to perform another transplant surgery and instead returned to his research on mechanical circulatory support systems.[62]

After more than a decade of laboratory experience with transplantation, Shumway performed his first human transplant operation at Stanford University Medical Center on 54-year-old steelworker Mike Kasperak on January 6, 1968. Weeks previously, Shumway had announced his intention to proceed with a series of clinical cases, stating that the time was right because he and his team had worked out the surgical technique and had reduced toxicity levels of rejection drugs to attain longer (by months) survival rates in dogs. He also said that the "ideal" transplant recipient should be facing imminent death and should have no unrelated heart disease incapacity and no other medical options.[63] Kasperak was not an ideal candidate; he was a very ill man who Shumway told reporters was a "terminal patient . . . with no hope of living more than a few days without a heart transplant."[64] Kasperak received the healthy, but much smaller, heart of 43-year-old Virginia Mae White, who had suffered a massive brain hemorrhage. While the heart appeared to function, Kasperak battled a range of problems based on preexisting conditions, including respiratory complications from years of working in a steel mill and being a heavy smoker, liver and kidney problems caused by a shortage of oxygenated blood from the small donor heart, and stomach and gastrointestinal tract bleeding that required blood transfusions. Shumway described it to *New York Times* reporter Lawrence Davies as "a fantastic galaxy of complications."[65] Additional surgical interventions did not resolve the problems completely, and two weeks after the initial transplant operation, Kasperak died as a result of gastrointestinal bleeding and sepsis (infection).[66]

In May, Shumway performed a second transplant surgery. He implanted the heart of 43-year-old Rudolph Anderson, who died of a brain hemorrhage, into 40-year-old carpenter Joseph Rizor, who thereafter battled serious lung problems. When asked about the lung problems by reporters, Shumway said that Rizor's lungs "were 'confused' by the new heart's better pumping power."[67] It seemed that Rizor's compromised organs had great difficulty adjusting to this donor heart, which apparently pumped six times more blood per minute (cardiac output) than had Rizor's diseased heart. Rizor lived only three days with his new heart, dying not of organ rejection but of respiratory failure.[68] Given Shumway's criteria that only patients "facing imminent death" were eligible candidates for transplant surgery, these results could hardly have been surprising. Shumway persevered, hopeful that a better selection of recipients would result in better clinical results.

In the late summer and fall of 1968, Shumway performed eight more cardiac transplant operations that did produce better clinical outcomes, extending the lives of some of these patients by several months.[69] These clinical cases allowed the team to adapt techniques and observations from the animal laboratory to the operating room, such as the operative technique and indicators of acute cardiac rejection. This clinical series also highlighted problems that were going to be more difficult to resolve, specifically the ongoing and serious challenges of patient infection, continuous acute rejection, and chronic rejection of the donor heart. As cardiologist-historian Bruce Fye points out, transplant surgeons constantly battled rejection and infection; the attempt to blunt the patient's immunologic reaction to the foreign organ significantly increased the likelihood of death by infection.[70] Shumway reported promising early results but advocated caution even as he predicted better results to come with more clinical experience.[71]

In the same period, Cooley and DeBakey also attempted numerous heart transplant operations and, like Shumway, reported varied results. In May 1968 Cooley conducted his first heart transplant operation, transplanting the heart of a 15-year-old girl, who had died of a gunshot wound to the brain, into 47-year-old Everett Thomas.[72] Within the week, Cooley performed two more heart transplants, and by April 1969 he had done more heart transplants (19) than any other surgeon in the world. Cooley's patients died within a matter of days or weeks. In his group of transplant cases, Cooley operated on adults, children, and infants, and he even transplanted a sheep's heart into a patient as a desperate measure to ward off death.[73] But all patients succumbed to organ rejection or infection. Cooley remained frustrated with his mortality rate in comparison with the much better results of the Stanford team; Shumway reported 42 percent patient survival at six months in contrast to the 10 percent survival rate recounted by most other surgeons.[74]

DeBakey was also in this elite group of surgeons daring to push the surgical boundaries through cardiac transplantation. Like everyone else, DeBakey battled organ rejection and infection in his transplant patients. However, he reported two remarkable cases. DeBakey transplanted his first heart on August 31, 1968, as part of a spectacular multiple transplant in which the donor's heart, lung, and both kidneys were transplanted into four different people in four different operating rooms at Methodist Hospital simultaneously. DeBakey implanted the heart of 20-year-old Nelva Lou Hernandez, who had died of a gunshot wound to the head, into 50-year-old William C. Carroll, who survived three years and almost nine months with his new heart.[75] DeBakey's third transplant patient was 16-year-old Duson Vlaco, who lived six years and almost two months with his new heart.[76] DeBakey performed six more transplant operations during the fall of 1968, but then the number of his transplant cases declined noticeably as the medical field reevaluated the procedure at this time.[77]

In 1968 more than 100 transplant operations were done worldwide, with Cooley, Shumway and DeBakey performing the greatest number of the operations.[78] Transplant surgery took place in 20 countries around the world, but the majority of the operations occurred in the United States. The incredible number of operations within this year reflected the enthusiasm and optimism shared by surgeons, patients, and the general public for this procedure. Laypeople wrote letters to these surgeons, in which they congratulated and occasionally offered "helpful" advice. Many asked for more information on cardiac transplantation and mechanical heart devices.[79] But these early transplant patients typically measured their survival in only days and weeks. With a more than 75 percent mortality rate, it was clear that heart transplantation was still an experimental procedure; medical and public disillusionment with it set in.[80] Perhaps surgeons had been too eager to perform this procedure on less than ideal candidates. Perhaps surgeons, feeling helpless, unwisely attempted the risky operation as a desperate measure to save patients who would certainly die otherwise. Perhaps surgeons, who were part of the new era of open-heart surgery, merely embraced transplant surgery as yet another exciting surgical innovation to be mastered, and they did not want to miss out. Social scientists Renée Fox and Judith Swazey labeled the year 1968 the "bandwagon" period in the history of heart transplantation.[81] Dr. Irvine Page referred to it as "an international race to be a member of the me-too brigade."[82] Shumway's Stanford team commented that initial enthusiasm for cardiac transplantation had "approached hysteria" but later was "replaced by a generally pessimistic outlook."[83]

It became clear that the Stanford team's decade of research work was a factor contributing to their better results. Dr. Edward Stinson, a member of Shumway's transplant team, bluntly stated, "Many centers took up clinical transplantation without the laboratory experience or profound support in clinically related areas such as immunosuppression. They didn't expect the difficulties that occurred after the operation. We did, from the decade of laboratory experience."[84] After Barnard, more than 60 surgical teams in nearly two dozen different countries around the world began performing heart transplant surgery; certainly not all were prepared to deal with the problems of rejection and infection that killed patients.[85] Shumway told a journalist, "People were performing transplants who had no idea what the hell they were doing. It wrecked the field for a good five years."[86] The Stanford team's research investment in transplantation prepared them to achieve better patient results and to weather the hype and disillusionment that came with this investigative high-risk procedure.

By the end of 1968, mounting medical criticism and poor patient outcomes deterred many cardiac specialists (and patients) from encouraging heart transplant operations. While some might agree upon the technical ability of surgeons to transplant hearts, both the medical and the popular press criticized the procedure as being premature; there was inadequate immunological knowledge to prevent organ rejection, and there were no alternative means to sustain life in the event of failure. Cardiologists had good reason to hesitate to refer patients to their surgical colleagues for this procedure, given its experimental nature; it was a radical heart failure treatment, and its therapeutic value had yet to be demonstrated for the majority of patients who underwent the procedure.[87] It illustrated "the experiment-therapy dilemma" that, according to Fox and Swazey, comes with the research physician's burden of reconciling the roles of clinician and investigator.[88] The field had criticized Barnard for his limited research in heart transplantation before brazenly attempting the procedure clinically, wary of his reasons for doing this. Research was meant to prevent investigators from moving recklessly into the clinic, to arm them with knowledge from which to make the crucial judgement call that the time was right. They were not to experiment on humans, but to offer a plausible treatment alternative. Clinical investigation required clear purpose and objectives, an attempt, derived from lab research, to minimize the uncertainty surrounding clinical use. The stronger the uncertainty, the stronger the proclivity to research should intuitively become. The pendulum swung in favor of returning to the lab.

At the 1969 meeting of the Society of Thoracic Surgeons, members discussed the dismal outcomes of transplant cases, some expressing clear doubts whether these operations should continue.[89] In Canada, such operations were halted; a suspension of the procedure occurred at the Montreal Heart Institute, where cardiac surgeon Pierre Grondin, who had trained with DeBakey and Cooley in Houston, had performed nine heart transplant operations. The decision to stop transplanting hearts in Montreal fueled the debate within the medical community on whether an overall moratorium ought to be called.[90] The medical community and the press more openly acknowledged the difficulties associated with heart transplantation, and as Fox and Swazey state, there was a "jumping off the bandwagon" by surgical teams in this period.[91] Cooley, Shumway, and DeBakey supported the lessening number of such operations but not necessarily the abandonment of heart transplantation. In 1970 the American College of Cardiology encouraged an unofficial moratorium on heart transplants, with which most medical centers agreed; cardiologists were clearly discouraged by low survival rates linked to organ rejection.[92] Shumway ignored the moratorium, determined that his survival rates, which were better than most, would continue to improve with better patient selection and immunosuppression management.[93] Consciously maintaining a low public profile, Shumway continued a cautious clinical research program, performing no more than two heart transplants a month during the 1970s and grappling with ongoing problems of organ rejection and patient infection.[94] As heart specialists debated the wisdom of pursuing transplant operations, the spotlight on cardiac replacement broadened sensationally from human hearts to mechanical ones with the first clinical implantation of a TAH.

Notoriety for the Mechanical Heart: Haskell Karp

In 1961, after spending three months at the Cleveland Clinic observing the artificial heart work of Willem Kolff's team, Argentinian surgeon Domingo Liotta moved to Houston to begin a three-year cardiovascular surgical fellowship under DeBakey. It was a tremendous surgical training opportunity for Liotta as well as the chance to extend his TAH research beyond the rudimentary work he had completed at the University of Cordoba.[95] In 1964 Liotta joined DeBakey's artificial heart program full-time, as a researcher under program director C. William Hall, and an NIH research grant paid Liotta's salary.[96] By this time, DeBakey's group at Baylor College of Medicine was collaborating with Rice University physical scientists and engineers on various pump designs, materials, power units, and drive consoles, as a result of companion grants from the National Heart Institute for this purpose.[97] The many problems associated with building a TAH convinced them to focus on ventricular assist pumps, or partial artificial hearts, to better understand and resolve technical, surgical, and biocompatibility issues. Over the next several years, the Baylor-Rice team developed different types of assist pumps, many of which were studied in animals and a few implanted clinically with limited success. In 1968 the team returned to TAH research with a new biventricular pump design, conducting work at both Baylor and Rice University research sites.[98]

In early 1969, DeBakey authorized Liotta to implant the Baylor-Rice TAH device in animals at Baylor's Surgical Research Laboratories to test device feasibility, to determine proper anatomical attachment, and to collect physiological data.[99] From January to March 1969, Liotta implanted the Baylor-Rice TAH in seven calves with poor results. The first four calves died on the operating table from implantation and device problems. DeBakey advised Liotta to replace the tissue valves with mechanical valves in the TAH and to improve the surgical technique for better attachment of the pump in the animal. The next three calves survived between 8 and 44 hours before expiring from renal failure and respiratory failure, among other problems.[100] Prudently, DeBakey contended that this device was not ready for use in humans.[101]

Just prior to these animal experiments, Cooley contacted Liotta to discuss moving forward with the clinical implantation of the TAH.[102] This excited Liotta, who had always been interested in TAH research but had been forced to sideline this work in favor of assist pump research in DeBakey's artificial heart program. He immediately began working double-duty for DeBakey and Cooley in their respective artificial heart research programs.[103] In early 1969, Cooley established the Cullen Cardiovascular Laboratories at THI, where work on constructing and testing artificial hearts could take place. Funding came from THI as well as from donations by patients and local heart associations.[104] At Cooley's request, Liotta did not inform his Baylor boss, since DeBakey would almost certainly have prevented Liotta from working on both research teams simultaneously.[105] In contrast, Rice University engineer William O'Bannon did communicate openly with his boss, Dr. J. David Hellums, the director of the Rice end of the joint Baylor-Rice artificial heart program, about moonlighting. O'Bannon told Hellums about receiving "a confidential inquiry" to build a duplicate of the drive console (power and control unit) that Rice University had developed for the Baylor heart device. When asked, O'Bannon refused to tell Hellums that it was Cooley who had approached him. Hellums granted O'Bannon permission to make this duplicate outside of his work at Rice University, so O'Bannon built the unit on his own time, in his garage, during February and March of 1969.[106]

During this period, Cooley, at the time the most prolific heart transplant surgeon, complained to the press about the problem of the supply of donor hearts.[107] Cooley had dozens of sick heart patients waiting in the wards of St. Luke's Hospital or in nearby motels in Houston, who, according to him, were eager to undergo a transplant operation. Many patients died before a donor heart became available. Cooley contended that an artificial heart might extend a patient's life, by sustaining mechanical circulatory support and providing more time to find a donor organ. By the end of March 1969, Cooley instructed his team to prepare for the possible clinical use of an artificial heart; Liotta fabricated and sterilized three TAHs at Baylor Surgical Laboratories while Cooley arranged his surgical team at St. Luke's Hospital.[108]

On April 2, 1969, O'Bannon delivered the TAH power and control unit to the hospital.[109] The next day, Cooley requested movie footage and still photography of Karp's impending operation from Baylor's Medical Communications staff.[110] It was a daring and desperate "bridge" operation that Cooley proposed, and he would be the first to perform it.

On April 4, 1969, Cooley operated on the severely damaged heart of 47-year-old Haskell Karp, an Illinois printing estimator suffering from end-stage heart disease, who became the first recipient of a TAH. According to Cooley, he had never seen a "worse-looking heart."[111] Karp had suffered from extensive coronary heart disease and numerous myocardial infarctions (heart attacks) for more than 10 years. He had been hospitalized 13 times previously for heart problems and had received a cardiac pacemaker in May 1968. His heart was greatly enlarged as a result of advanced coronary arterial occlusive disease (closed blood vessels to the heart) and myocardial fibrosis (heart muscle scarring), and there was a complete heart block (an obstruction of electrical impulses in the heart).[112] Cooley suggested cardiac transplantation, but Karp resisted, showing a reluctance increasingly shared by many other patients (and physicians) in response to the poor outcomes associated with heart transplantation in the previous year. Karp wanted Cooley to perform a myocardial excision with ventriculoplasty, or "wedge operation," with extensive restructuring of the ventricle. That is, the surgeon would cut out the damaged segment of the heart muscle and then rebuild the pumping chamber of the heart. Before going into surgery, Karp agreed to a heart transplantation, consenting to the use of the mechanical heart as a bridge device if necessary, should the ventriculoplasty operation fail. During the cardiac restructuring procedure, Cooley found the damage to Karp's heart to be too severe, and after the excisions, there was not enough healthy heart muscle left to complete the operation successfully. Karp's heart was fatally compromised, and the patient would not survive once disconnected from cardiopulmonary bypass support. So Cooley removed Karp's remaining heart ventricles and implanted a TAH to keep him alive until a transplant operation could be performed.[113]

Inside Karp's chest was a two-ventricle, pneumatically driven artificial heart, which was lined with Dacron and encased in a Silastic shell. It was the approximate size of a human heart. A diaphragm, modified to resist stress and wear, pumped each inner chamber shell. Inside the chambers, the lining, when forced inward, moved blood out of the heart. When relaxed against the outer shell, the lax lining opened to allow the heart to fill up with blood before then pushing it forward again. To facilitate blood flow, the device contained four Wada-Cutter valves, described as allowing a more open flow of blood that reduced thromboembolic, or clotting, complications better than other mechanical valves or animal grafts. The device attached to the patient via Dacron cuffs and grafts to the upper chambers and vessels of Karp's natural heart, respectively, specifically the right and left atria, pulmonary artery and aorta, to allow blood to flow through the lungs and then into the body. Most visible, four long tubes connected the implanted device to a large power console, roughly

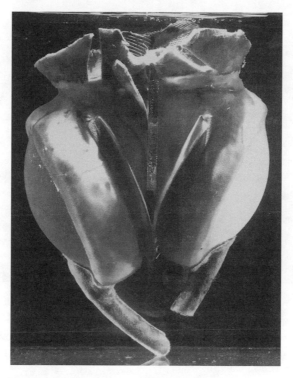

The Liotta-Cooley artificial heart, used in the first artificial heart implant case, in Houston, Texas, April 1969. Photo courtesy of the Division of Medicine & Science, National Museum of American History, Smithsonian Institution.

the size of chest freezer, which sat at the bedside. The power console had two major subsystems, namely the pneumatic pressure sources, which generated the pressure and vacuum needed for pulsing the prosthesis, and the monitor-control unit, which consisted of a display oscilloscope, four pressure preamplifiers, and the pulse unit. Physicians monitored the device's performance, recorded arterial and chamber blood pressures, and adjusted the pressure as needed.[114]

Once implanted with the artificial heart, Karp was disconnected from cardiopulmonary bypass support, but he still required intensive monitoring, respiratory support, and isolation. Karp temporarily regained consciousness shortly after the surgery, responding to verbal commands, moving his hands, and opening his eyes, although he was unable to speak because of a breathing tube inserted through his mouth, according to newspaper accounts.[115] Cooley told reporters that the artificial heart would remain in the patient only until a donor heart could be found for transplantation. Cooley's narrative to journalists, that the artificial heart was implanted out of desperation—as a stop-gap measure—to save the life of his patient after the failed reparative surgery, is perhaps more after-the-fact rationalization than a full

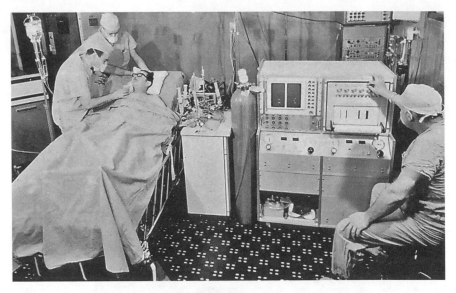

Cardiac surgeon Denton Cooley and Argentinian surgeon-researcher Domingo Liotta (*left*) with artificial heart recipient Haskell Karp at St. Luke's Hospital, Houston, Texas, April 4, 1969. Note the bulky external equipment required to power and regulate the implanted artificial heart, monitored by biomedical engineer John Jurgens (*far right*). Courtesy of the Texas Heart Institute.

disclosure of his intent. The extent to which Cooley's use of the mechanical heart was "premediated" is difficult to determine, although the fact that the equipment, the research team, and the Baylor medical photography group were in place on April 4 suggests Cooley was indeed planning on using the device (and was more than just being prepared for multiple scenarios if the ventriculoplasty failed).[116]

No doubt distraught and worried for her husband, Mrs. Shirley Karp spoke directly to the media, at the urging of Cooley, to make a nationwide plea for a donor heart. "I see him [Haskell Karp] lying there, breathing and knowing that within his chest is a man-made implement where there should be a God-given heart," stated Mrs. Karp.[117] Two days after the implant, a donor heart was found. A medical team flew Mrs. Barbara Evans, who had suffered irreparable brain damage, from Lawrence, Massachusetts, to Houston, where she was pronounced dead and her heart removed for transplantation.[118] After living for 64 hours with a mechanical heart, Karp returned to the operating room for removal of the device and transplantation of the newly acquired donor heart.[119]

After Cooley's research team removed the artificial heart from Karp's chest, they closely examined the device for signs of mechanical failure. They reported none; the interior surfaces and valves were free of thrombi (blood clots) with a smooth lining that consisted of fibrin and platelet deposits, suggesting adequate blood flow through the device. This appeared remarkable since the patient had received no anticoagulants (blood thinners) during the period.[120] Liotta told journalists that the explanted device "looked really wonderful"; he believed that Karp "could have lived six months with it."[121] In published case reports, Cooley appraised the prosthesis as providing "a commendable performance as a simple mechanical pump."[122] He added that some hemolysis (blood damage) in the patient had occurred, possibly from the bubble oxygenator used during the surgery or perhaps owing to the mechanical heart. In the end, neither the device implant nor the heart transplant worked well enough to reverse Karp's multiple problems. While implanted with the mechanical heart, Karp battled serious renal and respiratory complications that accompanied end-stage heart disease. Cooley stated that Karp's renal problems increased while living with the mechanical heart, putting the patient in critical condition to receive the heart transplant. Karp's kidney and lung problems were evident when he received the donor heart, which necessitated substantial doses of immunosuppressive drugs, increasing his risk of infection.[123]

On April 8, 1969, Karp died from pneumonia and kidney failure, having survived only 32 hours after his transplant operation. Karp lived longer with the artificial heart than with the donor heart, yet it was hardly evidence of the superiority of mechanical devices. The consensus was that Karp's terminal disease was the ultimate cause of his death. His body suffered the fatal consequences of living with severe, chronic heart disease, and neither cardiac replacement therapy was able to compensate for years of damage at this late stage. Arguably, the use of the mechanical heart contributed to Karp's death. The device did not alleviate any of Karp's medical issues, but instead increased his renal problems and put him in a state of semiconsciousness with the need for continuous ventilator assistance. At the time of the donor heart transplant on April 7, Karp was in very critical condition; as a result of implanting the artificial heart, there was now a much higher risk of failure than if he had undergone the transplant surgery on April 4 (instead of the ventriculoplasty procedure).[124]

The media printed details of Karp's artificial heart operation, the search for a donor heart, the follow-up transplant surgery, and then Karp's death, all the while praising the artificial heart as a breakthrough device that promised to extend the lives of dying patients who needed transplants.[125] According to one *New York Times* article, "heart surgeons have long wanted an effective artificial device to remove some of the terrible time pressure from heart transplantation," and "Dr Cooley proved that just a few days can suffice."[126] The media celebrated the implant surgery as a triumph—the device had worked for 64 hours—and framed the event with the typical cast of characters: the heroic surgeon, the brave patient, and the distraught family of the dying man. The media did not reveal medical details that would have implied that the mechanical heart placed Karp in a weaker position to receive a donor heart. Journalists presented both procedures as experimental, rescue-oriented operations to save the life of a dying man. These had been "last-resort" options that had not resulted in a miracle recovery, and there was no blame attributed to Cooley for Karp's death at this time. The media focus then shifted quickly to the drama unfolding concerning allegations of device theft and lack of authorization to perform this procedure.

The development and implant of Cooley's device used in the Karp case had occurred in relative secrecy with obvious disregard for institutional guidelines in the use of experimental procedures. As a result, national and local investigations were immediately launched. Without delay, Theodore Cooper, director of the National Heart Institute at the NIH, wrote a terse letter to DeBakey: Was the device used in the Karp case developed with the assistance of NIH research money? If so, did surgical researchers adhere to federal guidelines relating to the collection of experimental data and the decision to move forward to clinical use?[127] DeBakey led the largest federally funded artificial heart research program in the country, and most assumed that the device had emerged out of his laboratory. However, DeBakey had no knowledge of Cooley and Liotta's collaboration on the development of an artificial heart, and he only learned about the surgery after the fact while he was in Washington, ironically, for a meeting at the NHI. Cooper, who had visited DeBakey's lab only two weeks previously in preparation for an upcoming NIH program review necessary for a $3 million grant renewal, expressed concern that Cooley had implanted the still-quite-experimental device that was being funded by NIH research money. Cooper had many concerns and questions, particularly owing to press attention and media accounts of the "first" artificial heart implant.[128] As president of the Baylor College of Medicine, DeBakey was no doubt embarrassed and angry that he had been caught unaware and unable to answer Cooper's questions. He returned to Houston and immediately initiated a formal Baylor investigation; at DeBakey's urging, Leonard F. McCollum, chairman of the Board of Trustees of Baylor College of Medicine, appointed a Special Committee, chaired by Hebbel E. Hoff, associate dean for faculty and clinical affairs, to investigate the Karp case to determine if Baylor had violated NIH guidelines in the development and use of the artificial heart. The Karp case threatened to tarnish the reputation of the college and to end federal funding of DeBakey's artificial heart research program.[129]

Cooley, more than Liotta, drew the attention of committee investigations, each seeking to ascertain whether any professional transgressions had occurred in this sensational case. In response to questions posed by Cooper, Cooley stated that he had developed the artificial heart used in the Karp case from private funding, not federal funding, and so NIH guidelines did not apply.[130] This was true. Cooley had not applied for, nor received, NIH research grant funding for this work. But after investigating the matter, members of Baylor's Special Committee concluded that NIH funds had been used in the development of the artificial heart implanted in Karp and that guidelines for use of experimental devices in humans had not been followed.[131] Cooley had not gained permission to use the device from the Baylor College of Medicine Committee on Research Involving Human Beings, a group of doctors who could have easily assembled for this emergency decision. Cooley stated that he had never consulted with this group in the past when it came to the use of new devices; furthermore, through recent bench and animal research, he was sufficiently satisfied with the performance and efficiency of the TAH to use the device clinically.[132] Cooley also defended himself by stating that he had secured informed consent from Karp's family and needed to act quickly to save the life of his patient. Cooley acknowledged that the surgery was a desperate act, but his actions reflected his surgeon's obligation to save the patient and to do everything possible. He had not been motivated to perform the operation for the sake of testing the artificial heart to see if it worked in humans.[133] Cooley later commented that if he had sought the Baylor College of Medicine committee's approval, the group would have notified DeBakey, who would have surely denied the request. In the end, the committee recommended censuring Cooley for ignoring institutional policy that was in place to protect the rights of patients. Likewise, the American College of Surgeons and the Harris County Medical Society censured Cooley for actions deemed "unprofessional" during this case.[134]

During Baylor College of Medicine's investigation of the Karp case, DeBakey remained out of the limelight on purpose. To the executive committee of the Board of Trustees at Baylor College of Medicine, DeBakey stated, "I am in a rather difficult position to make any public statements, since I am not only the Principal Investigator of the Artificial Heart Program, but, as President of the College, am also the responsible Executive Officer of the College. I therefore consider it necessary for me to remain aloof from the public controversy and make no public comments or statements."[135] But he was involved in making sure that a detailed Baylor College of Medicine investigation took place and that a mechanism for clinical investigation was well established to appease NIH administrators. As one way to avoid another incident like the one involving Haskell Karp, the Board of Trustees approved a new Baylor College of Medicine appointment form that required mandatory faculty compliance with the rules of the Committee on Research Involving Human Beings.[136] A defiant Cooley commented that he would do it again, refusing to bend to the will of a committee that, in his opinion, was controlled by DeBakey. Cooley did not sign the form and resigned from the Baylor College of Medicine over the issue.[137] Losing his affiliation with the Baylor College of Medicine was of minimal significance to Cooley; he simply continued his surgical practice and research at THI.

Liotta's involvement made DeBakey's accusation of theft quite plausible. Liotta was the connecting player between the two research programs, and he, unlike O'Bannon and Hellums, had ignored a professional courtesy, if not obligation, to inform DeBakey of his actions to facilitate Cooley's clinical use of the experimental device. Without Liotta, Cooley would not have had a device to implant. While O'Bannon did provide the power unit, he then refused to attend the operation. On April 3, Cooley asked O'Bannon to operate the power unit in the operating room at St. Luke's Hospital. O'Bannon was uneasy with this request, having told Cooley that he had built the unit for animal experimentation only and not for human use. O'Bannon called Hellums for permission to participate in the operation but was denied, based on "sincere doubts as to whether this pump has been properly tested."[138] When Cooley phoned Hellums directly, Hellums refused permission, since neither of them had DeBakey's authorization to proceed. O'Bannon was not present at Karp's operation on April 4.[139] O'Bannon's actions infer that Cooley's artificial heart was almost certainly a duplicate of the Baylor-Rice artificial heart, that Cooley had made the decision in advance of Karp's surgery to implant the experimental device if the occasion arose, and that Cooley and Liotta wanted to conceal their activities from Baylor College of Medicine administrators (notably DeBakey).

Liotta defended his secrecy by stating that he was developing a different device in Cooley's lab, but no one believed this. The Liotta-Cooley artificial heart was practically identical to the Baylor-Rice artificial heart, with only minimal changes. Descriptions and photos of the Baylor-Rice heart in comparison to the Liotta-Cooley heart support this conclusion.[140] As a second-year Baylor College of Medicine student, O. H. Frazier had worked with Liotta on the development of this mechanical heart. Frazier stated that "it was that [Baylor] pump that resulted in the first implantation of a TAH. That was a pump that Cooley implanted in 1969 that we were working on in the lab. There weren't a lot of changes. There were some. I think [Liotta] changed the valve a bit."[141] One associate stated, "It's the same damn heart we've been working on for years."[142] When asked about the three pumps that Liotta instructed his Baylor lab colleagues to fabricate, plastics technician Suzanne Anderson testified in court that "they had been making this type of pump in the lab for some six to eight months" (that is, many months previous to Liotta and Cooley's initial meeting).[143] According to Anderson,

> We had been given a deadline by Dr Liotta . . . approximately March 20 . . . and he said he must have three perfect pumps with the dacron lining. . . . [Then] Dr Liotta came and said that the tubing must be longer—about 7½ inches longer. . . . We did not use elastic adhesive but regular silastic so there would be no leakage. These are all ways in which I could determine that these three pumps were intended for human use rather than animal use. On the last Saturday in March I gave Dr Liotta the various parts for the fabricating of these three pumps, the domes and bodies with lining. He personally put in the valves, the diaphragms and assembled the three pumps. . . . It was unusual for Dr Liotta to assemble the component parts into the total heart. We normally do that in the plastics fabrication shop and have always; this was the exception.[144]

Anderson told social scientists Fox and Swazey that individuals in the lab suspected that "something was up" but were intimidated to confront the physicians—Liotta and Cooley—despite strong reservations that the device was not ready for human implantation.[145] (This sense of obligation and conformity to the demands of their medical superiors disturbed Fox and Swazey, who called for greater training in professional ethics.)[146]

Liotta's involvement of Baylor lab members supports the implausibility of Liotta's building a new device independently in just four months. Liotta admitted to *Life* reporter Thomas Thompson that he "stuffed parts of the DeBakey artificial heart into his briefcase and took them to St. Luke's."[147] (The extent to which Cooley was aware of Liotta's device theft—most flagrantly appropriating device parts from the Baylor lab to be used in Cooley's operating room—is uncertain.) Fuming, DeBakey openly charged Cooley and Liotta for "covertly taking" the Baylor-Rice artificial heart from the Baylor College of Medicine Surgical Laboratory to St. Luke's Hospital for implantation in Karp.[148] The Board of Trustees suspended Liotta from the artificial heart program at Baylor and stopped his salary.[149] Cooley then hired Liotta as the director of the Surgical Research Division at THI, where Liotta worked for two years before returning to Argentina.[150]

Accusations of wrongdoing also came from Shirley Karp, the wife of Haskell Karp, who filed a medical malpractice suit against Cooley and Liotta for wrongful death in 1971. She asked for $4.5 million in compensation for damages sustained by her family.[151] The case came to trial in Texas in 1972. At the center of the lawsuit were accusations of lack of informed consent and brazen human experimentation. Shirley Karp testified that she had not understood that her husband's heart would be removed and replaced by a mechanical one, and thus she had certainly not given consent to the surgeons to do this. The defendants presented the consent form signed by Haskell Karp as well as testimony from medical staff and a rabbi (who had seen Haskell Karp several times before the surgery), which indicated that Haskell Karp had indeed understood the surgery. In light of this, the judge ruled that the wife's understanding and consent were not legally necessary.[152]

The charge of human experimentation was equally difficult to prove, and in particular, Mrs. Karp's claim that her husband had died as a result of the artificial heart implant. The Karp family needed to provide expert medical testimony to substantiate the claim that Cooley and Liotta had deviated from normal practices and procedures when using an experimental device in clinical practice for the first time. Typically, once medical researchers had collected encouraging animal data, they cautiously introduced new procedures or devices into limited use in humans, as a last therapeutic step. Many institutions, such as schools of medicine, had some form of a review board in place to oversee this shift from animal to human use and to guide medical researchers through the process. The plaintiffs wanted DeBakey to testify that the artificial heart was not ready for use in humans and that he (and most likely any reputable medical review board) would not have recommended its implantation in Haskell Karp.

Such testimony from DeBakey would have made Mrs. Karp's case; DeBakey led the program that had developed the "covertly taken" device, and he could speak to the terrible results compiled from animal implant tests. To the executive committee of the Board of Trustees at Baylor College of Medicine, DeBakey stated, "The patient's clinical response to the artificial heart was much the same as observed previously in animals, with progressive damage to the kidneys and even to the brain, resulting in complete renal failure at the time the transplant was performed and complete brain failure, since this was developing progressively and the patient never regained consciousness after the heart transplantation was performed." It had been a desperate measure with an experimental device known to have too many problems for it to work effectively in a patient. The committee bluntly asked if the device might work well enough to buy time to secure a donor heart for the patient. DeBakey replied, "It is not possible that this artificial heart can keep a patient alive in sufficiently good condition for two days to permit recuperability of the damage that takes place over this period to the vital organs, such as the brain, kidneys, and lungs." It had simply been a bad call. Ethically, DeBakey pointed out, the procedure was a problem because of the lack of animal evidence of its safety and effectiveness as well as the uncertainty of securing a donor heart. DeBakey argued that "the application of an untried procedure to sustain life for 12 to 24 hours is worthless when the damage done by the procedure during this time would vitiate recuperability even if a donor heart became available. What is a more justifiable procedure is to wait until the donor heart becomes available before attempting a corrective operation that might fail. The patient in question, Mr Karp, had been in the hospital for more than a month, and it would have been better to defer the operation until a suitable donor became available for a heart transplantation."[153]

In a July 1969 letter to Dr. Harold Brown, chairman of the Baylor College of Medicine Faculty Committee on Research Involving Human Beings, DeBakey again bluntly stated that the clinical use of this experimental device had not been warranted, its use did not help the patient, and, in fact, it had thwarted the possibility of a successful heart transplant. DeBakey wrote that "the progressive deterioration in that patient from the time of insertion of the orthotopic cardiac prosthesis until its removal for cardiac transplantation was obviously irreversible, and these irreversible changes precluded the patient's survival." In this case, according to DeBakey, the risks to the individual were not outweighed by the potential benefit to him or by the importance of the knowledge to be gained.[154] With statements like this from DeBakey, Mrs. Karp's case would have been a slam dunk.

But DeBakey did not testify in the case, nor were any Baylor College of Medicine materials, amassed during the investigation of the Karp case, permitted to be used, owing to Judge Singleton's decision that this material "would serve no useful purpose."[155] Lawyers for the Karp family subpoenaed DeBakey to testify, and in a private deposition, DeBakey stated that the device was "not ready to use clinically," was very high-risk, and was "not acceptable medical practice in April of 1969." But the Karp family lawyers were blocked from using these statements in court and from making DeBakey testify in court. After a private hearing with DeBakey, the judge ruled that DeBakey's testimony would be more inflammatory and prejudicial than useful, given the well-publicized hostility between DeBakey and Cooley. To the judge, DeBakey made it clear that he had "never examined Haskell Karp," he would "not express any medical opinion based upon hypothetical questions even if asked to do so," and he "would refuse to express an in-court expert opinion concerning [the Liotta-Cooley mechanical heart used in Haskell Karp.]"[156] The judge then declared that "DeBakey had no evidence of any probative value to present to the jury," and he dismissed DeBakey.[157] The judge legally sealed DeBakey's deposition and all Baylor College of Medicine records related to the Haskell case. This action cut the knees out from under the Karp family case. With no expert medical testimony to establish "proof," the judge ruled against the wrongful death charges. The Karp family appealed the decision but lost again.[158] Cooley and Liotta did not pay any damages to the family, and the artificial heart research community undoubtedly let out a collective sigh of relief. As Fox and Swazey point out, Judge Singleton's decision to exclude DeBakey's testimony is "hard to understand or justify" and suggests a disturbing compliancy to conceal possible medical wrongdoing and to prevent legal punishment.[159] It was more than just a bad break for the Karp family; Fox and Swazey question whether the legal system adequately protected patients like Haskell Karp.[160] The verdict neither blamed nor exonerated Cooley and Liotta but stated that the Karp family had not made their case of wrongful death.

In general, the medical community did not agree with Cooley's maverick actions of implanting the stolen device in a secret operation, and most agreed that the use of the device clinically had been premature. Yet they recognized and respected Cooley's enormous surgical skill; if any surgeon was capable of pulling this off, it would be Cooley. The community's reaction of admiration yet disapproval of Cooley's implant case presented itself in different ways. Only two weeks after the Karp implant, Cooley spoke about the bridge-to-transplant case at the annual American Society for Artificial Internal Organs meeting with the permission of ASAIO president Adrian Kantrowitz and panelist Willem Kolff. It reflected the community's interest in the recent procedure and their respect for Cooley as a surgeon that they altered the formal program in this way, yet it also confounded others. DeBakey directly questioned Kantrowitz's decision to grant Cooley this platform, which arguably was tantamount to ASAIO's affirmation of Cooley's professional actions.[161] In the end, Cooley's peers and professional community did lay sanctions. But they amounted to nothing more than a slap on the wrist to Cooley and Liotta, although the incident somewhat tarnished their reputations. The Liotta-Cooley artificial heart was never implanted in another human case, and Liotta's research career in the United States fizzled out.[162] For researchers, the Karp case had only confirmed the device's mechanical and biological problems already identified in calves. For clinicians, it supported the dominant medical opinion that TAHs were not yet ready for patient use and that university hospital review board processes had to be respected when introducing new procedures clinically. The Karp case did not immediately set off more human implant cases with other devices but reinforced the imperative role of careful lab research, prudent bench-to-bedside transitions, and inclusive decision-making processes when it came to the clinical introduction of novel treatments.

The "success" of the device, as characterized by Cooley and Liotta, was that its implantation had not immediately killed Karp and that it had worked in pumping blood for 64 hours, thus providing "enough success" to continue device development. The priority was to establish device efficacy—building an artificial heart that did not cause blood damage or aggravate other compromised organs—rather than to debate therapeutic effectiveness. The 1969 implant case was about testing an experimental device in a human as much as it was about "doing everything possible" to save the life of a moribund patient. It fed into the allure of mechanical replacement parts as viable treatment options. DeBakey's research program continued to secure NIH funding for its artificial heart work, and Cooley expanded his research program with the recruitment of several key innovative individuals, including Japanese medical researcher Tetsuzo Akutsu, who had worked in the laboratories of Kolff and Kantrowitz, and cardiac surgeon-researcher O. H. Frazier, who had trained under both DeBakey and Cooley. Arguably the most consequential result, the Karp case reinforced the important function of medical review boards in the transition of experimental procedures from animals to humans. The Karp case was a cautionary tale, and the next implant of a TAH in a human did not occur for another 12 years.

Debating the Better Course: Human or Mechanical Hearts?

For days after Karp's death, the artificial heart news stories continued, focusing on the accusations of device theft and the clash between the two famous surgeons—the Texas Tornado and Dr. Wonderful, as one *Life* reporter dubbed DeBakey and Cooley, respectively.[163] The news coverage focused on the surgical and technological first of the artificial heart implant and the dramatic flight of a donor heart across the country. The more complex issues of medical effectiveness (a new therapy to be repeated?) and medical ethics (questions of informed consent and human experimentation) were not raised by journalists in any meaningful way.[164] But the medical community did discuss these issues, informally and formally, at professional meetings and in the medical literature.[165] One of the biggest questions was, Which cardiac replacement procedure—heart transplantation or artificial heart implantation—promised to be the better therapy? Should human or mechanical parts be used to save patients dying of heart failure? Few heart specialists or investigators suggested abandoning either research line, but they did want to discuss and guide the clinical practice of each procedure.

DeBakey, Kantrowitz, and Cooley advocated mechanical hearts over human transplantation. Arguably, DeBakey was simply defending his multi-million-dollar NIH-supported research empire. In the *Journal of Thoracic and Cardiovascular Surgery,* DeBakey stated that artificial hearts, similar to the artificial kidney, would provide necessary patient backup when cardiac transplant operations fail. Also, he continued, mechanical hearts overcome the problem of supply (donor heart availability) and circumvent the ethical and legal debates surrounding new organ procurement policies (brain death as opposed to cardiac death) as safeguards against removal of organs prematurely.[166] Investigators at the Cleveland Clinic, the University of Utah, and elsewhere, who were similarly invested in the continuation of artificial heart research, supported DeBakey's position.[167]

Many practitioners in the medical community questioned the benefit of heart transplantation, particularly since the record of transplant surgery was far from encouraging. The British medical community supported a moratorium on transplant surgery, stating that heart transplants had been attempted too soon. In 1969 the editor of the prestigious medical journal *Lancet* bluntly stated that while the surgical technique of heart transplant had been established, postoperative patient management problems still needed to be solved before the surgery offered any real therapeutic benefit.[168] A total of only six heart transplant operations took place in Britain over the next decade.[169] In New York, Kantrowitz walked away from doing any more transplant operations after his second failed attempt. With renewed conviction, he returned to his research on mechanical heart devices, certain that many more lives could be saved with mechanical assist devices than with transplant surgery. In this period, Kantrowitz received a $3 million NIH grant (second-largest to DeBakey's approximately $4.5 million NIH grant) for an ambitious ventricular assist research program.[170] Worldwide, Kantrowitz was recognized as a leading expert and innovator in both fields of research.[171] Many other cardiac surgeons also chose to stop performing heart transplant operations at this time because of the high mortality rates.

Cooley defiantly confronted the critics, and at a medical conference in Chicago in 1969, he stated that cardiac transplantation should be considered a "stepping stone" toward a mechanical heart, which would be the more practical treatment for heart failure patients.[172] Several years later, he softened his position when asked to compare various aspects of transplantation against the mechanical replacement of the heart, yet he grumbled about the "delays and procrastination" in the clinical testing of artificial hearts.[173] In terms of procurement, the artificial heart was easier to obtain than human donor hearts; in terms of performance, cardiac transplantation had the better clinical experience and record (although still poor in the mid-1970s). Artificial hearts and human hearts faced different rejection problems in the patient. If the artificial heart was used as a bridge-to-transplant device, it seemed unfair for the artificial heart implant patient to be given priority on the donor organ list, and issues of cost and access for this technology had yet to be worked out. Neither procedure was without problems, so neither was entirely ruled out. In the end, Cooley advocated a two-staged cardiac replacement approach—the temporary use of mechanical devices followed by transplantation of a human heart, as he had done in the Haskell Karp case—which might lead to its use as a permanent implant with future device improvement.[174]

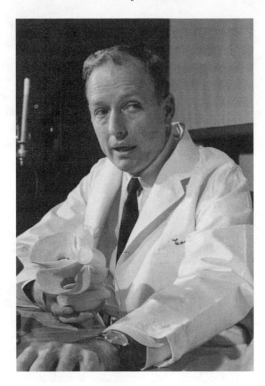

Cardiac surgeon Denton Cooley, holding an artificial heart, talks to reporters about the Haskell Karp case at a press conference at St. Luke's Hospital, Houston, Texas, April 7, 1969. (AP Photo/Ed Kolenovsky)

In opposition to DeBakey, Kantrowitz, and Cooley, Shumway and Lower argued for the abandonment of artificial heart research in favor of cardiac transplantation. After years of research on transplantation, Shumway and Lower had gained significant information about the immune system and organ rejection, and they had refined surgical techniques and organ preservation methods. This knowledge and experience bolstered their belief that heart transplantation would be clinically useful long before researchers would be able to overcome the bioengineering challenges associated with a mechanical heart, notably the need for biocompatible materials and an implantable power source.[175] At a transplantation symposium, Shumway speculated that the loud noise of a mechanical heart would make the recipient feel conspicuous. He even went so far as to suggest that with an artificial heart a person might even question his identity as a human owing to the mechanical part implanted in his chest.[176] Shumway also did not support the use of an artificial heart as a temporary measure, such as in the two-staged approach to a heart transplant that Cooley suggested. Like DeBakey, Shumway was often asked which cardiac replacement procedure should be pursued. In 1968 he told Congress, "Only heart transplants really offer exciting and real possibilities."[177]

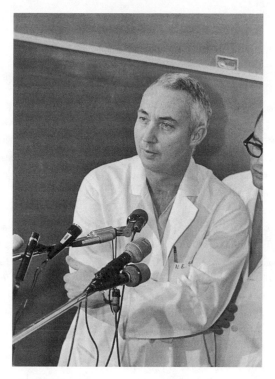

Cardiac surgeon and transplant researcher Norman Shumway addresses a crowded room of journalists after performing his first human heart transplant at the Stanford University Medical Center on January 6, 1968. Courtesy of Stanford University, Special Collections and University Archives.

Shumway's position on the artificial heart was clear; the use of a mechanical heart as a bridge device was more of a problem than a solution for the end-stage heart failure patient. He told an audience of the Commonwealth Club of San Francisco that the concept of an artificial heart was "marvelous," supplying "something you could go to the shelf and take down and place it [in a patient] . . . but it's just not that simple."[178] He called it "dangerous" owing to problems with device materials and the threat of blood clotting that could kill the patient before the transplant surgery.[179] Moreover, the use of an artificial heart as a bridge device simply intensified the donor shortage, according to Shumway. It did not eliminate the problem of too few donor hearts, but instead shifted the patient with an artificial heart (given the anticipation of complications soon after implant) to the top of the priority list for a transplant, thus inserting issues of access and fairness into the process.[180] For Shumway, the artificial heart remained a "crude device with no future," and he referred to it as "a sort of gimmick to get a donor."[181] Among artificial heart supporters, Shumway became well known for his disparaging remarks about the artificial heart.[182] Yet, recognizing that more than 20 percent of heart patients died while awaiting cardiac transplantation in the early 1980s, Shumway found a way to support both replacement approaches.

During the 1970s and 1980s, Shumway supported the clinical research of Stanford colleague Philip Oyer with the Novacor cardiac assist device for two reasons: first, the Novacor device was driven by an electrical power source, as opposed to compressed air, permitting much smaller external lines exiting from the chest wall; second, the device was intended to be a permanent implant. These were key characteristics of the Stanford device that distinguished it from other devices in development, according to Shumway.[183] He continued to focus on device valve problems, fatal blood clots, and power sources with troublesome exit lines. He argued that the devices for bridge-to-transplant use did not resolve donor organ shortages; they allowed implant patients to leap-frog to the top of waiting lists, possibly even jeopardizing a patient's status as healthy enough to receive a donor heart.[184] Device problems related to materials, durability, and power source were great, and he repeatedly told audiences during the 1970s that there were "almost no clinical results worth reporting, even with use of the partial or left ventricular assist device implanted in a few patients across the land."[185]

Still, there was a role for these devices in cardiac replacement, which even Shumway had to concede. Stanford favored heart transplantation, with no plans to implant TAHs, but an assist device might serve limited uses in its program.[186] At a 1992 Stanford medical forum, Shumway told the audience, "It is our feeling at Stanford that there can be no serious transplant program without an artificial heart component. It is just as important for the artificial heart to stand by for critically ill patients as it is for cardiac surgeons to back up the angioplastic efforts of our cardiological colleagues."[187] For Shumway, the artificial heart played a supportive role, and specific assist devices "may be all we need."[188]

A consensus emerged within the medical profession that cardiac transplantation and mechanical hearts were complementary, rather than competing, lines of investigation in the broader research endeavor of combating heart failure at this time.[189] In the 1970s, neither of these approaches to cardiac replacement secured the results wanted by the medical profession; all patients in heart failure died at this time, as neither therapy was yet perfected. The obstacles to heart transplantation and mechanical replacement of the heart appeared to be "of approximately equal magnitude."[190] Both cardiac transplantation and TAHs remained experimental procedures, and medical societies pleaded that investigation be left to those few institutions possessing the specialized units and expertise to support its development.[191] After the initial rush of transplants in 1968 and 1969, surgeons practically stopped doing heart transplant operations for the next decade as a result of the dismal patient outcomes.

In the 1980s, the introduction of the immunosuppressant drug cyclosporine began to reverse this trend, but the reversal was not immediate, nor did heart transplant surgery become commonplace, despite increasing rates of patient survival.[192]

With more than 4 million Americans suffering heart failure at this time, only a small number of patients received heart transplants.[193] According to the voluntary Organ Transplant Registry of the American College of Surgeons, less than 100 heart transplants occurred in 1980, and in 1985 the annual number of cardiac transplant operations was 844, with roughly 71 American medical centers reporting at least one transplant operation performed.[194] Thereafter the annual number of transplant operations rose, cresting at just over 4,400 operations worldwide in 1994, according to the registry of the International Society for Heart and Lung Transplantation.[195] Prompting this increase in transplant operations were the new antirejection drugs, such as FK-506 and rapamycin, which promised to be more potent and effective than the conventional regimen of cyclosporine, prednisone, and/or azathioprine; and as Shumway had predicted, transplant patients benefited from a combination of drugs.[196] Again it was Shumway's program at Stanford that was conducting leading research in transplantation immunology, further evidence that Shumway, rather than Barnard, was the heart transplant innovator; Barnard succumbed to the media attention of his early transplant surgery and never really engaged with any robust research thereafter. The magnanimous Shumway, however, commended Barnard for "awakening the neurosurgical community to the concept of brain death," which led to changing laws regarding the definition of death and the greater viability of donor hearts for transplantation.[197] In the end, Shumway had been right; researchers overcame the central limitations of transplant surgery before those of the artificial heart.

A Complementary, Not Competing Relationship

In this period, the fledgling field of mechanical circulatory support systems gained greater stabilization as a result of overlapping events and debates within the cardiac transplantation community. Dubbed the "ultimate operation" by the press, heart transplantation added hearts to the list of body organs that could be replaced by spare human or mechanical parts.[198] It is not surprising that DeBakey and Cooley, as cardiovascular surgical leaders in the field, became entangled in the broader professional debate surrounding cardiac replacement in the late 1960s. But the drama over the "covertly taken" device that was used in the first artificial heart implant case added another dimension, and the surgeons' feud became its own story, rivaling the medical feat of cardiac replacement.[199] For the media, both heart transplantation and artificial heart development provided dramatic story lines of life and death issues, alongside hero personas, which became embedded in the medical and technological optimism of the period. This sensational media reporting shaped public understanding of organ replacement therapy, which included the hopefulness of spare parts surgery, and offered an introduction to the medical and ethical complexities of clinical investigation.

The experimental procedures of heart transplantation and artificial heart implantation were intertwined in the 1960s, traversing similar issues, surgeons, and patient populations. How best to replace the damaged heart that could not be surgically repaired—with a transplanted human heart or with an artificial heart implant? Some researchers in the field preferred one approach over the other, but in the end, the two procedures were used in complementary, rather than competing, ways. Artificial heart researchers envisioned these devices as an independent therapy, either temporarily as a bridge to recovery after surgery or permanently as a replacement device for the failing natural heart. The initial challenges and uncertainties of heart transplant surgery, which kept it from emerging as the dominant procedure during the 1960s and 1970s, nonetheless strengthened legitimacy for cardiac replacement therapy. There was room for mechanical replacement alongside human replacement in the emerging field of cardiac replacement. This relationship became tighter with the creation of a new role for artificial hearts as bridge-to-transplant devices. It was a contentious role for mechanical devices, which complicated, rather than resolved, several issues raised by heart transplant operations, most notably the shortage of donor organs and priority status for device-implant patients on long waiting lists. But for most artificial heart researchers, the use of mechanical devices as bridge-to-transplantation helped to support their grander aims of developing artificial hearts for longer-term and permanent use. Allied with the heart transplant community in these ways, artificial heart researchers sustained funding, expectations, and a broader medical base, reinforcing the imagining and promise of heart replacement.

DeBakey and Cooley's well-publicized rift over the April 1969 implant case revealed that device authority and its clinical use does not, and should not, lie with one individual. Individual innovation and ownership of a medical technology as complex as artificial hearts cannot be defended, given the institutional and team structure necessary to develop and marshal an investigational device from the laboratory to clinical use. The justifiability of trying an unproven device in a patient is a process shared among medical, political, and social groups, with varying degrees of influence. Cooley's assertion that a surgeon must do everything possible to save the life of the patient is both reassuring to the patient and reflective of the commitment of clinicians who face often complex and impossible medical situations. Without diminishing those two things, institutional review boards function as safeguards for both patients and medical practitioners and are guided by strict research protocols that have been endorsed by the medical science community at large. A clinician's decision to use an investigational treatment is guided by her judgment regarding its potential benefit over its risk and by her sense of competency in offering it to her patient. Yet when such therapies are delivered in hospitals, which are regulated to some extent by internal policies, it involves others. Whether the device was stolen from the Baylor College of Medicine or not (and there is overwhelming evidence that it was), the other professional transgression was Cooley's decision to proceed independently without consultation or transparency, inciting concerns of human experimentation with a controversial technology, battling to establish its feasibility.

The fallout of the Karp implant case for the various individuals involved in the drama was varied: it was disastrous for the patient, his family, and Domingo Liotta; it

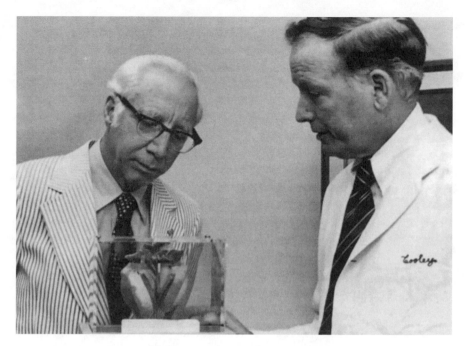

Cardiac surgeon Denton Cooley with visiting colleague physician-researcher Willem Kolff (*left*), at the Texas Heart Institute in the mid-1970s, admiring the Liotta-Cooley artificial heart that had been implanted in Haskell Karp and was subsequently encased in a Lucite box filled with a formaldehyde-type solution. In 1978 Cooley donated this device to the Smithsonian Institution's National Museum of American History, where it is considered one of the treasures of the national collection. Courtesy of the Texas Heart Institute.

was embarrassing for DeBakey, the Baylor-Rice research program, and the NIH; it was exhilarating and then blinding for Cooley, who may have initially enjoyed the surgical challenge and media attention of the case, but less so when it got nasty and the Karp family filed their lawsuit. Artificial heart technology gained media exposure as a result of the Karp case, although the "hype" soon led to a "crash" similar to the narrative trajectory of heart transplant surgery in this period. This event affected expectations, and there was a cooling off of public pronouncements of success with either heart replacement procedure. By this time, the budget for the Artificial Heart Program had leveled off to about $8 million a year, and administrators shifted more, but not all, of this funding to the development of cardiac assist devices.[200] The Karp case did not detonate the Artificial Heart Program nor discourage the small but dedicated core of artificial heart researchers who more or less dismissed Cooley's implant as a one-off.

Work on artificial hearts continued, quietly and less dramatically but with no less commitment and belief in its eventual fruition on the part of a handful of researchers in the field. DeBakey resumed his research on the Baylor-Rice artificial heart as well as on cardiac assist pumps, but he refused to speak to, or even acknowledge, Cooley for almost four decades.[201] (In 2007 Cooley, age 87, and DeBakey, age 99, formally reconciled their differences when their respective surgical societies, established by their former trainees—the Denton A. Cooley Cardiovascular Surgical Society and the Michael E. DeBakey International Surgical Society—exchanged lifetime achievements in surgery awards to DeBakey and Cooley, respectively.)[202] The goal of developing artificial hearts, as permanent or temporary, assist or replacement devices, to extend the lives of patients dying of heart failure remained. One of the most ardent advocates of this goal was Willem Kolff, who became involved in a different and contentious line of research during the 1970s—the development of a nuclear-powered artificial heart.

CHAPTER THREE

Technology and Risk

Nuclear-Powered Artificial Hearts and Medical Device Regulation

If there's a chance, any chance at all, that problems caused by technology could outweigh the benefits, we should stop. Trouble is, I hardly know any scientists who will dare say, "Stop."

Dr. William Bradfield, in *Heart Beat* (1978)

Heart Beat is a medical disaster novel, published in 1978, that predicts the perils of an atomic artificial heart. It is a story of Dr. William Bradfield's daring efforts to save the life of a dying patient through the implantation of a mechanical heart powered by plutonium. His patient, Henry Gray, survives the experimental procedure, makes an impressive recovery, and is discharged from the hospital to resume life with his fiancée. Both Bradfield and Gray enjoy their newfound celebrity status as guest speakers describing their experience with the radioisotope-powered artificial heart, and Bradfield goes on to implant more hearts with similar success. But then Gray is kidnapped by a madman who intends to remove the hundred grams of plutonium that power Gray's heart and spray the substance into the air, exposing thousands of people to dangerous levels of radiation. The FBI and local police begin a manhunt, while the National Heart Institute, government officials, and emergency-services personnel discuss contingency plans in the event that plutonium contaminates the area. A life-saving technology for one has now become a threat to society at large.

It is this issue of technology and risk, rather than an endorsement of heroic therapies, skilled surgeons, or triumphs of medical science, that the authors direct readers to reflect upon. Written by Eugene Dong, a cardiovascular surgeon, and Spyros Andreopoulos, the information officer of the Stanford Medical Center, this book tells an unlikely tale, yet it raises an intriguing question: Should technologies that pose society-wide risks be developed to save individual lives?[1] *Heart Beat* is fiction, but the technology it depicts is not. Between 1967 and 1977, medical researchers and engineers in two separate federally funded US programs tackled the technological complexity of designing a radioisotope-powered mechanical heart, one in which the heat generated by radioactive decay is the primary power source. When Dong and Andreopoulos speculated "what if" in *Heart Beat,* they reflected public anxiety about the risks associated with atomic power. In asking whether risky technologies could or should be developed to save lives, they invoked the classic conundrum of how to balance individual and collective good in a liberal society.

In a century replete with celebrated advances in science and technology, the 1970s emerged as a decade in which many individuals, as well as environmental groups, the consumer movement, and others speculated on the risks and unintended consequences for society that had resulted. Sociologist Dorothy Nelkin argues that the public's understanding of these risks came most often from journalists who had to "cope with complex and uncertain technical information and sort out conflicting scientific interpretations."[2] Risk reporting was often sensational and confusing, and at times it was misinformed; it reflected the competing interests and disputed meanings that surrounded controversial technologies. According to Nelkin, many journalists tended to grant authority to scientists over others in their reporting of evidence and definitive solutions.[3] As a result, science and technology news was put forth as predominantly good news, according to journalist Daniel Greenberg. In medicine, optimistic reporting of advances in disease understanding, cures, and devices tended to outnumber the stories that highlighted public dangers. Greenberg criticized the lack of scrutiny and the minimal accountability that surrounded many federally sponsored, large-scale science and technology projects of this period, such as the Apollo program or the Superconducting Super Collider project.[4] Yet the government maintained steadfast confidence in science and technology, bolstered by reports from the scientific community and its assertions of future benefits for Americans.[5] One such federally funded project was the development of atomic-powered artificial hearts.

Most scholarship on the development of artificial hearts—including the work of social scientists Renée Fox and Judith Swazey; historians Barton Bernstein and Barron H. Lerner; and bioethicists George Annas, Arthur Caplan, and Albert Jonsen—does not examine the development of atomic hearts but focuses on the sensational artificial-heart implant cases of the 1980s that highlight issues of human experimentation, patient celebrity, excessive socioeconomic costs, and misplaced confidence in technology.[6] Yet comparable debates about atomic heart research had occurred years earlier. For example, scholars studying the 1980s cases describe the remarkable technological optimism and research zeal that supported work on artificial hearts.[7] Earlier studies of atomic hearts may be characterized in the same way, with nuclear power fitting into Howard Segal's description of technological utopianism as a possible solution to many problems.[8] Historian Angela Creager describes how the US federal government promoted the use of radioisotopes in research, bolstered by scientific claims that radioisotopes would revolutionize medicine.[9] In both decades, queries from inside and outside the scientific community checked that zeal.

This chapter explores the overlooked atomic heart that emerged from the ambitious Artificial Heart Program of 1964. I highlight the technological optimism of scientists and engineers, the intersection of science and government, and the broader context of the public debates about risk and uncertainty that were occurring at the time.[10] Medical researchers and engineers claimed that atomic hearts were feasible and practical and the technological complexities surmountable. But political and social apprehension challenged these assertions. During the late 1940s and the 1950s, research into atomic medicine expanded, most notably the development of radioisotopes as a replacement therapy for radium.[11] Yet by the late 1950s and the 1960s, medical scientists reluctantly began to acknowledge the limits of radioisotopes.[12] As Soraya Boudia argues, a combination of scientific and social discourse articulated the hazards of radiation and public anxieties surrounding the use of radioisotopes.[13] The parallel development of atomic pacemakers, which were being implanted in patients in the early 1970s, strengthened the position that plutonium-238 was the superior power source available in this period. But the atomic heart required more than a hundred times the amount of plutonium used in atomic pacemakers, and society was not convinced that sufficient encapsulation and shielding would protect them from involuntary radiation exposure. Public concern regarding medical technologies and risk was not unwarranted. Litigation and publicity raised awareness of defective pacemakers, intrauterine devices (IUDs), and other medical devices in the late 1960s and the 1970s. The Medical Device Amendments of 1976 reflected political and public support for an increased federal role in protecting consumers against faulty devices, without negating the benefits of innovative medical technologies. The failed development of atomic hearts during this period was due to political and social concerns regarding the uncertainty and risk of radioisotopes in medicine, within the broader context of faulty medical devices. Ultimately, such concerns trumped the scientific community's assertion of the atomic heart's safety and efficacy.

Developing Atomic Hearts: The Emergence of Competing Programs

In 1964, after much lobbying by cardiovascular surgeon-researcher Michael De-Bakey, the Congress established the Artificial Heart Program at the NHI, part of the National Institutes of Health in Bethesda, Maryland. Shortly thereafter, NIH director James Shannon persuaded surgeon-researcher Frank Hastings, who several years earlier had developed a crude mechanical heart device, to administer the new program.[14] The Artificial Heart Program was the NHI's first targeted, extramural (contract) development program, created to lure both academic and industry investigators to pursue development of mechanical circulatory support systems. The NHI funded various lines of research related to design, materials, construction, blood interface, and biocompatibility issues, as well as energy sources and control and driving systems, for mechanical heart application. In this period, one of the greatest engineering challenges was finding the right implantable power source for an artificial heart. The power source needed to operate the heart pump sufficiently and had to be able to fit inside, and be tolerated by, the human body. Could atomic energy be a possible solution?

Thermo Electron Engineering Corporation of Boston proposed a radioisotopic power source for circulatory support systems to both the NHI and the Atomic Energy

Commission (AEC), hoping to tap into funding from both agencies. The AEC, under chairman Glenn Seaborg, was actively engaged in developing a series of isotopic power units, the most common of which, the radioisotope thermoelectric generator (RTG), produces electricity from the heat of radioactive decay. William Mott, chief of the AEC's Thermal Applications Branch, who became the lead project coordinator for the AEC radioisotope-powered mechanical heart, explained, "We were always on the alert for new problems to match with our solutions."[15] Indeed, RTG was a solution looking for a problem, as industry sought applications beyond spacecraft and remote-navigation beacons. Both the NHI and the AEC expressed interest in pursuing this research, although both rejected the Thermo Corporation's bid, citing the proposal's lack of understanding of the complexity of artificial heart systems.[16]

Neither agency rejected the concept, however. The possibility of building an atomic heart appealed to the political aims of both agencies; the NHI sought to expand its fledgling Artificial Heart Program, building on the Lyndon Johnson administration's interest in heart disease, while the AEC, typically involved with nuclear power, welcomed this project as contiguous to its work on radioisotope-powered space and medical applications and thus bolstering its role in development and regulation of all things nuclear.[17] Both agencies viewed the project as within their scope of activities: the NHI promoted heart disease research and the development of cardiac devices, while the AEC supported the use of nuclear power (radioisotopes) and regulated its safety.

Over the next several years, Seaborg and the NHI's director, Donald Fredrickson, worked collaboratively to explore the feasibility of a radioisotope-powered engine by sharing the cost of four separate conceptual design studies. In 1967 they jointly funded Aerojet-General, Thermo-Electron Engineering, Westinghouse Electric, and McDonnell-Douglas to conduct parallel design studies of an isotopic engine that would power pumps to assist or replace functions of a diseased heart. Unlike RTG technology, which converted heat to electricity, the isotopic power source for the artificial heart heated a thermal engine that used the expanding action of a gas to drive a hydraulic blood pump. Both vapor-cycle and gas-cycle thermal engines had the potential for the efficiency, reliability, and compactness necessary for an artificial heart system. Other components of the engine included a heat exchanger using blood as the cooling medium and a control system to regulate the power output of the engine.[18] Each of the corporations involved proposed different engine designs. More importantly, each of the four studies stated that there was a sufficiently large population of potential recipients to justify a large-scale research effort; of the 700,000 persons who had died of heart disease in 1963, approximately 12 percent would have been considered candidates for heart replacement.[19] Each proposal declared that the radioisotope-powered engine was the only possible energy solution for a completely implantable device. The ideal implantable device had to have no external lines or connections from the patient to outside power sources and must last for at least 10 years. By comparison, conventional batteries required recharging multiple times each day from an external source and would need to be explanted from pa-tients every two years.[20] Experts judged that the difficult engineering problems with the atomic heart, most notably the weight and safety of a radioisotope-powered engine for implantation in the human body, were surmountable obstacles.[21] Based on these favorable reports, the NHI and the AEC described the prospect for devel-oping a radioisotope engine for mechanical hearts as "good."[22]

However, NHI and AEC collaboration ended before the next phase of the proj-ect was initiated. Despite the instruction of the Joint Committee on Atomic Energy (JCAE)—a congressional committee that monitored atomic energy development, use, and control from 1946 to 1977—that the two agencies were to negotiate an in-tegrated, interagency plan for development of an atomic heart, the NHI and the AEC launched independent programs. The AEC's Isotope Development director, Eugene Fowler, detailed the NHI's lack of cooperation in a four-page report.[23] Ac-cording to Fowler, the agencies could not agree on management jurisdiction or the approach for engine development, making a collaborative venture practically impos-sible. The NHI's new director, Theodore Cooper (who had succeeded Fredrickson), proposed to develop the engine in two stages: first, a non-radioisotope-powered device, followed by a radioisotopic engine. Since the first system would not be radioisotope-powered, Cooper asserted that the NHI was the appropriate agency to direct, as well as fund, all heart engine development. In 1968 the NHI awarded contracts to five companies to develop different thermal engines, these firms re-porting back only to NHI administrators.[24] The NHI directed its contract recipi-ents to produce a workable non-radioisotope-powered device, reflecting the practical orientation of the Artificial Heart Program.

The AEC strongly disagreed with this approach, arguing that integrating radio-isotope power into an engine designed to be powered otherwise would not be straight-forward.[25] Furthermore, the NHI program priorities conflicted with the AEC's aim for this device: the NHI supported short-term heart assistance devices, while the AEC sought to develop an implantable, complete artificial heart to replace the diseased one on a long-term basis—a loftier, and more expensive, goal.[26] Thus the AEC proposed a separate, parallel effort to develop a radioisotope engine for mechanical hearts.

Since the two agencies were politically and scientifically motivated, neither one was willing to concede direction or management of atomic hearts. For the NHI, the development of atomic hearts was one of various projects in its newly launched Artificial Heart Program, which had been established as part of the institute's broad mandate of developing basic scientific knowledge about cardiovascular disease, as well as transferring that knowledge to practical application via pharmaceuticals, surgical techniques, or medical devices for the practicing physician. The AEC, on the other hand, welcomed various projects promoting the peaceful uses of nuclear energy, including, for example, the irradiation of sewage to reduce it to a sanitized solid for use as a building material, as well as atomic explosions to release trapped natural gas locked within rocks.[27] The prospect of developing an atomic heart constituted a much more dramatic peaceful use of nuclear energy. Early in his career, Seaborg had developed more than 100 atomic isotopes, including the isolation of plutonium-238 as a fuel, hoping to find medical applications for these substances. Nuclear medicine, in its infancy in the 1960s, was an emerging medical specialty, utilizing radioactive substances (ingested by the patient) to image the body to detect such problems as tumors, aneurysms, and irregular blood flow and to treat diseases like cancer.[28] Seaborg and others at the AEC were undoubtedly eager to contribute to this budding field of nuclear medicine by using their expertise on engine components and radioisotopes for atomic hearts; they refused to be squeezed out by the NHI.

The problems for the AEC in implementing its program were a lack of funds and the limited view of its role in this area of development.[29] In 1968 the Bureau of the Budget (renamed the Office of Management and Budget [OMB] in 1970) denied Seaborg's request for $1 million to continue work on a nuclear-powered source for heart devices. The bureau, driven by Republican reappraisals of the value of federal research and development, considered the NHI the best agency to efficiently manage the development of an atomic heart and thus granted it jurisdiction over research on heart disease and related projects, reflecting the shift from the generous funding of 1960s science and technology positivism to tougher, new congressional oversight in the 1970s.[30] The AEC would maintain control over the radioisotope fuel, while the NHI would manage the atomic heart project, although the bureau assumed that the NHI would seek the AEC's assistance and collaboration in the development of an isotopic engine.[31] Because of the NHI's plans to develop a nonradioisotopic, intermediate-stage device, the NHI refused to transfer funds to the AEC. Cooper hoped that the AEC would readily supply medical grade radioisotopes for related NHI research on heat dissipation and radiation emissions (which the AEC in fact did), but otherwise the AEC would not be consulted until the intermediate-stage device successfully advanced to the stage of incorporating a radioisotope. Seaborg complained about the NHI's lack of cooperation, but Cooper asserted that the cooperation between the two agencies was adequate.[32]

The frustrated Seaborg made a case before the JCAE for the AEC's continuing involvement in this research.[33] Citing the agency's previous experience in power sources and engines, as well as its broad authority for nuclear applications of all kinds, Seaborg argued for the appropriateness of the AEC's involvement in the atomic heart project.[34] He also argued that the NHI was "going down a dead-end road," because it supported a hardware-oriented program with in vivo studies (animal implants) to provide physiological-effects data that could be fed back into the program to produce more hardware. In contrast, the AEC team proposed an analytical evaluation that would assess the practicality of a nuclear-powered artificial heart without having to "bend tin," or produce hardware.[35]

Seaborg told the JCAE that the idea of an isotopic engine was technically feasible: an isotopic heat source would generate heat, which would then increase the temperature of a gas or generate steam; gas heated to the proper temperature could operate a Stirling engine or steam could run a Rankine cycle; and finally, such engines could operate a blood pump for use in humans. But was it practical? Applications of these basic ideas differed by duty cycles, load profiles, or varying power demands. A radar set, an automobile, and the human body each possess different power demands, including intermittent calls for power. How flexible or controllable was nuclear energy for its use in a mechanical heart implanted in a human? According to AEC expert Mott, the key issue was whether a completely implantable, radioisotope-powered artificial heart was practical: could a device of the requisite weight, volume, shape, performance, isotope inventory, reliability, durability, and cost be developed within a reasonable time and at reasonable expense?[36] Reflecting its practical concerns, the AEC proposed conceptual designs modeling these challenges, culminating in one design for production as a working model for bench testing. There were no AEC plans for in vivo studies at this stage.[37]

In addition to the AEC's criticism of the NHI's premature animal implants, the AEC's project members challenged the NHI's two-stage approach. The AEC team maintained that the radioisotope fuel and its containment and conversion system needed to be developed together with the device from the outset. Furthermore, they argued, only the AEC possessed the unique expertise and capability required. Countering this argument, Cooper and his NHI team contended that they should be responsible for total system development because of as yet poorly understood physiological factors affecting it. Consequently, AEC-NHI collaboration meetings always ended in impasse, and hence Seaborg pleaded with the JCAE to allow his team to lead its own development program.[38]

Initially, Cooper and his NHI team had no intention of altering their development program despite this AEC criticism and the decision by Seaborg for the AEC to pursue a different approach. But in mid-1970 the NHI, now renamed the National Heart and Lung Institute (NHLI), softened its position. After reviewing the AEC's critical assessment of its atomic heart program, the NHLI team conceded, granting the expediency of an independent AEC device development program. Fowler, who was one of the leaders of the NHLI team, reported that the NHLI would no longer oppose an AEC program, because "the proposed AEC work would neither duplicate NHLI's ongoing *in vivo* test program nor depend upon it."[39] In fact, the NHLI later came to regard the AEC's work as complementary to its own.[40] However, Fowler suggested that this new position represented less an "appreciation" of the proposed AEC work than an NHLI strategy to end a shaky collaboration.[41] In early 1971 the OMB, per the recommendation of the JCAE, acknowledged the irreconcilable differences between the two agencies and released $800,000 to the AEC, as well as additional funds to the NHLI for its program.[42]

The AEC Atomic Heart

After securing its funds, the AEC awarded contracts to Westinghouse Electric and Thompson Ramo Wooldridge Inc. (TRW) to conduct parallel analytical studies for a radioisotope-powered thermal converter, a device that would convert thermal to mechanical energy. Upon evaluating many thermal energy-conversion alternatives, each firm submitted a design of an artificial heart system with its preferred thermal converter. Each one asserted that its system design, if developed, would lead to a practical and fully implantable ten-year device to replace the human heart. Only intending to fund the development of one artificial heart system, the AEC selected Westinghouse's Stirling mechanical converter because its approach had a better understood and better developed technological basis. The Stirling mechanical converter was the most efficient in the size range desired; had greater potential reliability, owing to a reduced number of rubbing seals and bearings; and required the least nuclear-energy wattage. The AEC then awarded Westinghouse another contract to develop a complete radioisotope-powered artificial heart system.[43]

Over the next two years, Westinghouse completed additional theoretical and experimental work and then coordinated the fabrication of a realistically sized bench model of the full system.[44] The envisioned prototype of the AEC-Westinghouse nuclear-powered artificial heart system consisted of two main subsystems: the thermal converter, or power supply, and the blood pump mechanism. The work of fabricating the artificial heart necessitated the expertise of both engineers and medical scientists. Westinghouse subcontracted the construction of the thermal converter to the engineering firm Philips of North America, which was the leading expert in the Stirling engine.

The thermal converter produced by Philips was a gas-driven Stirling cycle engine, powered by 60 grams of plutonium-238, or Pu-238 (as a 33 watt nuclear-energy source), that was triply encapsulated in high-strength, high-temperature-bearing metal alloys (platinum-rhodium, tantalum, and Pt-20 Rh) for safety and durability.[45] After considering such radioisotopes as promethum-147 and thulium-171, Philips chose Pu-238 because of its low radiation-emission rate with high power density, its long half-life at 87.7 years, and its availability. Recognizing the toxicity of Pu-238, the Philips engineers designed durable encapsulation and containment of the radioisotope and provided sufficient thermal insulation for the converter to reduce heat dissipation (and hence tissue damage) in the body.[46]

To assemble the blood pump, Westinghouse worked with the artificial heart team of Willem Kolff at the Institute for Biomedical Engineering at the University of Utah.[47] Kolff's team proposed a pusher-plate blood pump with a flexible drive shaft to connect to the thermal converter. The blood pump consisted of two ventricles, which received and flushed out the body's blood by the compression of a roll-sock diaphragm on pusher plates attached to a Scotch-yoke mechanism. The blood pump's drive mechanism took the rotating drive-shaft output of 1,800 rpm from the Stirling engine, and through reduction gearing and the Scotch-yoke mechanism actuated the pump diaphragms at 120 beats per minute.[48] Blood came in contact with the Silastic rubber ventricles, whose coating of Dacron fibrils would reduce blood clotting.[49] This mechanical blood pump would be fitted orthotopically in the

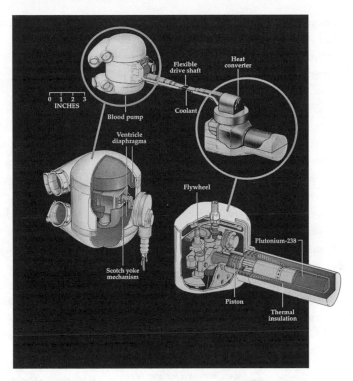

Schematic diagram of the Atomic Energy Commission nuclear-powered heart. The blood pump connected via a drive shaft to the thermal converter, intended to be implanted in the patient's chest and abdomen, respectively. Special Collections, J. Willard Marriott Library, University of Utah. Reproduced from *Physics Today* 69, no. 5 (2016): 38, with the permission of the American Institute of Physics.

chest (after removal of the diseased biological heart) and connected via the flexible draft shaft to the thermal converter implanted in the abdomen.

During this period the Philips engineers, Westinghouse's Astronuclear Lab researchers, and Kolff's team managed a coordinated and cooperative effort, capitalizing on their respective expertise and producing encouraging results. For example, medical researchers at the University of Utah supplied Philips with suggested practicability criteria, such as power and control requirements for a blood pump and surgical-implantation factors that facilitated successful component integration for the device.[50] But in 1972 the AEC-Westinghouse artificial heart was far from ideal, because both the Philips converter and Kolff's blood pump needed to be reduced in size and weight and improved in efficiency and reliability; also needed was greater system responsiveness to the needs of the body (called the load profile). Nevertheless, Westinghouse officials were encouraged, and they committed the next several years to improving the fabrication and to testing of the entire system, with eventual animal implants scheduled for 1974.[51] Their optimism and confidence in their atomic heart, however, was exceeded by that of NHLI officials in their own device, and the NHLI team beat their rivals to the punch. The first animal implantation of a nuclear-powered artificial heart system did not involve the AEC-Westinghouse device, but instead an assist device developed by the NHLI program.

The NHLI Atomic Heart

In February 1972 cardiac surgeon John C. Norman, of Harvard Medical School's Surgical Laboratories and Boston City Hospital, implanted a NHLI-sponsored heart assist system powered by Pu-238 in a calf. The ventricular assist pump attaches to the natural heart to assist in the pumping of the blood into the body's circulatory system. Norman was the first to test an atomic heart (albeit an assist pump) in an animal. He reported that the device worked for eight hours, keeping the calf alive, until a kinked inflow tube terminated the experiment.[52] NHLI director Theodore Cooper issued a press release to announce the achievement, and the story was front-page news nationwide, including images of the nuclear-powered assist device and photos of the implanted calf.[53]

There were key similarities and differences between the AEC-sponsored and the NHLI-sponsored nuclear-powered hearts at this time. Like the AEC-Westinghouse device, the NHLI's assist system consisted of two main parts: the thermal converter,

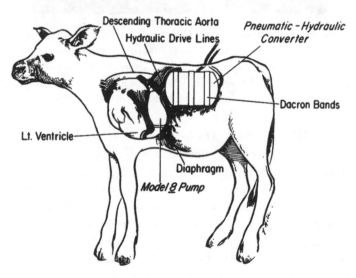

Illustration of a nuclear-powered heart-assist device, sponsored by the National Heart and Lung Institute, positioned in a calf. Reproduced with permission from J. C. Norman, F. A. Molokhia, L. T. Harmison, R. L. Whalen, and F. N. Huffman, "An Implantable Nuclear-Fueled Circulatory Support System: I. Systems Analysis of Conception, Design, Fabrication and Initial in vivo Testing," *Ann Surg* 176, no. 4 (1972): 492–501, fig. 11, p. 500, http://journals.lww.com/annalsofsurgery/Citation/1972/10000 /An_Implantable_Nuclear_Fueled_Circulatory_Support.7.aspx © Wolters Kluwer.

or nuclear-powered engine, and the blood pump mechanism. But there were significant design differences with these two systems. Most obviously, the NHLI system used an assist device—Thermo's Model VIII Left Ventricular Assist Pump—and not a complete replacement device for the heart. The Model VIII pump connected to the left ventricular apex of the heart and to the descending thoracic aorta, thereby helping the left side of the heart pump oxygenated blood into the greater heart vessels for circulation throughout the body. Like the AEC-Westinghouse pump, the Model VIII was made of Silastic and the blood moved through the bladder by action of a pusher plate. Also like the AEC-Westinghouse pump, the blood surface areas of the Model VIII contained Dacron fibrils to produce a smooth lining and prevent blood clot formation. The pump bladder was clamped in stainless steel housing, and this pump unit was hydraulically driven from the attached six-pound cylinder (situated in the abdomen), which contained a miniature thermal engine with a nuclear heat source.[54]

The thermal converter of the NHLI's heart assist system was developed by the Thermo Electron Engineering Corporation, an NHLI contractee, and it differed from Philips's thermal converter in its mechanics and in its need for double the amount of plutonium. The Thermo converter was a tidal-regenerator engine, or a regenerative gas-cycle engine, that combined the advantages of the Rankine engine with those of the Stirling engine. It was a thermodynamic machine in which heat was converted to work by means of a cyclic process whereby the working fluid was vaporized and condensed.[55] The familiar steam engine is an example of a vapor-cycle engine. (Interestingly, AEC's Mott, in his comparison of the AEC and the NHLI devices, reminded his team that they had evaluated and eliminated both the thermocompressor engine and the tidal-regenerator engine in favor of the Stirling mechanical converter during their Phase I Thermal Converter Practicability Study.)[56] In contrast, NHLI supporters of the tidal-regenerator engine argued that the few moving parts of this system—it had no valves or sliding seals—constituted an advantage in comparison with other nuclear engines under development. Mechanical differences like this were used by the squabbling researchers as the AEC and the NHLI fought for congressional attention and funding within a research program that supported multiple approaches to overcome engineering difficulties that were thought to be insurmountable.

Like the AEC-Westinghouse device, the NHLI-Thermo engine employed a Pu-238 fuel capsule, triply encapsulated; however, the NHLI-Thermo engine required 120 grams of Pu-238 to generate 52 watts of energy of converted hydraulic power to drive the pump, which was twice the amount of plutonium required in the AEC-Westinghouse device.[57] This greater amount of plutonium and energy wattage was not inconsequential; it contributed to the uncertainty regarding which pump design and its required power would be the more viable and lower-risk device. For both public and scientific communities, shifting thresholds of risk in medical innovation began tempering the appeal of radioisotope power. Combating potential opposition, atomic heart researchers pointed to such technical safeguards as triply encapsulated containment of the radioisotope and highlighted the energy advantage of plutonium. According to Thermo engineer Victor Poirier, nuclear energy was very attractive owing to the density of energy that could be created; a radioisotope-powered implantable device eliminated concerns of recharging or replacing batteries in electrically driven devices.[58]

The NHLI embraced the timing of Norman's animal implant case to release a status report on its nuclear-powered heart program. Acting program chief Lowell Harmison (who succeeded Frank Hastings after his sudden death in 1971) wrote a 63-page report outlining the "substantial progress" in both nuclear-engine development and blood pump systems as a result of five years of NHLI-funded research.[59] Most likely, this report, with its simplified presentation of contributions, its pronouncement of successes, and its confident tone of overcoming the remaining challenges, was designed to reassure senior management and public officials. Written for lay rather than scientific consumption, the report was dismissed by many in the field as a political document. Moreover, for many scientists and engineers, it also smacked of conflict-of-interest issues concerning its author, who, as an NHLI researcher (who had only recently moved into administration), was very much involved in the development of the H-TAH (Harmison-TECO Assist Heart) and the Model VIII Left Ventricular Assist Pump that was currently being used (and promoted) in the NHLI atomic heart system.[60]

Many of the scientific and technological gains declared in the report as NHLI "successes" were hardly exclusive to NHLI's nuclear-powered heart program. First, blood pump development had certainly improved by 1972, with advancements in device mechanisms and biomaterials having been reached by many in the field. The NHLI report highlighted the NHLI "flocked" interface of Dacron fibers bonded to blood-contacting surfaces of these pumps as an important contribution to controlling the problem of blood clotting and reducing blood damage (hemolysis) when the positive-displacement pumps of this device were used. The AEC-Westinghouse device also incorporated positive displacement and similar blood-interface design and materials. Second, research on the effects of radioisotope heat and radiation in dogs and primates supported scientific claims that the body could tolerate prolonged exposure with minimal effects. Again, AEC-funded research at Cornell University presented similar results. Third, the NHLI reported on its various nuclear-engine systems. Whereas the AEC program concentrated on one design—a standard pattern of a Stirling engine with a Scotch yoke-type of crankshaft, a flywheel, and a mechanical delivery of power from the engine to the actuator of the pump—the NHLI program supported multiple engine designs: a tidal-regenerator engine, a modified Rankine engine, a thermocompressor engine, a modified Stirling engine, and a high pressure Stirling engine.[61] But rather than offering a comparative analysis of these different engines, the report simply described the independent work completed to date by each contractee. All engines were "technically feasible," but their size, weight, and coupling to the blood-pump systems needed refinement before achieving a functional circulatory support system. Nevertheless, the overall message of the NHLI report was clear: five years of NHLI-sponsored research had culminated in the "successful" development of a nuclear-powered artificial heart system.[62]

The AEC's artificial heart researchers and other critics of the NHLI program challenged the announced success of the NHLI-sponsored nuclear-powered heart assist system, noting that the results were overstated. There was no NHLI atomic heart nearing clinical use, nor was any other such device supported by NHLI funds.[63] One anonymous critic (possibly Mott) denounced the NHLI statement as "full of deceit" and delivered for the purpose of obtaining more money from Congress.[64] AEC researchers like Fowler feared that the NHLI report might threaten their own congressional support; they warned Congress not to be misled, because the NHLI engine technology showed no major advancement since the NHLI atomic heart program's last review in June 1970.[65] According to Mott, the NHLI report was "the greatest piece of technology charlatanism that has come down the pike in a long time." He pointed the finger at Harmison, who "operated unchecked, without knowledgeable peers and superiors."[66] Indeed, Harmison had exaggerated the research innovation and performance of the NHLI's nuclear-powered artificial hearts. In response to all this criticism, the NHLI released another statement conceding the "technical bugs" in its system, admitting to the problems that the engine overheated and blood clotted in the pump.[67] After only four animal implants in early 1972, Norman stopped his testing until mechanical modifications improved device efficiency and reduced heat losses in the surrounding tissue. In 1973 and 1974, Norman implanted another 11 calves, but according to him, while "significant progress [had] been made, many problems remain[ed] to be solved."[68] Obvious technical problems aside, media reports and lawsuits against faulty medical devices currently in commercial use also contributed to researchers' reluctance to prematurely announce artificial heart devices' readiness for patient use.

Defective Devices and New Medical Device Legislation

The US Food and Drug Administration possessed authority over medical devices well before the beginning of artificial heart research. Early federal acts such as the Food and Drugs Act of 1906 simply defined the term *drug* to include medical devices.[69] In 1938 the Food, Drug, and Cosmetic Act defined devices as distinct from drugs and enabled the FDA to police and remove fraudulent devices from the marketplace.[70] By the 1960s, medical devices constituted a $3 billion to $5 billion industry, about half the size of the pharmaceutical industry, and it was still being monitored under the 1938 act.[71] Developments in electronic miniaturization, biomedical engineering, and plastics contributed to an increase in the number of new and sophisticated medical devices, from surgical implants to intensive care monitoring equipment. Hence, the FDA lobbied to expand its authority to review the pre-market safety and effectiveness of all new medical devices. As stated by historian

Kirk Jeffrey, the FDA's timing coincided with "the broader push by consumer and environmental groups to project the national government into safeguarding Americans in the workplace, the consumer marketplace, and the shared natural environment."[72] The enactment of the Kefauver-Harris drug amendments in 1962, spurred on by the thalidomide tragedy, strengthened the FDA's regulation of the drug industry. The lack of any provision for medical devices in this legislation further encouraged FDA administrators to act.

Faulty medical devices contributed to more than 700 deaths and 10,000 injuries in the United States during the 1960s, according to the Study Group on Medical Devices, chaired by NHLI director Cooper (it was also known as the Cooper Committee).[73] Consumer advocates reported on anesthesia machines that burst into flames, cardiac pacemaker malfunctions, and ineffective emergency respirators as only "the tip of the iceberg" of defective medical equipment "needlessly killing" Americans.[74] The Cooper Committee consulted extensively with doctors, manufacturers, engineers, trade associations, and consumer groups, reporting alarming cases of contaminated intraocular lenses that caused patients' vision loss; unsafe intrauterine contraceptive devices that caused infection, sterility, or death for thousands of women; and hearing aids that resulted in further hearing damage. Heart valve failures caused hundreds of deaths and radiation equipment resulted in thousands of injuries, as did a variety of prosthetic and orthopedic devices, dental equipment, sutures, syringes, and heating pads and blankets.[75] "Medical device problems too often are related to faults in the design and manufacture," the committee's report asserted.[76] The committee was distressed "by the lack of data in many areas related to the interaction of medical devices with the human body, and by the seemingly unquestioning acceptance of claims for medical device safety and performance unsubstantiated or inadequately supported by scientific fact."[77] The report also acknowledged that some of the problems were caused by improper use, but this factor was downplayed. The Cooper Committee concluded that the problem of medical device hazards related mainly to problems of design and manufacture, areas that legislation could ameliorate.[78]

In 1970 the committee submitted 17 recommendations to Congress intended to shape new medical device legislation. The most significant recommendations addressed the process of premarket evaluation, provided an inventory and classification of current medical devices, and created device standards. Most importantly, the committee recommended that medical devices needed a different regulatory approach than drugs and that, given the breadth and diversity of such devices, such regulation should be carefully tailored to the type of device involved.[79] It proposed that medical devices be classified according to their comparative risk and regulated accordingly, suggesting a three-tiered classification that the FDA could use: Class III, devices of high risk (such as artificial hearts), which required expert review prior to marketing; Class II, devices of moderate risk (such as powered wheelchairs), for which standards could be established to protect the public health and safety; and

Class I, devices of low risk (such as tongue depressors), which required neither standards nor expert premarket testing. At the time, no such inventory of medical devices in clinical use existed. The Cooper Committee also recommended that the government establish or encourage development of device standards and compliance testing for all new instruments or machines and that the FDA be given authority to audit manufacturers to ensure compliance. It was hoped that new regulation would protect patients from faulty devices, while still fostering the continued development of new devices.

Less than one month after the submission of the report, Representative Paul Rogers (D-Fla.) introduced a bill that incorporated almost all of the committee's recommendations.[80] While politicians wrangled over its language and contents, the FDA immediately began compiling an inventory of medical devices on the US market. It cataloged a staggering 8,000 devices produced by approximately 1,000 manufacturers and, with the help of appropriate experts, classified each device according to the proposed three-tiered system.[81] The FDA's activity kept pressure on Congress not to bury the bill. More importantly, however, publicity from defective device mishaps underscored the need for increased regulation.

Public outrage over deaths and injuries from defective heart valves, pacemakers, and IUDs rallied support for the passage of medical device legislation. Many patients reported heart valve problems caused by poor surgical implantation and flawed device design.[82] At the same time, several manufacturers, including Medtronic, General Electric, Cordis, Biotronik, and Vitatron, initiated a series of pacemaker recalls based on a variety of causes, such as premature battery failure, moisture seepage into the pacemaker case, and faulty leads that stopped transmitting electrical current to the heart. These problems resulted in some deaths, including among children.[83] Garnering even greater media coverage, thousands of women sought damages through the courts after experiencing excessive bleeding, uterine perforation, septic abortions, and pelvic infection from faulty IUDs.[84] Battling thousands of lawsuits, the manufacturer of the Dalkon Shield IUD withdrew it from the market in 1974 and eventually went bankrupt.[85] Increased litigation fueled public pressure for the federal government to safeguard the health of Americans, but without denying them the benefits of new technologies.

In response to these court cases, Congress held hearings to discuss the need for increased federal regulation of medical devices. It was, as noted by the health policy analyst Susan Foote, a period of strong consumer activism during which women's groups, the elderly, Ralph Nader's Health Research Group, and others pressured the government to protect consumers.[86] They argued that the burden of proof to establish products as unsafe should not lie with the FDA, but rather, that manufacturers were responsible to demonstrate their products' safety and effectiveness. These consumer activists suggested that increased regulation brought a "preventive approach" to ensure quality products and reduce malpractice suits. But medical professionals and manufacturers warned that their own judgements would be eliminated in the bureaucratic process and their expertise hamstrung by inflexible procedures. They argued that increased regulation could stifle innovation and hamper development, delaying the entry of valuable devices into the marketplace, and they pleaded with the government to refrain from safety "overkill" and to bear in mind that the majority of imperfect heart valves and pacemakers had extended many lives. Surgeon Arthur Beall emphasized the risk-benefit ratio of new devices: "Although about 500 people have died from imperfections in artificial valves, over 200,000 are alive who would have died without the artificial valves."[87] Researchers and manufacturers bristled at the intervention of the federal government and the concomitant burden of meeting new regulations. Both disliked the added preclinical scientific testing and burdensome record-keeping being proposed for FDA approval, stating, for example, that self-regulation by manufacturers of pacemakers had led to their voluntarily modifying their devices to accommodate the American Heart Association's recommendations for standardizing leads and instrument specifications.[88] Manufacturers also reminded Congress that unsafe use of their devices was part of the problem; professional training and user education needed to be part of the solution as well. At this time, however, the medical device industry was an unorganized collection of large and small groups who could do little to slow the momentum toward increased federal regulation; their arguments against regulation were overshadowed by the publicity surrounding faulty devices and patient risk.[89]

President Gerald Ford enacted the Medical Device Amendments of 1976, which contained many of the recommendations in the Cooper Committee's report.[90] The new legislation established a complicated regulatory scheme that would remain basically unaltered for decades.[91] Congress, siding with consumer groups, wanted to ensure the FDA's authority to regulate medical devices and therefore outlined the agency's responsibilities and actions. The intention was to strike a balance between protecting the public and promoting research and development of innovative life-saving medical devices. Risk would be contained without delaying the benefits of new medical technology to Americans in need. Some medical researchers disagreed, contending that the regulations would discourage clinical investigation and ruin the innovative small-scale manufacturer, who, with limited resources, would be unable to meet FDA's new requirements. FDA personnel were "well-meaning and intense young people," asserted one physician, but they "were inherently suspicious of private enterprise and somewhat crusading in their approach."[92] Furthermore, the critics contended that the legislation would force many US device manufacturers to conduct their initial clinical trials abroad, where less rigid European oversight was more attractive both financially and administratively. They predicted that the new federal regulations would neither improve the scientific database nor noticeably decrease the risk of high-technology devices.[93]

Under this legislation, atomic hearts were classified as high risk Class III devices, and new safety and efficacy standards for patient use would have to be met later when pursuing commercialization of the device. Yet it was the faulty-device reports and political discussions leading up to the passage of the regulations that were more significant for the future of atomic hearts, because they underscored both public and scientific concerns surrounding the exposure of patients and society to risky medical technologies. As the public became more fretful, questions of acceptable risk and unintended consequences of medical technology captured people's attention. Supporters of atomic hearts found themselves situated within a milieu of risk awareness or consciousness; that is, as scholars Anthony Giddens and Ulrich Beck argue, modern society seemed fixed on managing or containing risk during this era.[94] Politicians, bioethicists, journalists, and others became more directly involved in shaping the development of atomic hearts.

Should Atomic Hearts Be Built?

Even if experts resolved the technological problems, were nuclear-powered artificial hearts desirable? Were the risks acceptable, given the potential medical benefits? And who should make these judgments? Experts, government officials, and bioethicists alike began to ask such questions in the wake of controversies over medical device safety. Individuals working in both the NHLI and the AEC programs anticipated this line of questioning. As Mott commented, "Without question a plutonium-238 powered heart, regardless of its technological assets, will stir many more emotions and evoke much stronger criticism than would a heart powered by any other means."[95] Perhaps naively expecting technical expertise to mollify public anxiety, Mott was irked when critics with "no direct competency" challenged the ability of experts like himself and his conviction regarding the nuclear safety of atomic hearts.[96] By the early 1970s, the critiques of large-scale government-funded science and technology projects by antinuclear and environmental groups made nuclear energy projects increasingly difficult to justify.

Political scientist Robert Duffy points out that by the 1970s, discussions of nuclear power had shifted to the potentially harmful effects associated with its use owing, in part, to outsiders or nonscientists who emphasized the political and social dimensions of the technology.[97] Environmental groups may initially have hoped that nuclear power would be better than conventional fuels for the environment; however, for many Americans, nuclear waste issues, nuclear plant meltdowns, radiation risks, and a growing distrust of the nuclear industry created an overall uneasiness about nuclear power. Likewise, in matters of clinical research, bioethicists raised political, economic, and social questions associated with medical innovation. Historian David Rothman calls the emergence of bioethics at this time a "movement," or a shift to collective rather than individual decision making. Bioethicists aimed to ensure that researchers would assess risks and benefits to human subjects in ways that were not self-serving, and that physicians would reach critical medical judgments that were not idiosyncratic.[98] In this environment of reform, exotic new technologies like atomic hearts concerned bioethicists, consumer groups, politicians, and others.

The NHLI attempted to lead this debate by convening a mixed panel of medical and lay persons to examine the broader ethical aspects of its artificial heart program. The agency deemed this move prudent because of the approaching clinical use of mechanical hearts, the unresolved moral and legal implications of heart transplants that were evident from recent experiences, and the need to understand the consequences of technology, specifically nuclear power.[99] In July 1972 the NHLI's Artificial Heart Assessment Panel explored the social, ethical, legal, and economic implications of the development and use of artificial hearts in humans. Its discussions were not limited to the atomic heart, although that device figured prominently in the panel's resulting report. The panel consisted of three physicians (a cardiologist, an internist, and a psychiatrist), two economists, two lawyers, one sociologist, one priest-ethicist, and one political scientist. No members were artificial heart specialists or engineers; in fact, most of the panel admitted to knowing very little about the medical and technical requirements of artificial hearts. This, however, did not deter the panel from asking about the medical need for such hearts and the present state of artificial heart technology. Panel members met with members of the NHLI atomic heart team and the AEC atomic heart team; numerous artificial heart researchers, including John C. Norman, Willem Kolff, Michael DeBakey, and Tetsuzo Akutsu; and individuals from the Institute of Society, Ethics and the Life Sciences in New York (later renamed the Hastings Center), the Kennedy Institute for Bioethics at Georgetown University, and the Health Policy Program at the University of California–San Francisco.

Nearly two years later, the panel submitted a 250-page assessment of NHLI's artificial heart program, recommending that research on all types of MCSSs should continue with NHLI funding and concluding that artificial hearts (if successful) would contribute to a healthier population. The report covered issues of access, including potential shortfalls in supply, cost, and quality of life. It identified larger issues, but these were discussed only superficially: namely, the relationship between experimentation and therapy and the conditions for human experimentation and informed consent.[100] The report concluded that the nuclear-powered approach to artificial hearts was the better power source option compared to biological fuel cells, which were decades away from practical use, and battery systems, which tended to overheat, required daily recharging, multiple times, from an external energy source, and had a limited life span of only two years.[101] A plutonium fuel capsule would provide a reliable source of energy for a period of 10 years, with no dependence on external sources of energy. In short, said the report, "The nuclear system is far more advantageous to the recipient in terms of his sense of well-being and personal convenience."[102]

However, the panel was uneasy about the toxicity of the plutonium, the possibility of accidents or criminal acts relating to the device, and the radiation exposure to recipients, their families, and the public at large.[103] This latter issue of radiation exposure raised the most serious concerns, since there was little scientific data about the biological effects of continuous exposure to low doses and therefore exposure guidelines were somewhat nebulous. In 1971 the National Council on Radiation Protection and Measurements (NCRP) recommended different allowable levels of whole-body exposure. It proposed an occupational level of 5 rem per year for nuclear workers, but a much lower general public exposure of 0.5 rem per year.[104] Atomic heart recipients would be exposed to 55 rem of radiation annually, and their spouses risked annual exposures ranging from 0.7 to 9.0 rem, depending on interactions, such as whether recipient and spouse slept in the same bed or not.[105] This exposure constituted a significant increase and range of radiation exposure when considering that typically the average person received about a hundred millirems of cosmic-background radiation per year.[106] Medical personnel performing atomic heart implants potentially faced exposure to more than the occupational limit of 5 rem annually. According to the recommendations of the NCRP, the estimated combined exposure during the plutonium implant itself and for the recipient's life thereafter was too high, causing individuals to be at risk of sterilization and development of leukemia or other cancers, among other possible health problems. The panel acknowledged, however, that recipients and their families might choose to accept these risks rather than face certain death.[107] Similar questions of risk and safety arose during the parallel development of atomic pacemakers in this period.

In the early 1970s, the first human implants of nuclear-powered pacemakers took place in Europe and the United States. At about the same time that the AEC had been approached by Thermo to investigate nuclear energy to power heart pumps, cardiac surgeon Victor Parsonnet contacted the AEC with a similar nuclear energy proposal to power pacemakers.[108] Mercury batteries caused pacemakers to fail within 18 months of implantation, prompting the search for a better energy source. The AEC contracted the Nuclear Materials and Equipment Corporation (NUMEC) to develop an atomic pacemaker, utilizing Pu-238, as a better, long-term power source for these devices.[109] By 1969 the AEC reported encouraging animal implants that showed great promise for heart patients in the not-too-distant future.[110] The following year in Paris, French doctors performed the first human implant of a nuclear-powered pacemaker, utilizing the French-made Medtronic-Alcatel device.[111] Some Americans demanded this new nuclear technology; for example, Carole Wilson, writing to her US senator, asked: "Why the delay? Especially since the British and French already have put nuclear pacemakers in patients. . . . I live in constant fear of a sudden failure of my batteries which at present must be surgically changed every 18–22 months as opposed to the 11–20 years medical scientists believe the nuclear powered pacemaker can give me. (I am 31 years old.) . . . Please help me and others like myself by taking an immediate active interest in this matter to rectify this situation. NUCLEAR CAN KILL! NUCLEAR CAN CURE! WHICH SHALL IT BE?"[112] Wilson was not alone in writing to her elected officials about this matter. Such letters prompted some senators to make inquiries on behalf of their constituents. The AEC replied that once reliability and safety standards had been met, the device would be available for general use.[113] Not long thereafter, Parsonnet implanted the first US-built NUMEC nuclear-powered pacemaker in a patient in New Jersey in 1973.[114]

According to historian Kirk Jeffrey, the nuclear-powered pacemaker was an "effective technology," using a superior power source that rarely needed replacement in comparison to the unsatisfactory life of the mercury battery.[115] The NUMEC nuclear-powered pacemaker converted the heat from a small amount of plutonium-238, which was triply encapsulated inside the pulse generator, to an electric current to pace or regulate the beating of the heart. By the end of the decade, there were seven different models in clinical use—four American and three European designs—that met international safety standards.[116] Environmental impact studies reported that the radiation exposure from atomic pacemakers was well within acceptable levels for recipients, spouses, and the public.[117] According to one pacemaker inventor, it was "the most reliable pacing system ever built."[118] Many recipients praised the device; Simone Fouquet of Maryland wrote in 1976: "I have been one of the recipients of the nuclear pacemaker since July 24, 1973 and in my gratitude I must express my admiration for this great invention. I can climb two or three flights of stairs which I could not do with the other pacemakers that I wore before. The other pacemakers had to be changed within two years and for a person my age, the surgery involved was exhausting."[119] A nuclear reactor physicist said this about his nuclear pacemaker: "The only hazard that I can see would be . . . being blown up by a bomb that would rupture the pacemaker and disperse the plutonium into the environment. I am well aware of the highly toxic nature of plutonium, but I am also aware of the extremely low probability that a catastrophic accident will happen to me or to anyone else wearing a nuclear pacemaker. . . . Let me extend my heartfelt thanks to those who developed the nuclear pacemaker, and to the AEC for its foresight in licensing the device."[120] Another recipient simply wrote, "Please accept this letter as a layman's vote for continued use of the nuclear pacemaker."[121]

Still others opposed the use of this device. One woman blamed the atomic pacemaker for the death of her adult daughter, who before this had managed her heart problem successfully with traditional battery pacemakers. She asked her senator to "check into the matter of atomic pacemakers because some are defective, and their radiation will kill the patient [and] that's what I feel is happening to my poor daughter."[122] Alfred Mann expressed his skepticism regarding the AEC's ability to control and to supervise the use of the nuclear material, as well as the claims of scientists that the plutonium casing was "indestructible." He stated, "There is no way in which a prudent citizen could be convinced that the nuclear pacer is necessary or acceptably safe."[123] In addition, the high cost of the nuclear pacemaker at $5,000, in comparison to the $1,500 battery pacemaker, dissuaded many from using it.[124]

By the end of the 1970s, fewer than 3,000 atomic pacemakers had been implanted worldwide.[125] The device's use declined for two reasons. First, strict AEC licensing requirements regarding hospital acquisition and monitoring, as well as patient compliance for safe travel and ultimate nuclear material disposal, deterred many from using it. Second, the introduction of new lithium-powered pacemakers, with an eight-to-ten-year life span, matched the longevity of atomic pacemakers, offering a viable alternative at lower cost and risk. By the mid-1980s, the atomic devices were no longer available for implantation.[126] According to Parsonnet, however, there may still have been individuals in the United States with implanted nuclear-powered pacemakers in 2006.[127]

The development of artificial hearts (MCSSs) and pacemakers (clinical cardiac pacing and electrophysiology) are set in two distinct research and clinical areas, with separate professional meetings and journals. However, the exploration of nuclear energy to power these devices provided some crossover. Atomic heart researchers, including Kolff, were aware of the parallel development of atomic pacemakers but understood that significant technical differences between them and artificial hearts meant the two could not be directly compared. Most obviously, the atomic artificial heart required more than 100 times the amount of plutonium used in the nuclear-powered pacemaker, and thus the magnitude of the risk was significantly different. Issues of nuclear material licensing and regulation and of radiation emission were more prominent in the artificial heart discussions. More plutonium also meant that the artificial heart device would be significantly more costly than the pacemaker. The AEC estimated the cost of medical grade plutonium at $1,000 per gram, with the hope that, with increased production, the price would drop to $430 per gram.[128] It was also evident that the artificial heart was a much more complex system than the pacemaker. The artificial heart required more energy, generated more heat that needed to be dissipated, contained many movable parts that came into contact with the blood, and had a more demanding duty cycle and load profile. Overall, the artificial heart had a greater potential for technical failure, and such failure would almost always be fatal for the recipient.

There is no evidence that atomic heart and atomic pacemaker researchers collaborated in the development of their respective devices. However, the political and social aspects associated with using atomic energy did overlap. Atomic pacemakers shared the question of individual benefits versus public safety and risk, which made such information as radioisotope management, device registration, and public concerns regarding involuntarily exposure to radiation of interest to researchers of both types of devices. AEC administrators and NHLI program directors read development reports on nuclear-powered pacemakers and retained documents that might have been useful for artificial heart systems, such as patient agreements and instructions about self-identifying as a nuclear-powered pacemaker recipient.[129] No doubt many program administrators anticipated the contrasting positions of those Americans who would support and others who would oppose any device powered by atomic energy. Focusing exclusively on artificial hearts, the NHLI Artificial Heart Assessment Panel's report did not address any research or clinical experiences regarding the nuclear-powered pacemaker.

The End of Atomic Heart Research Programs

The Artificial Heart Assessment Panel, in its recommendations, attempted to balance the aggregate benefits to society of this technology against the aggregate risks. The report concluded that the benefits of an atomic artificial heart appeared to outweigh its low or acceptable risks; the possibility of accidents or criminal acts involving patients with atomic hearts was remote; the radiation exposure could be lowered; and the regulation and licensing of Pu-238 would contribute to controlled management of this potentially harmful material. It appeared confusing that the panel would deem atomic hearts of "low or acceptable risks"; this judgment spoke to the panel's desire to continue exploring the medical potential of atomic energy and its hope that the risks could be responsibly managed and reduced. Members did not dismiss the atomic heart's high levels of radiation exposure, well aware that its exposure exceeded NCRP recommendations, thus raising the question whether the risk-benefit analysis was an ethically appropriate measurement tool. The panel's report wanted to play both sides: to encourage further device research and to acknowledge the risks of clinical use. The report could have explicitly recommended to bury atomic hearts, given their radiation risks, but it did not. Instead the report concluded that atomic power was the superior energy source and that its aggregate benefits outweighed its risks but that atomic hearts should not be implanted in humans until it was scientifically established that there would be no significant risk of injury involuntarily imposed on nonrecipients. It was a bewildering conclusion, further muddled by the report's plea for greater efforts to develop alternative energy sources—specifically, better battery technology.[130]

Atomic heart researchers like Kolff contested the panel's recommended ban on clinical use. Investigators experimenting with animals fully expected to move forward to human implants, contending that human tests could supply data that was impossible to obtain from animal experiments. The panel members were not persuaded; here they drew the line: continue with animal experiments, but no human implants. They pointed to the danger of a "slippery slope": namely, more widespread use of atomic systems could not be controlled once human implants, experimental or otherwise, began.[131] The AEC's Mott, shocked by what he considered to be baseless conclusions by the panel, challenged its members' technical competence and commented that they were "preoccupied with the nuclear system and its risks."[132] Indeed, the panel was uneasy about the nuclear system, questioning the claims of AEC and NHLI scientists that the nuclear fuel capsule was indestructible. Since this assertion was not grounded in actual experience, the panel chose to err on the side of caution.

Administrators, government officials, and the public seemed to agree. The public was especially apprehensive about radiation exposure during this period—whether from nuclear power plants, other atomic energy applications, or even medical and dental X-rays.[133] Acceptability of atomic hearts by recipients and their families with no other options was one thing, but acceptability by the general public was quite another. When the Artificial Heart Assessment Panel asked members of the Subcommittee on Somatic Effects of the NAS-NRC Advisory Committee on the Biological Effects of Ionizing Radiation about the risk of a radioisotope-powered artificial heart, one scientist replied: "My main worry about a Pu-238 powered heart pump is that one day on a Trans-Pacific flight, economy class, I will be seated between two of them."[134] As sociologist Lee Clarke has pointed out, the public is often more tolerant of risks when exposure is regarded as voluntary, instead of involuntary.[135] The panel anticipated that the public would not find the risks associated with radioisotope-powered artificial hearts acceptable; it decided therefore to limit experimental implants to animals, hoping that safer nonnuclear energy sources would be forthcoming soon, thus rendering the nuclear option moot.

The Artificial Heart Assessment Panel's report influenced both the NHLI's and AEC's atomic heart projects. NHLI administrators responded immediately to almost all of its recommendations, discontinuing support for the atomic heart and redirecting its attention to other energy sources. By this time, unsatisfactory animal testing of three different agency-sponsored thermal engines with various ventricular assist devices resulted in a discouraging outlook for nuclear-powered devices. Norman had implanted a total of 15 calves with plutonium between 1972 and 1974, and the survival rates had been measured in hours, not days. The average animal lived less than 48 hours until various technological problems with both the pump and the engine, including device leaks, breaks, and thermal exposure to the animal, terminated the tests. Mechanical modifications made after each animal implant demonstrated improved system efficiency and reduced heat losses to the surrounding tissue, but many problems still remained to be solved.[136]

Clarence Dennis, who had succeeded Harmison as administrator of the NHLI's artificial heart program, moved to stop the "unproductive, extravagant experiments" linked to the atomic heart. Dennis stated, "In contrast to the AEC, which in 1970 embarked upon development of a single thermal engine, the NHLI Program was launched without sufficiently thorough investigation and funded several contractors and designs. . . . The multiple approach with insufficient prior investigation has resulted in a funding of patterns of thermal drives which should have been rejected outright on the basis of the physiological implications."[137] The budget of the NHLI's atomic heart program was four times that of the AEC's. NHLI administrators had awarded contracts to six different engineering companies, totaling more than $14.3 million, in comparison to the AEC's one contract to Westinghouse for the sum of $3.5 million. Calling for a return to basic science, Dennis advocated ending the NHLI's atomic heart program and redirecting funding toward the development of alternative energy sources.[138]

In 1974 the incumbent AEC chairman, Dixy Lee Ray, announced that the AEC would phase out the development of its atomic heart program over the next three years. AEC officials admitted that the questions raised regarding public acceptability by the Artificial Heart Assessment Panel partly influenced this decision, as did general uncertainty about the ultimate success of the program.[139] A 1974 review of the AEC's atomic heart program by a group of seven independent engineers and research physicians criticized the device as "immensely complicated with more than a dozen gears and heaven knows how many bellows and bearings. It is difficult for most to conceive of such a device working successfully for 10 years without service."[140] They also expressed concern over the device's radiation levels. Contributing to this pessimism was the budget crunch of the mid-1970s. Many government officials deemed the atomic heart program too long-term and costly to continue, and thus drastic budget cuts seemed imminent.[141] Meanwhile the AEC, under public pressure because of its perceived conflict between dual missions to promote and regulate nuclear power, split into two new agencies: the Energy Research and Development Administration (ERDA), which directed all research and development programs, and the Nuclear Regulatory Commission, which assumed all regulatory functions.[142] Atomic heart researchers now working for ERDA fought to keep their program alive, arguing that they had developed a viable system for thermal energy conversion, but it was too late. Mott, a key AEC/ERDA project coordinator, left the program after being reassigned to a different area, and Donald Cole took over as project coordinator. Senior AEC administrators commented that they were reviewing "future directions and priorities within the program," which meant they were transferring the atomic heart program to the NHLI.[143]

Having invested considerably in the AEC atomic heart, Kolff lobbied politicians and pleaded with the JCAE to reinstate ERDA's program, thus prompting another review of it.[144] Expert bioengineers and medical researchers recommended that ERDA continue funding its atomic heart program, arguing that the advantages of the plutonium source outweighed its risks, making plutonium the energy source of choice.[145] Yet the OMB allocated no money to ERDA for continued research on the artificial heart during the next fiscal year, thus effectively terminating the program.[146]

In his final report, the disappointed Kolff defiantly declared the AEC-Westinghouse artificial heart a "success," although it had never been tested with plutonium. Denied access to plutonium, Kolff replaced the Stirling engine with a small electromotor on the pump and implanted this device in calves, of which one survived for 35 days.[147] But like the NHLI's heart assist systems, Kolff's artificial heart also wrestled with problems regarding biocompatibility and device performance. The NHLI's Dennis commented, "One might say that AEC has suffered from putting all eggs in one basket while the NHLI has suffered from trying to carry too many baskets at one time."[148] In his observation, Dennis correctly pointed out that neither program had produced a viable atomic heart, but that it had less to do with approach than with technological problems. In a 1977 review of the NHLI's circulatory support program, scientific assessors identified numerous remaining bioengineering challenges of current blood pump designs, including the threat of thrombosis and embolization (blood clots leading to strokes), problems of hemocompatibility with pump materials (suitable blood-interface materials), and infections with percutaneous (through the skin) drive lines. Yet, for all of these pump difficulties, the many problems of nuclear power as an energy source appeared greater.[149] By 1977 institutional support for atomic heart programs ended.

Navigating Uncertainty and Risk

When the Medical Device Amendments of 1976 came into effect, critics argued that the new legislation would stifle technological innovation and retard the delivery of potentially life-saving medical devices, but the amendments did not. The new act took effect in December 1978, after which the FDA approved hundreds of new devices, ranging from stent systems to brain stimulators to artificial sphincters.[150] Further legislation, in the form of the Safe Medical Devices Act of 1990, expanded FDA authority to require postmarket surveillance of medical devices by industry and medical professionals, in the wake of well-publicized defective pacemakers and ruptured silicone breast implants.[151] The public's demand for increased federal oversight for protection against faulty devices was met without denying Americans the benefits of new, innovative medical technologies. The 1976 legislation succeeded in placating public anxiety, answering its call for federal oversight to mediate risks, although it certainly did not remove all device risk.[152] The FDA never reviewed the safety and effectiveness of atomic hearts, since these devices were never commercialized.

Medical scientists and engineers did not develop atomic hearts beyond limited animal testing. Despite their assertions that the technological complexity of this device was surmountable, public concern and political responses to the uncertainty and risks associated with medical devices in general, and the use of radioisotopes in the body in particular, contributed to the government's decision to withdraw funding, effectively ending this line of investigation. From 1967 to 1977, as the public was beginning to demonstrate greater consciousness of risks in medical technologies, the development of atomic hearts vacillated between being a potentially positive and valuable nuclear-powered product and being a medical device that was risky to the wider public. Laypersons, such as bioethicists, journalists, consumer groups, and politicians, became more vocal, calling attention to the broader political, economic, and social issues surrounding complex medical technologies. Society and the state—outsiders as opposed to predominantly scientific experts—influenced how the boundaries around artificial heart research would be constructed. The concerns raised by bioethicists and other laypersons and the FDA both increased federal management of the risks associated with medical devices and effectively ended the scientific research on atomic hearts.[153]

New legislation classified the artificial heart as a high risk Class III device, and FDA approval was now mandatory for its clinical use or testing. The development of nuclear-powered artificial hearts ended before the Medical Device Amendments of 1976 came into effect. Almost certainly, atomic hearts would not have met the new FDA standards of patient safety and effectiveness. In sharp contrast were the air-powered artificial hearts under development, poised for clinical testing in the early 1980s. Some cardiac surgeons, like William DeVries at the University of Utah, adhered to the regulations, while others, such as Denton Cooley at the Texas Heart Institute and Jack Copeland at the University of Arizona, did not always do so, prompting the FDA to create a category of one-time emergency use of nonapproved devices. The new legislation did not inhibit artificial heart research and development, although many industry researchers shifted early testing of their experimental devices to European venues before returning to the United States for FDA approval. The American market was too significant economically for device manufacturers to ignore FDA procedures. In the United States, the federal government mediated the risk associated with such high risk devices as artificial hearts without denying the public of the potential benefit of new technologies.

The risk debate surrounding the development of the nuclear-powered artificial heart played no direct role in the passage of the 1976 amendments. However, the connection is the concern over risk—individual and larger societal risk—that pervaded discussions of medical devices in this period and the public consensus for increased federal oversight in these matters. With the ongoing reporting of defective pacemakers and IUDs, a wary society questioned all investigational devices introduced clinically. The Medical Device Amendments of 1976 now required peer review and collective surveillance of devices, in an attempt to prevent harmful contraptions from reaching the public. As a result of the 1976 amendments, approximately 10 percent of all medical devices received Class III status (such as artificial hips, pacemakers, replacement heart valves, and artificial hearts), while more than half of all devices earned Class II status (for example, x-ray machines, powered wheelchairs, infusion pumps, and other noninvasive equipment).[154] In the end, the benefits of the regulations included better preclinical and clinical testing protocols, both of which almost certainly resulted in lower risks to patients.[155]

To be sure, the ambitious pursuit of developing the atomic heart experienced significant technological difficulties during the period studied here. One major bioengineering obstacle in constructing viable artificial hearts concerned finding an implantable power source. The aim of utilizing nuclear energy as a potential implantable power source for mechanical hearts not only encompassed technical challenges but also stirred political and social complications. Most researchers, such as Kolff, remained steadfast in their view that, given time, all technical problems could be overcome, but they were less capable of navigating the political and social issues surrounding atomic heart development. These issues complicated the situation, expanding the debate beyond the technological issues and consequently reducing the authority of these researchers.

In the competing AEC and NHLI programs, neither research team produced a satisfactory atomic heart. The significance of the parallel agency work is not that it demonstrated the task of building atomic hearts as too great, or that one development approach was better, or that the split approach hindered meaningful research gains. Instead, it speaks to the circumstances that facilitated the implementation of two federally funded programs, specifically: the nascent young field of artificial hearts in these years (who knew which device design and power source would prove most viable?); the development course, established by the Artificial Heart Program in 1964, of multiple approaches supporting collaborative industry and government agency teams; and the interdisciplinary nature of building artificial hearts, with its required expertise in physiology, bioengineering, energy sources, and other matters. I argue that the competing atomic heart programs of the AEC and the NHLI did not bolster political or scientific momentum for artificial heart development but contributed to scientific dispute and public skepticism regarding device feasibility, scientific authority, and tolerable risk levels relating to medical innovation. In the case of atomic hearts, the energy source triggered significant political and social concerns. The scientific community was not unified in its support of either the development of an atomic heart or the role of outsiders in assessing research programs. Moreover, a discernible political shift in the NIH's circulatory support program promoted attention to alternate technological solutions, including greater support for the development of VADs instead of complete mechanical hearts and greater support for nonnuclear power sources for implantable devices. Declining congressional financial support accompanied this change in program orientation.[156] The fact that atomic heart research continued for 10 years (1967–77) is testimony to the commitment of a handful of researchers, including Kolff, to developing the technology as well as the peril of entrenchment of specific research pursuits in regard to individual and government investment.

Despite the attempts of many individuals during the late 1960s and the 1970s to explore avenues in which atomic energy might be used in a positive way, radioisotope-powered artificial hearts did not fulfill these hopes. The risk scenarios surrounding atomic hearts, such as damaging radiation exposures and stolen plutonium incidents, never had the opportunity to become reality, remaining fictionalized in the novel *Heart Beat.* The book received some attention, but it was not a bestselling novel; reviewers liked its powerful and authentic operating-room sequences but criticized its stilted dialogue and one-dimensional characters.[157] Nevertheless, its significance is as an artifact of a society wrestling with risks and anxieties, articulating one fear rooted in the science and technology pursuits of the period. Although the nuclear power source was abandoned, work on the artificial heart did continue, benefiting from earlier research on biomaterials, pump mechanisms, and other aspects of the device. Kolff, for example, achieved better clinical results with a pneumatically driven, rather than a radioisotope-powered, artificial heart in the early 1980s.[158] Political and social concerns arising in the context of a heightened sense of risk awareness in the 1970s ultimately played the biggest role in shutting down the atomic heart programs, as strong public support for increased government control of both atomic energy and medical devices overrode scientific assertions that further development could produce a safe and efficacious atomic heart.

To be clear, what was abandoned was the atomic energy source, not the development of a mechanical heart. Most researchers continued their work on artificial hearts, and within the next several years, investigational clinical use of both total artificial hearts and heart assist systems took place. But one device, more than any other, garnered medical and public attention. In the early 1980s, mechanical hearts were front page news once again; this time it was due to the controversial implants of the Utah TAH, also known as the Jarvik-7 TAH. The ambiguous clinical results of the Jarvik-7 heart raised vociferous debate about continued federal support for the development of artificial hearts, dubbed by one critic "The Dracula of Medical Technology."[159]

CHAPTER FOUR

Media Spotlight

The Utah Total Artificial Heart and the Charge
of Bioethics

The pioneer recipients of the artificial heart, people like Barney Clark and Bill Schroeder, have inspired all Americans with their courage. But the difficulties they have experienced raise questions that cannot be ignored regarding the quality of life for recipients of the artificial heart in its present stage of development.

Congressman Harold Volkmer (D-MO), chairman of the Subcommittee
on Investigations and Oversight (1986)

The Utah total artificial heart, first implanted in a human in 1982, emerged as one of the best known medical devices of the twentieth century, owing to the extensive media coverage of its experimental use during the 1980s. Journalists celebrated the Utah heart as a turning point in the development of artificial heart technology and applauded the researchers, surgeons, and patients who so valiantly battled heart disease. The well-publicized implant cases of the 1980s, reminiscent of the dramatic heart transplant cases of the 1960s, raised the profile of artificial hearts as a prospective therapy for individuals dying of heart failure. An organ donor shortage meant that heart transplantation was not always an option, but now the artificial heart appeared to be a device strategy to potentially alleviate that problem. The clinical use of the Utah heart at this time appeared to signal a major therapeutic advance, and it was sensationalized as a "medical breakthrough."

Indeed, it held all the attributes of a breakthrough device. As historian Bert Hansen states, "An invention is in general more likely to become a breakthrough to the extent that the advance is seen as large, sudden, useful, already realized rather than just potential, and of interest to a wide public."[1] The Utah heart exemplified many of these characteristics. It was a landmark device for its technological achievement as a mechanical circulatory support system that had seemingly overcome the material and engineering challenges of replicating the human heart. Early reports of its success in keeping patients alive led many to endorse the breakthrough status of this device and fueled tremendous public interest.

The media spotlight on the Utah heart contributed to the notoriety of the device as well as the American public's dissonance with the technology. Through the media, Americans followed the progress of artificial heart recipients and, at the same time, gained an education on the broader issues surrounding the use of experimental devices. Newspapers often printed dramatic headlines and photos to convey the clinical feat of the Utah heart, but journalists also provided their readers with information on the prevalence of heart disease in America, the costs and regulation of medical devices, medical management challenges, and the uncertainty surrounding experimental therapy. As stated by physician-historian Barron Lerner, the 1980s implant cases "provided Americans with an unexpected crash course in medical technology and human experimentation."[2] In addition to keeping the public informed on each case, the media provided one of the forums through which the political, economic, and social aspects of the artificial heart were debated.

A study of the 1980s clinical cases, with a focus on the Utah heart, can be informative in three ways toward understanding this extremely contentious period in the history of artificial hearts. First, the Utah heart cases generated enormous public interest, providing an opportunity to examine the role of the media in shaping public understanding of this device and reflecting public concern with its use. Media reporting was initially enthusiastic and celebratory. Then journalists adopted a more ambivalent tone by middecade, in response to the turbulent medical courses of implant patients as well as growing medical and bioethical criticism of the experimental technology. Second, an examination of the Utah heart during its transition from research to clinical use highlights the regulation and business of medical devices, which affected how and where it was utilized. The transition of the Utah heart from an investigational device to a commercial product created significant tensions among research team members as the privately formed and later publicly owned company grappled with the regulation and commercialization stages involved in device development. Third, the experiences of the Utah heart patients did not meet hoped-for expectations held by clinicians and the public, thus fueling vociferous debate among bioethicists, members of the medical community, and others and leading to public disillusionment. In this period, dissension focused less on the feasibility of developing an artificial heart and more on the desirability of a clinically acceptable device (perfected or otherwise) when its costly and experimental nature was taken into account. In the end, a lack of consensus emerged regarding the success and meaning of these 1980s clinical cases and created an ambiguous and difficult environment for the development of TAHs thereafter.

Inside Kolff's Lab: Designing and Testing the Utah Heart

The Utah TAH came from Willem Kolff's laboratory at the University of Utah, where Kolff directed a robust artificial organ research program. After years of butting heads with Cleveland Clinic administrators, Kolff shifted his work to Salt Lake City in 1967. At the Cleveland Clinic, Kolff had had a stormy relationship with administrators as he constantly demanded more money, more space, and more people for his research program. Kolff accused his Cleveland Clinic bosses of trying to limit his work despite the promise of artificial heart research, as substantiated by Congress's recent establishment of the Artificial Heart Program. Funding for artificial heart research was expanding at the very time Kolff felt that institutional support for his research was diminishing.[3] He was not entirely mistaken; reflecting their priorities, Cleveland Clinic administrators wanted Kolff to return to clinical kidney research and give less attention to artificial hearts. Kolff issued an ultimatum to the Board of Governors: "You must make up your mind whether the administrative difficulties I put you through outweigh my value to the Clinic past, present and future. I must consider whether you offer me sufficient opportunity to do my work."[4] Feeling frustrated and constrained, Kolff made inquiries elsewhere; a colleague in DeBakey's program connected Kolff with University of Utah officials who were keen to expand their renal transplant program and also launch a new artificial organ program.[5]

After some negotiation, Kolff accepted Utah's offer, which included less money but more autonomy and less bureaucracy, to build an interdisciplinary institute devoted to artificial organ research and development in Salt Lake City.[6] To University of Utah president James Fletcher, Kolff pledged "to apply all of his energy" to build a world-class program, and Fletcher responded that the university would "do everything in our power to make it possible."[7] Just as Michael DeBakey had transformed Baylor College of Medicine into a formidable cardiovascular center, Kolff was poised to build the leading artificial organ program in the country and put the University of Utah on the map. Kolff's future success creating something from nothing (or from very little) at the University of Utah can be attributed to his individual persistence, his vision, his talents, and his ability to motivate and mentor good people in his research program. Of secondary importance, but still important, was an institutional environment that fostered, rather than hampered, a productive laboratory. The University of Utah provided space, staff, and some equipment for the new Institute for Biomedical Engineering and the new Division of Artificial Organs; Kolff secured necessary research funding through government grants, contracts, and private donations, among other sources. Several researchers followed Kolff to Utah. The new institute promised to bring together medical research with science and engineering disciplines in a concrete way that they had not enjoyed in Cleveland, and many were committed to Kolff and his vision.

The institute developed rapidly, supporting a broad research program that encompassed artificial kidneys, artificial limbs, artificial ears, and artificial eyes in addition to artificial hearts and circulatory assist devices. Kolff recruited and welcomed any researcher who had creative and feasible ideas. Within a few short years, his team numbered more than 100 individuals and included cardiologists, surgeons, engineers, chemists, physicists, machinists, medical students, veterinarians, and others. Kolff convened regular morning conferences in which members of this diverse group gave brief reports of their work, generating discussion and inspiring different approaches to solving research problems. Known as a domineering taskmaster, Kolff nonetheless encouraged young investigators to pursue their own ideas within the confines of the Utah research program objectives and available funding.

During the late 1960s and the 1970s, Kolff secured funding from National Institutes of Health grants and contracts and other sources and managed a productive research program that introduced numerous device innovations, such as the wearable artificial kidney (WAK).

Made available to dialysis patients in 1979, the WAK promised to give these individuals greater mobility to travel, take a vacation, or treat themselves at home. It was a bulky 37-pound unit—a wearable unit with a combined blood and dialysate pump, rechargeable batteries, and tubing, as well as a carrying case that held dialysate supplies for one week's operation.[8] WAK dialysis offered freedom and lifestyle advantages, in addition to potentially being more cost effective than in-hospital dialysis sessions. Kolff took great pride in Utah's WAK and the institute's "Dialysis in Wonderland" program, a vacation and recreation therapy trip program for WAK patients to Lake Powell, Canyonlands National Park, and other local areas.[9] Kolff boasted, "These were people who once felt that they were dependent on dialysis for the rest of their lives—that is, treatment with an artificial kidney, three times per week for four hours and being constrained to be dialyzed either in a hospital, a limited care facility or at home. Now, these people suddenly are able to go in a raft down the rapids of the Colorado River and are dialyzed on shore. They see a whole new world and begin to realize that life still has a lot to offer."[10] The development of Utah's WAK did not advance beyond investigational prototype stages.[11] Nonetheless, it was this aim of restoring patients to an enjoyable lifestyle, returning them to activities in the community, that motivated Kolff in his artificial organ research.[12]

Kolff's main research project was the development of an implantable TAH. For the next three decades, Kolff directed the design and production of many different Utah hearts, often simultaneously. To avoid confusion, Kolff named each device after its designer, assigning sequential numbers to altered versions.[13] Some of the Utah hearts developed in Kolff's lab included the Kralios artificial heart (1970), the Lyman artificial heart (1972–73), the Donovan artificial heart (1973), and the Unger artificial heart (1974). The absence of a Kolff heart reflects Kolff's mentoring leadership and generous spirit toward the researchers in his lab.

Kolff was an inspirational lab director. He held weekly roundtable meetings to promote open and shared discussions of researchers' work. He engaged with everyone's project, offered suggestions and directions to overcome challenges, and encouraged his team to brainstorm and to test novel ideas to resolve device challenges. He supervised every aspect of the design and fabrication of prototype devices. Sometimes he asked one researcher to test or improve another's device. In Kolff's view, this was healthy competition to stimulate new directions. But this tactic, as well as the naming of devices after their designer, led to animosity on the part of some researchers. In the 1980s, Clifford Kwan-Gett challenged Robert Jarvik's alleged sole credit for the Jarvik-7 heart, stating that it had been developed from the Kwan-Gett heart.[14] The squabble over credit bothered Kolff, who responded by producing a list of 247 people from all over the world who had worked on the development of artificial hearts in his lab up to that time.[15] Thereafter, all new artificial heart devices created in Kolff's lab were simply named Utah hearts. According to cardiac surgeon William DeVries, who started in Kolff's lab as a medical student, the working environment was competitive, collegial, and productive.[16]

The number and variety of experimental devices that emerged from Kolff's lab during the 1970s and the 1980s was second to none.[17] The majority of the Utah hearts were short-lived, however, owing to design and biomaterial problems. Still, their initial development demonstrated Kolff's open approach to experimenting in different directions. If it worked, it was pursued; if it did not work, it was abandoned. Some projects Kolff stopped reluctantly, as in the case of the nuclear-powered artificial heart during the 1970s.[18] The most promising artificial hearts from Kolff's lab were two pneumatically driven devices: the Kwan-Gett artificial heart (1967–71) and the Jarvik artificial heart (1972–90).

The design and construction of the celebrated Utah heart of the 1980s may be attributed to the work of two key researchers, Clifford Kwan-Gett and Robert Jarvik. Kwan-Gett was an Australian engineer and physician who joined Kolff's team in

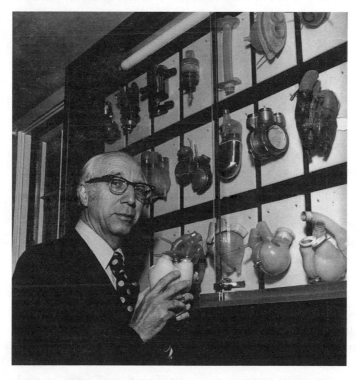

Physician-researcher Willem Kolff, dubbed "the father of artificial organs," standing next to a case display of artificial heart models developed in his laboratory during his career of more than 40 years. Courtesy of Special Collections, J. Willard Marriott Library, University of Utah.

1966 as a research fellow to build and test artificial hearts. In Cleveland and in Salt Lake City, Kwan-Gett performed surgical implants of artificial hearts in animals, supervised engineers in the research program, designed a heart monitoring system that could regulate cardiac output, and invented a diaphragm-type mechanical heart—the Kwan-Gett TAH.[19] He laid the groundwork for the artificial heart system that was used in the first permanent device-implant case in a human.

The Kwan-Gett heart was big and round, slightly larger than a grapefruit, and functioned by air power. It had two ventricles, each hemispherical in shape, which connected at the base to form a spherical device. The outer casing or housing of the pump was made of Dacron-reinforced Silastic. There were inflow and outflow connections with valves that were continuous with the housing, positioned so as to permit the surgeon to stitch these connections to the patient's remaining heart tissue and surrounding vessels. Within each ventricle, a diaphragm made of a thin layer of Dacron-reinforced Silastic expanded and collapsed by means of compressed air delivered through a metal tube at the base of the device. The driving system used pulses of compressed air applied to each ventricle through two 6 foot drive lines. Compressed air passed between the diaphragm and the base, expanding the diaphragm toward the housing and moving blood through the outflow valve. The diaphragm collapsed when air in the heart and the connecting lines was vented to the atmosphere, thus allowing blood to enter the device through the inflow valve.[20]

Kwan-Gett's innovation was the use of a diaphragm as the pumping element to move the blood through the device. This technique marked a significant development in the Utah artificial heart program. In the early 1970s, the Kwan-Gett heart tested well in mock circulation systems, demonstrating no problems with mechanical breakage or blood damage (hemolysis). In animal implant cases, the Kwan-Gett heart functioned for one week in 1971, then improved to two weeks in 1972, leading the field with these survival records. But problems did emerge with this device. First, the device caused excessive clotting of the blood; small clots formed when blood came in contact with the device, and these clots then circulated throughout the body, with sometimes fatal results. To address this problem, Kwan-Gett altered the smooth silicone rubber material of the inside of the heart. He made it a nonsmooth surface by attaching tiny fibers of Dacron to anchor the small clots. The clots would form a smooth layer of fibrin (a protein that helps to create a weblike mesh that traps platelets and red blood cells and holds a clot together), hopefully preventing clots from dislodging into the blood stream, where they could cause serious problems. More significantly, "right heart failure syndrome" (a problem attributed to imperfect fit that obstructed venous return of blood into the heart) occurred in calves that lived more than 10 days with the Kwan-Gett heart. When Kwan-Gett left in 1971 to complete a cardiothoracic residency, Kolff challenged a new researcher, Robert Jarvik, to overcome these device problems.[21]

Jarvik, who had some training in biomechanics and medicine, joined the Utah lab as an assistant design engineer in 1971. After completing an undergraduate degree in zoology at Syracuse University, Jarvik attended medical school at the University of Bologna from 1968 to 1970, but he did not finish the program. Abandoning his medical studies, he returned to the United States to complete graduate work in occupational biomechanics at New York University. A phone call to Kolff from an executive at a surgical supplies company marked a key turning point in Jarvik's career; Kolff hired the 25-year-old Jarvik and then doggedly pressured the University of Utah School of Medicine's chair of admissions to accept the young researcher into the program, despite past application rejections. In something like a father-son relationship, Kolff mentored Jarvik, both professionally and personally, from the beginning; perhaps Kolff was taken by Jarvik's propensity to challenge and be convinced about how and why things should work. Not always appreciated by everyone, this trait and other personality issues of Jarvik's led to conflicts with other researchers, which amplified when Jarvik started to work full-time in the lab after graduating from medical school in 1976.[22]

Under Kolff's direction, Jarvik worked on modifying the Kwan-Gett artificial heart, renaming the device as the Jarvik heart with various iterations (such as the Jarvik-III, the Jarvik-5, and the Jarvik-7). Like the Kwan-Gett heart, the Jarvik heart consisted of two ventricles with diaphragms, powered by compressed air. Inflow and outflow valves and connectors ensured the unidirectional flow of blood into the pump and back to the body. However, Jarvik decided to modify the shape of his mechanical heart; the Jarvik heart had an elliptical shape, which did not compromise the lung space, leaving plenty of room for the venous structures above the heart (thus avoiding right heart failure syndrome). In addition, Jarvik experimented with various blood surface materials other than Silastic in different models and eventually settled on the polyurethane Biomer to create surfaces on the inside housing that prevented thrombosis, or clotting of blood. For the diaphragm, Jarvik again used Biomer in three, and later four, thin-layer sheets, which improved the flexibility and durability of this component. Lastly, Jarvik designed a novel, quick-connect system in which the inflow and outflow cuffs joined coated rigid polycarbonate segments. Dacron vascular prosthetic grafts then connected the artificial heart to the patient's blood vessels.[23]

Jarvik's device was a significantly modified version of the Kwan-Gett artificial heart, and it continued to evolve. Learning from both bench and animal testing, Jarvik experimented with different materials and sizes for the device. The first heart that Jarvik designed in 1971 was never tested in an animal, but the third, fifth, and seventh versions were implanted in sheep and calves over the next 10 years.[24] Certainly important design changes contributed to the better survival rates of this evolving device; however, so did improved animal caretaking at the university.

In 1972 Don B. Olsen, a veterinarian who had earlier consulted for Kolff, joined the Utah artificial heart research team full-time to direct animal care and device implants. The animal barn and experimental surgery cases required improved management, since animals continued to die of infections, convulsion, hemorrhaging, and other preventable causes. Olsen imposed proper animal care protocols to be followed before, during, and after all animal operations. Calf sitters were hired to keep animals clean and fed. Often premed or science students at the university, calf sitters were trained to administer drugs, to take blood pressure readings and blood samples, and to be prepared for any emergency that might occur during their shift.[25] Animal survival rates dramatically improved thereafter.

In 1974 animal implants with the Jarvik-3 heart set new animal survival records: one calf named Bruce lived 18 days, and another, called Crocker, survived 24 days.[26] In 1975 calves Tony and Burk survived 36 and 94 days, respectively, with their Jarvik-3 hearts.[27] The increase in animal survival was due to a combination of factors: Jarvik's heart design was better than Kwan-Gett's; bioengineer Tom Kessler's new fabrication of smooth polyurethane reduced blood clotting issues in the device; and Olsen's new technique of implanting the device through the animal's side after moving the fourth rib, instead of splitting the thorax, resolved several surgical issues.[28] The lab soon discovered that their calves were outgrowing the device; calves grew from approximately 200 pounds at surgery to more than 300 pounds in five to six months. So Jarvik designed the larger Jarvik-5 heart, which pumped more blood with each stroke to meet the growth of calves. This model allowed the calf named Abebe to survive six months in 1976.[29] Still, at autopsy, recurring problems presented, including mechanical failures, infection, hemorrhaging, thromboemboli, and pannus (uncontrolled growth of connective tissue at suture points, which spread across inflow openings of the device). Jarvik observed a wearing of the diaphragm in the device, so he added another (fourth) thin layer to this component. He then evaluated the shape and fit of the device in human cadavers, made additional design modifications, and presented a smaller model—the Jarvik-7 TAH.[30] Beginning in 1978, researchers in Kolff's laboratory began implanting the Jarvik-7 heart in both calves and sheep to test device durability and performance.

A year later, cardiac surgeon William DeVries, who had worked in Kolff's lab as a medical student during the 1960s, returned from his nine-year surgical residency at Duke University and rejoined the research team.[31] DeVries accepted a position in the cardiovascular surgical division at the University of Utah Medical Center, which allowed him to build a practice and to hold hospital privileges. As the clinical surgeon on Kolff's research team, DeVries stepped into the role of implanting Jarvik hearts in lab animals to refine the procedure and device fit. Over the next several years, Kolff's team made various device improvements and reported incremental increases in animal survival rates. In 1980 and 1982, respectively, Phred (a calf) survived 169 days and Ted E. Bear (a sheep) remained alive for 297 days with their Jarvik-7 hearts.[32] During the early 1980s, the Utah artificial heart research team implanted their devices in more than 350 animals, and many calves survived months with the Jarvik-7 heart.[33] Over the years, the Utah team collected data of implanted animals on treadmills, recorded postsurgery complications, documented daily animal regimens, and meticulously analyzed explanted devices and animal bodies at

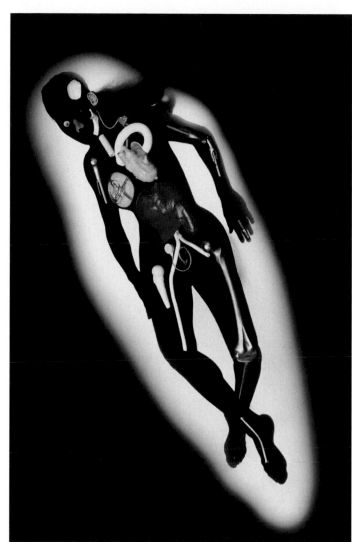

Plate 1. Touting an "era of rebuilt people," a 1965 *Life* magazine article marveled at the existence of numerous replaceable organs and tissues, shown superimposed on this image of a woman's body. All were synthetic parts, except the transplanted kidney and liver, pictured in red (*center*). A silicone rubber artificial heart and lung (*above right*, from transplanted organs) was still experimental, but a wide array of substitute parts had been introduced clinically by this time, including Dacron arteries; ceramic hip joints and jawbones; plastic corneas and eyeballs; silicone rubber tracheas, tendons, breasts, and nose and ear cartilages; electronic bladder stimulators and blood pressure regulators; metal thigh bones and shoulder, elbow, and finger joints; and animal bones used in the skull. Taken from *Life* magazine, September 24, 1965. Used with permission from Getty Images.

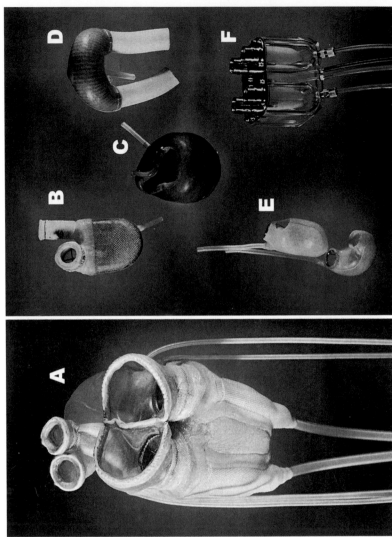

Plate 2. Six air-driven devices designed to replace or assist damaged hearts, under development during the early to mid 1960s: (*A*) A silicone rubber total artificial heart developed by Willem Kolff's team, Cleveland Clinic; (*B*) An assist pump built by the Baylor-Rice research group, Houston, Texas; (*C*) A National Heart Institute device that fits around the heart ventricle, expanding and contracting, to strengthen pumping action; (*D*) A Kantrowitz-Avco mechanical auxiliary ventricular or "booster" heart, Brooklyn, New York; (*E*) Two Baylor-Rice intraventricular pumps, Houston, Texas; (*F*) A total heart replacement pump, partially made of Lucite, developed by Harry Diamond Laboratories, Washington, DC. Taken from *Life* magazine, September 24, 1965. Used with permission from Getty Images.

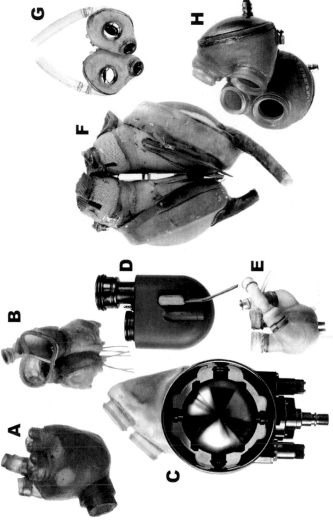

Plate 3. Collage of experimental total artificial hearts: (*A*) a polyvinyl chloride heart, designed by Willem Kolff and Tetsuzo Akutsu at the Cleveland Clinic, 1957; (*B*) a silicone rubber total artificial heart developed by Willem Kolff's team at the Cleveland Clinic, mid-1960s; (*C*) an AEC-Westinghouse radioisotope-powered total artificial heart, with pump developed by Willem Kolff's team at the University of Utah, mid-1970s; (*D*) a teflon-covered steel heart designed by Yukihiko Nosé at the Cleveland Clinic, late 1960s; (*E*) the Kwan-Gett total artificial heart, a diaphragm-type pump with two connecting hemispherical ventricles, developed in Willem Kolff's laboratory, University of Utah, roughly 1967–71; (*F*) the Liotta-Cooley artificial heart, used in the first total artificial heart case, in patient Haskell Karp, Houston, Texas, 1969; (*G*) the Akutsu III total artificial heart, implanted in Willebrordus Meuffels, Texas Heart Institute, 1981; (*H*) the Jarvik-7 total artificial heart, developed in Willem Kolff's lab at the University of Utah during the 1970s and 1980s, distributed by Kolff Medical–Symbion Inc., and first used clinically in patient Barney Clark, Salt Lake City, Utah, 1982. Taken from *Life* magazine, September 1981. Photographer: Enrico Ferorelli. Used with permission from Martha Saxton.

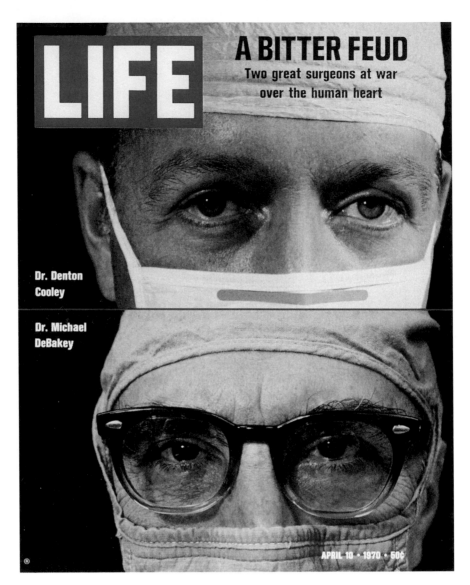

Plate 4. In 1970 *Life* magazine ran a cover story on the dramatic feud between Houston cardiovascular surgeons Michael DeBakey and Denton Cooley that ignited over the device used in the first artificial heart implant case, in 1969. The incident severed the professional relationship of DeBakey and Cooley because of allegations of device theft and lack of authorization to perform the implant procedure, and the two men did not speak to each other for nearly four decades thereafter. *Life* magazine, April 10, 1970, cover. Used with permission from Getty Images. LIFE logo and cover design ©Time Inc. LIFE and the LIFE logo are registered trademarks of Time Inc., used under license.

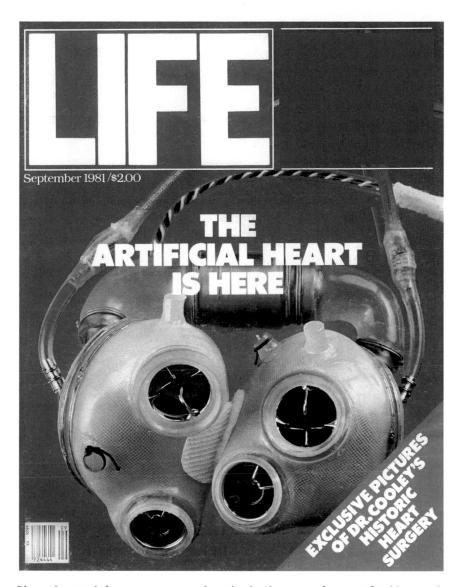

Plate 5. In 1981 *Life* magazine reported on the development of two artificial hearts: the recently implanted Akutsu III total artificial heart in Willebrordus Meuffels at the Texas Heart Institute, Houston, and the implant readiness of the Jarvik-7 total artificial heart at the University of Utah, Salt Lake City. The issue cover displayed an electrohydraulic Jarvik-7 total artificial heart, while vivid interior images presented the implanted and explanted Akutsu III total artificial heart, the Texas and Utah surgical teams, and profiles of the device designers. A year later, it was the pneumatic Jarvik-7 total artificial heart that came to dominate the media's attention in regard to this technology, particularly the Barney Clark case in 1982–83. *Life* magazine, September 1981, cover. Photographer: Enrico Ferorelli. Used with permission from Martha Saxton and from Time Inc. All rights reserved. LIFE logo and cover design ©Time Inc. LIFE and the LIFE logo are registered trademarks of Time Inc., used under license.

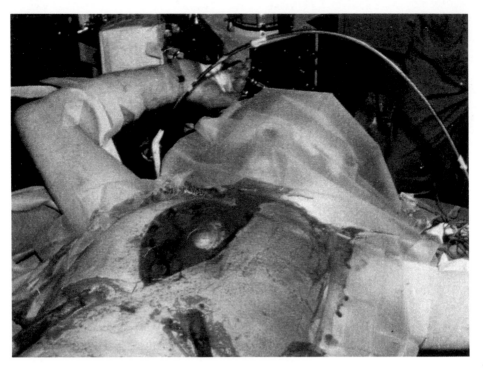

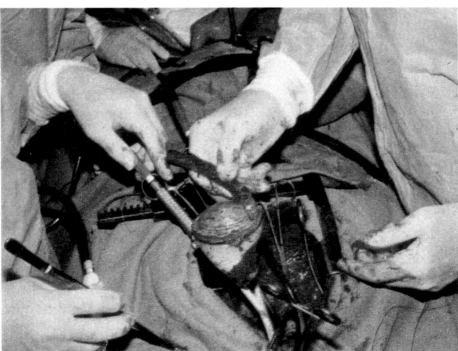

Plate 6. At the Texas Heart Institute, Willebrordus Meuffels lived for roughly 55 hours with an implanted Akutsu III total artificial heart (*top*), which was removed (*bottom*) upon the arrival of a donor heart. Meuffels died a week after his cardiac transplant operation from massive infection and organ failure. Taken from *Life* magazine, September 1981. Photographer: Enrico Ferorelli. Used with permission from Martha Saxton.

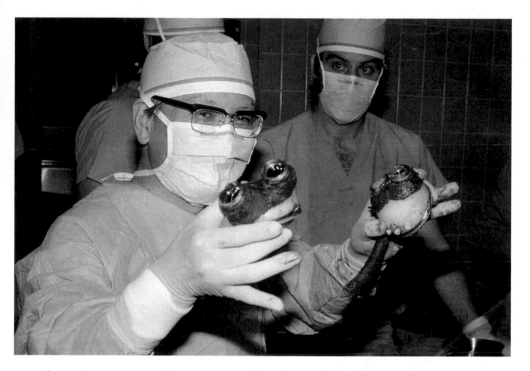

Plate 7. Device inventor Tetsuzo Akutsu holds the two halves of the Akutsu III total artificial heart, explanted from patient Willebrordus Meuffels, Texas Heart Institute, July 25, 1981. Despite the medical team's report of the "success" of the device, no Akutsu heart was ever used clinically again. Taken from *Life* magazine, September 1981. Photographer: Enrico Ferorelli. Used with permission from Martha Saxton.

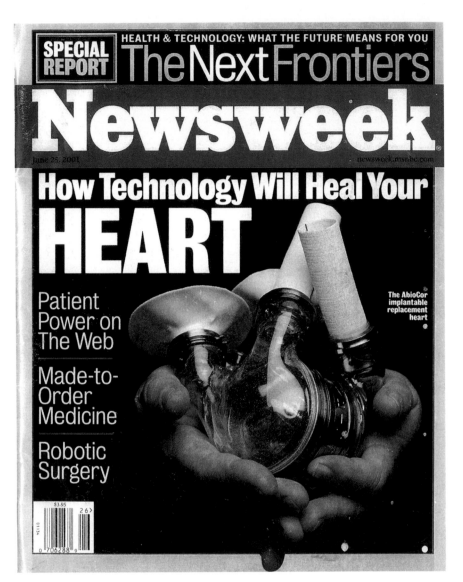

SPECIAL REPORT

HEALTH & TECHNOLOGY: WHAT THE FUTURE MEANS FOR YOU

The Next Frontiers

Newsweek

June 25, 2001

newsweek.msnbc.com

How Technology Will Heal Your HEART

Patient
Power on
The Web

Made-to-
Order
Medicine

Robotic
Surgery

The AbioCor
implantable
replacement
heart

$3.95

0 706288 9

Plate 8. Throughout the decades, the media shaped and reflected American society's fascination with artificial hearts, and the majority of the narratives promoted the feasibility and desirability of this technology. In 2001 the AbioCor total artificial heart, reverentially held in two hands in this image, was hyped as the future of cardiac medicine. Taken from *Newsweek,* June 25, 2001, © 2001 IBT Media. All rights reserved. Used by permission and protected by the copyright laws of the United States. The printing, copying, redistribution, or retransmission of this content without express written permission is prohibited.

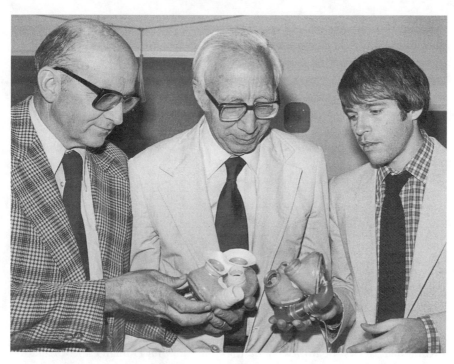

Members of the Utah artificial heart research team Don B. Olsen (*left*), Willem Kolff (*center*) and Robert Jarvik, posing with two Jarvik-7 total artificial hearts, each driven by a different power source: a pneumatic Jarvik-7 heart (*left*) and an electrohydraulic Jarvik-7 heart (*right*). Only the pneumatic device was ever implanted in patients. Courtesy of Special Collections, J. Willard Marriott Library, University of Utah.

autopsy, as they sought to improve device function and performance. The two dominant problems were blood clotting, leading to embolism, and infection at the exiting drive lines through the skin. As the Utah team recorded increasing animal survival rates, it appeared that these issues were manageable with strict postoperative care protocols. Was the timing right to move from animal to human implants?

Ready for Human Implantation? Tension and Debate

As argued by scholars Renée Fox and Judith Swazey, "the decision that 'the time is right' to move a new device, procedure, or drug from laboratory and animal testing to human testing is seldom an unambiguous, certain one, either at the time it is made or in retrospect."[34] The goal had always been to develop a device for human implant. During the late 1970s and early 1980s, the Utah artificial heart research team appeared close to implanting their device in a human, but key individuals—Kolff, Jarvik, Olsen, and DeVries—sent mixed signals to each other and to the public about their readiness to proceed. For example, Kolff wrote to leading cardiac surgery centers, asking them to consider using the Jarvik-7 heart in their hospitals.

Kolff wrote, "The implantation of an artificial heart in man is very close," and he said he would provide them with a Jarvik-7 heart and training for implantation in animals, and later humans.[35] Perhaps Kolff felt pressured to move to clinical cases to ensure continued funding and support of his artificial heart research in Utah. Government funding and support was shifting from research on TAHs to development of ventricular assist devices or partial artificial hearts that did not require the removal of the native heart.[36]

Newspaper reports drew public attention to the Jarvik-7 heart well before its first use in a human. In July 1980, headlines announced, "Utah Doctors to Try Mechanical Heart" and "Surgeons Are Ready for Mechanical Heart Transplant."[37] One month previously, DeVries submitted an application to the University of Utah Institutional Review Board to explore the possibility of implanting the Jarvik-7 heart in a patient. Once this application became public knowledge, Kolff, DeVries, and other team members received a barrage of inquiries, most significantly candid questions from NIH officials who had been supporting much of Utah's research. To John Watson, chief of NHI's Devices and Technology Branch and key administrator of the government-sponsored artificial heart program, Kolff wrote, "The unintentionally stated publicity is mostly incorrect, and regrettable. We are indeed talking with the Committee for Human Experimentation [University of Utah Medical Center Institutional Review Board]. We want the Committee for Human Experimentation to take their time and advise us. We are not ready."[38] Watson agreed, telling reporters that the use of Jarvik-7 hearts in humans was certainly premature.[39] Publicly, Kolff and DeVries admitted that they were not ready, but such statements were disingenuous; both envisioned their human implant case as occurring soon.[40] They saw that the device worked well enough to sustain animals for months, and they interpreted their animal survival rates as evidence of readiness; they began navigating the regulatory process to avoid delays in moving forward with human implants.

Jarvik and Olsen were against proceeding with human implantation anytime soon; they questioned device efficacy and human implant timing based on unresolved device complications in the implanted animals.[41] Jarvik stated, "Neither the Jarvik nor any of the several other TAHs being developed is yet ready to permanently replace a human heart, even on a trial basis, but the pace of improvement in the technology suggests that the day may not be long in coming."[42] Olsen, who was most familiar with the experimental animal results, wrote a colleague, "I can now say that we are closer to being ready to implant the artificial heart in man, but unfortunately we are not yet confident enough to do so."[43] The tension within the Utah artificial heart team surrounded the issue of acceptable risks in clinical research. To Kolff, the animal results suggested an acceptable level of risk for patients who would soon die. Jarvik and Olsen were not as accepting of this risk and were not swayed by the argument that these very ill patients would die regardless. They expected that device problems, such as clot formation, that had occurred in animals would also happen in humans, and this would not bode well for the clinical acceptance of mechanical circulatory support systems.

Had the two major engineering challenges of building an artificial heart—satisfactory blood-interface materials and a power source—truly been solved? Or at least, were the potential solutions good enough to proceed to human implants? There were still many unknowns regarding device performance in the human body; for example, while Utah researchers assessed test animals for evidence of organ damage and other systemic complications, there was hope that the human body would be more tolerant. Furthermore, researchers were using healthy animals as their test model, not seriously ill, compromised human bodies in severe heart failure. Although the disagreements were not explicitly drawn along researcher-against-clinician lines, those working most closely with the device in the laboratory expressed reservations more than either Kolff or DeVries, who saw the device as possibly helping a dying patient who had exhausted all other options. Eventually, the Utah research team united in the decision to proceed clinically. After "a lot of soul searching," Olsen supported implanting the device in a patient, stating, "If it were successful, it would be both a moral and financial stimulus to the artificial heart program."[44] Mixed emotions about the plan to proceed to human use nevertheless remained for many individuals involved in this first case.

In 1980 the Utah team initiated the process of securing institutional and FDA approval before implanting the Jarvik-7 heart in a patient, almost certainly because it was their intent to develop and use the device beyond just one clinical case. Such approval was not strictly necessary at this innovation stage, during which surgeons regulated their actions based on laboratory experience and their commitment to their patients, if and when a clinical case presented itself. However, complicated procedures performed in hospitals are regulated to some extent by internal hospital policies, through such mechanisms as credentialing, certification, privileges, and institutional review boards (IRBs), which in turn are regulated by state policies on hospital licensure. The larger, regulatory phase commences with the intent for wider clinical use and device commercialization, which involves mass production, marketing, and sales of new devices and the increased involvement of industry and the FDA.

Keen to move forward, DeVries signed on as the designated surgeon and the point person of the Utah team to write, and to secure approval of, the artificial heart protocol for its human use. To the University of Utah Medical Center IRB, he clearly stated that the implantation of the Jarvik-7 TAH would be a permanent therapy for dying cardiac patients; there would be no human heart transplant following the device implant, and the native diseased heart certainly could not be returned to the patient. DeVries's document submitted to the IRB for procedure approval was lengthy; he offered historical background information on the goal of artificial hearts, the Utah team's bench test and animal test results with the Jarvik-7 heart, his proposed patient selection criteria, a detailed description of the implant procedure, an outline of the postoperative care measures to be followed, and an informed consent form to be signed by the patient. But the document was terrible, triumphant in tone, with a Theodore Roosevelt quote thrown in to endorse the boldness of the proposal, and it irked the IRB members. In an interview with Fox and Swazey, one peeved IRB member recalled, "The protocol entered with trumpets and medieval trappings. It was like the entrance of Macbeth. It included a quote from Theodore Roosevelt, and we told Dr DeVries we wanted that page removed or we would not deal with the protocol."[45] It was clear that neither DeVries nor anyone else on the Utah research team had much experience with protocol design. According to another IRB member, "[It] had the mask or aura of science, but it was not a scientific protocol. . . . It basically said that the investigators want to implant the heart and see if it works."[46]

Multiple protocol drafts went back and forth between DeVries and the IRB committee until an acceptable document emerged. The IRB committee did not challenge the Utah research team's information related to the technical aspects of the device, but they did ask for substantive changes to the patient selection criteria and the informed consent form. For example, DeVries's patient criterion "virtually facing death" was amended to the Class IV New York Heart Association classification of seriously impaired heart function, with impending death and no further medical therapies available to arrest deterioration of the heart. A section was added to clarify that multiple physicians would be involved in the diagnosis of end-stage heart failure, perhaps an attempt to make clear that there would be additional medical judgment involved besides that of DeVries. The IRB committee asked why surgeons would not offer these patients a "less-radical" left ventricular assist device implant, which would not necessitate the removal of the native heart. At this time there was promising clinical data from the experimental use of these mechanical pumps, and a commitment to a TAH implant might deprive these patients of any LVAD benefits. It was clarified that only patients in severe biventricular failure, requiring functional replacement, not just assistance, would be offered the Jarvik-7 heart implant. Also, the IRB committee raised questions regarding patient lifestyle and operating costs, which they felt were not clearly presented in the consent form. What if a not-so-fully-informed patient awakened postoperatively to a drastically altered lifestyle with extremely limited mobility, not to mention enormous medical bills? The IRB committee was emphatic that the patient would have to understand what life might be like after the implant of a Jarvik-7 heart.[47] To address this concern, clear statements and details were added to the patient consent form, such as "my life style will be significantly different," "my activity will be severely limited because of the drive lines," and "I may have to remain bedridden due to pain, weakness or other problems." An entire section listing "substantial risks" was added, including device failure, emboli leading to stroke or other organ damage, hemorrhaging, and infection.[48] The intention of the form was to describe clearly all possible outcomes, including death, with no false hopes offered; it was a wonder that anyone agreed to sign the document, given the bleak scenarios!

The IRB committee raised many of the issues that bioethicists and others later debated in assessing these first clinical implants. The IRB committee would not rubberstamp the experimental operation; its members took seriously their duties as ethical medical professionals. There was much at stake for the committee. They served as protector of the rights and safety of patients and needed to uphold the professional and ethical standing of their institution. They also did not want to stifle innovation at their hospital, nor deny potentially life-saving treatments to dying patients. The committee members all agreed that a stricter protocol needed to be worked out, most significantly a limiting of the potential patient population eligible for this experimental procedure. DeVries complied and altered the application accordingly, with the help of the IRB committee. Fox and Swazey viewed the IRB committee as overstepping its role, which should have been limited to reviewing, not revising, the application.[49] It certainly seemed that the committee wanted to support the experimental operation, no doubt caught up in (even convinced by) the convictions of the Utah research team that the technology was ready for clinical use. After six months of meetings and amendments, the University of Utah Medical Center IRB approved the application with its now stricter protocol and granted permission for a Jarvik-7 heart implant in a patient in early 1981.[50]

Next, DeVries submitted an Investigational Device Exemption (IDE) application to the Food and Drug Administration as a first step on the long road to FDA approval for human testing, marketing, and eventual widespread clinical use of the Jarvik-7 heart. The recent Medical Device Amendments of 1976 required premarket review of all new devices to ensure their safety and effectiveness. Attempting to balance over- and underregulation, FDA administrators offered IDE status to some experimental devices for use in a limited clinical study in order to collect this safety and effectiveness data.[51] FDA administrators did not approve DeVries's first IDE application, instead responding with a long list of specific deficiencies. For example, the informed consent did not accurately present all possible complications, and the scientific protocols of assessing the adequacy of cardiac output needed to be tightened to produce sound data.[52] A six-person University of Utah Medical Center subcommittee, chaired by Dr. F. Ross Woolley, was formed to work with DeVries toward amending the FDA proposal for resubmission. After notable changes, FDA administrators approved the amended and resubmitted IDE application in September 1981.[53] Two months before this, however, a well-known surgeon chose to ignore the FDA process and implanted a different artificial heart in a patient in Houston, Texas.

Sharing the Spotlight: Denton Cooley and the Akutsu Heart

In July 1981, cardiac surgeon Denton Cooley implanted an Akutsu III TAH, as a bridge to transplantation, into a dying patient at the Texas Heart Institute, one of the world's leading cardiovascular treatment centers and the site of the first artificial heart implant case.[54] Medical researcher Tetsuzo Akutsu had joined THI in 1974 as assistant director of the Cullen Cardiovascular Surgical Research Laboratory, where he continued his work on the development of an artificial heart.[55] (In 1957 Kolff and Akutsu had successfully replaced a dog's healthy heart with a crude mechanical heart in Cleveland.)[56] At THI Akutsu tested his newest experimental artificial heart through extensive in vitro (bench testing for materials compatibility and device function) and select in vivo tests (cadaver implants for fit and animal implants for functionality). Reportedly, Akutsu destroyed the first two models of his mechanical heart because he was not satisfied with the workmanship.[57]

The Akutsu III artificial heart (the third model) was not unlike the Jarvik-7 heart in Utah. The Akutsu III heart was also an air-driven, double-chambered device that pumped blood by means of a reciprocating hemispherical diaphragm.[58] All blood-contact surfaces were fabricated from Silastic to reduce blood clotting, large disc valves (Bjork-Shiley) were used to facilitate blood flow, and detachable quick-connectors as part of the inflow and outflow conduits facilitated surgical implantation. Like the Jarvik-7 heart, the Akutsu heart was orthotopically positioned (situated in the exact location of the removed human heart) and required tubes to pass through the patient's abdominal wall to connect the device to an external drive console that powered, controlled, and monitored the artificial heart. Overall, the material and design differences were relatively minor between these two mechanical hearts; however, the Akutsu III heart had never been tested in animals.[59]

Certainly, Akutsu planned to test this device in animals before using the heart clinically. He had implanted earlier models of this device in calves and sheep and had also utilized cadavers to refine device fit in humans.[60] The Akutsu III heart had undergone rigorous bench testing but had yet to be implanted in animals. The lack of animal testing for this particular model did not bother Cooley, who, when presented with a heart failure case, pressed Akutsu for the device. It was an emergency clinical case, but it was not one well suited for the use of the Akutsu III heart.

No longer able to manage his heart condition with drugs alone, 36-year-old Willebrordus Meuffels traveled from his native Holland to Houston for heart surgery. On July 23, 1981, Meuffels underwent a triple coronary bypass operation, but he could not be weaned from the heart-lung machine. The surgical team implanted an intraaortic balloon pump to assist his damaged heart. After a few hours, Meuffels was back in the operating room owing to a massive infarction of both ventricles and cardiac arrest. The medical staff kept him alive through internal cardiac message. Given the "desperate condition of the patient," as characterized by Cooley and his surgical team, they decided that the only alternative to death was an artificial heart implant followed by a heart transplant.[61] Mrs. Meuffels provided written consent for the procedure.[62] Meuffels survived the implant operation, but was, at best, only semiconscious for the two days he lived with the artificial heart in his chest. A nationwide search for a donor heart was conducted. While waiting for a human heart, Meuffels suffered a pulmonary complication not unrelated to the artificial heart. According to the case report, there was a mechanical obstruction of the left pulmonary vein and possibly the right main pulmonary artery, which necessitated the use of an extracorporeal oxygenator to maintain adequate oxygenation of the blood. Greater urgency for a human heart probably led to the decision to accept a less-than-ideal donor heart. On July 25, Meuffels received the heart of a 27-year-old Tennessee man, at which time they discovered that the size of the slightly enlarged donor heart prevented surgeons from closing Meuffels's chest completely. A week after the transplant operation, Meuffels died as a result of massive infection and organ failure.[63]

Although the patient did not survive long after the transplant, the Texas group reported encouraging information on the use of the artificial heart in this case. For roughly 55 hours, the Akutsu III artificial heart had kept Meuffels alive, pumping blood to his lungs and through his body, but with some pulmonary complications. There were no valve failures, graft tears, obvious blood damage, or mechanical breakdown of the device while it functioned in the patient. Akutsu studied the artificial heart after its removal from Meuffels and reported that the internal surfaces were "smooth and glistening," with no evidence of thrombus or hemolysis. This pleased the Texas group, who reported it as a "gratifying feature" and in stark contrast to their first clinical experience, in which the Cooley-Liotta heart had presented extreme hemolysis.[64] As in the first clinical case, Meuffels died not long after the transplant operation, arguably too ill for this procedure to have any chance of succeeding. After the heart attack in which surgical personnel resorted to internal cardiac massage to keep him alive, Meuffels never fully regained consciousness. Perhaps it was better that he did not wake up to find himself with a mechanical heart, tethered to the large drive console at his bedside. Like Haskell Karp, who was implanted with the Liotta-Cooley heart, Meuffels had lived with three different hearts (his native heart, a mechanical heart, and the donor heart). However, he was never able to communicate that experience to family, doctors, or the public.

The Meuffels case drew moderate media attention that temporarily redirected the spotlight away from the Utah artificial heart. At the time of the Akutsu III heart implant, hospital spokespeople released only limited information, initially withholding the name of the patient. Newspaper articles dutifully reported events, pitching the story as a last-ditch effort to keep a very ill man alive until a donor heart was found. Journalists often included details of the earlier 1969 Cooley implant involving Haskell Karp as well as the artificial heart research at the University of Utah, but these reports lacked any real critical comparison.[65]

In September 1981, *Life* magazine ran the cover story "The Artificial Heart Is Here," with dramatic operation photos and ambivalent text. The article presented the artificial heart in a triumphant way, describing the remarkable performance of the device as well as the surgical team behind the event, while at the same time gently questioning the technology. "The artificial heart could be an invaluable interim step to transplants and, someday, might be able to take over permanently. The question is, should it?" But the article did not assess critically such heroic medical technologies, instead describing the controversy surrounding the device in a sensational way. Cooley was characterized as the surgeon doing what was needed to save the life of his patient, with "no time to bother with red tape."[66] Graphic photos of the operation, Meuffels's open chest, showing the artificial heart in place, and Akutsu proudly holding the bloody device after removal from the patient accompanied an hour-by-hour timeline of events that saved this man's life. The focus was the device, alongside the surgeons and researchers involved in its transition to clinical use. There was a two-page color montage of eight different models of artificial hearts, ranging from the historic 1957 device implanted in a dog to the current Akutsu III heart and the Jarvik-7 heart.

The Utah team was certainly not excluded from *Life*'s coverage of artificial heart developments. A large photo of the Jarvik-7 heart, not of a patient or a surgeon, dominated the cover of this issue. The focus was the technology, an exciting new medical device that was celebrated more than questioned. The technology, as presented, made it hard for readers to perceive the difference between therapy and experimentation. Inside, there were photos of DeVries's surgical team "standing ready for their implant of a Jarvik-7 heart," prepared to save lives, with the technology in the foreground. James Salter's article described Utah's animal success to date and hinted at the sense of competition within the field to develop the better device for use in humans. Salter's interest in artificial hearts emerged elsewhere at this time as well. He was a screenwriter for a Canadian movie entitled *Threshold,* starring Donald Sutherland as a cardiac surgeon who performs a daring artificial heart implant. Made in 1981 and released in the United States in 1983, the movie used a mechanical heart designed by Jarvik. Denton Cooley provided technical advice as well as briefly appearing in the film.[67]

Upon hearing the news of the Houston implant operation, Kolff proclaimed that "this was the second time Cooley had beaten him!"[68] He sent a congratulatory note to Cooley for "blazing the trail" once again.[69] To members of the Utah team, Kolff argued that Cooley's implant could help them gain federal and public approval to move ahead to their clinical cases.[70] Not wanting to repeat Cooley's bridge-to-transplant operation, the Utah team remained committed to implanting the Jarvik-7 heart as a permanent device in a cardiac patient ineligible for a heart transplant. Cooley responded to Kolff's congratulations with words of encouragement: "I only hope that the FDA will lift their restrictions on your project so we can learn how much practical knowledge we can gain now without waiting for years or until subsequent generations have the experience. I wish you and your team success when you get the green light."[71] That green light did not come for another 17 months.

Dying to Be the First: Barney Clark
and the Jarvik-7 Heart, 1982–1983

In late 1981, the Utah team secured permission to implant a Jarvik-7 heart in a human. However, the University of Utah Medical Center IRB committee and FDA administrators approved only a narrow, select patient population for this procedure: only a surgical patient whose heart had stopped while on the operating table and could not be restarted would be eligible for a Jarvik-7 implant. The first implant would take place in a patient facing imminent death. Over the next six months, several possible recipients for a Jarvik-7 heart consented to the implant, should their operations result in such a failure to restart their hearts. None of these cases provided these circumstances; all recovered from their surgery without the need of an artificial heart. As a result, DeVries was anxious to expand the patient category to include nonsurgical patients dying of severe heart disease with no other options. At this time, a publicized case with a patient who was demanding a Jarvik-7 heart assisted DeVries by providing the impetus for an expanded protocol.[72]

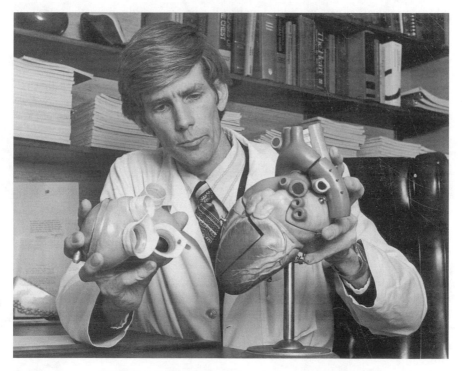

Cardiac surgeon William DeVries, holding a Jarvik-7 artificial heart next to a model of the human heart. Courtesy of Special Collections, J. Willard Marriott Library, University of Utah.

In March 1982, Dale Lott begged the University of Utah Medical Center IRB committee and FDA administrators to allow him to become the first recipient of the Jarvik-7 heart.[73] A 37-year-old Florida fireman, Lott was dying from cardiomyopathy, a progressive degeneration of the heart muscle that cannot be repaired surgically. Both the IRB committee and FDA administrators restated that the criteria for an artificial heart implant included only those patients whose heart stopped on the operating table. Lott threatened to sue the university for denying him this treatment, urging the IRB committee and FDA administrators to expand the patient category to those, like him, who suffered cardiomyopathy. University officials accused Lott of attempting to circumvent clinical research protocol by using the news media and intimidating legal proceedings to access treatment. Furthermore, he was not qualified as a candidate even under the expanded criteria, because he had respiratory problems.[74] Nonetheless, the media championed Lott's case, emphasizing bureaucratic obstruction as the reason he was being prevented from receiving a potentially lifesaving treatment.[75] His case maintained public awareness about the artificial heart. Lott never sued the university, but for DeVries, Lott's plea and its resulting media attention was timely. It supported DeVries's push to expand patient category eligibility for Jarvik-7 heart implants, and the IRB committee eventually agreed.[76] In addition to surgical patients, individuals suffering from cardiomyopathy were now added as possible device recipients. In June 1982 FDA administrators also approved this expanded protocol.[77] Despite this approval, many members of the Utah State Medical Association voiced concern and reservation about the clinical use of the Jarvik-7 heart, specifically that certain issues, such as cost, had not been fully addressed by the University of Utah Medical Center.[78] By this time, however, Dale Lott had withdrawn his request for the Jarvik-7 heart; his condition had deteriorated and multiple complications made him ineligible.[79]

Dale Lott was not the only heart patient to request a Jarvik-7 implant.[80] Many individuals in poor health as a result of heart disease requested more information on the device. Family members contacted DeVries, Kolff, and other Utah team members directly asking if their loved ones might be considered candidates.[81] One woman wrote, "My husband would like very much for you to try the plastic heart on him. . . . We both understand the chances he would be taking and we are still willing to try anything."[82] Many of these desperate people were responding to favorable media coverage of the device, most notably the 1981 *Life* cover story.[83] *People* magazine announced, "Utah Surgeon William DeVries Seeks a Patient Who Could Live with a Man-Made Heart."[84] Although such publicity captured the imagination of many families and individuals, most patients did not meet the strict criteria for candidates.[85] Finally, in late 1982, someone did meet the criteria and agreed to the experimental procedure.

In December 1982, 61-year-old Barney Clark, a retired Seattle dentist, became the first recipient of a Jarvik-7 TAH. The University of Utah Medical Center evaluation committee, which was chaired by DeVries and included two cardiologists, a psychiatrist, a social worker, and a nurse, approved Clark as a candidate for the permanent device implant. Several years earlier, Clark had been diagnosed with cardiomyopathy by his local cardiologist, who treated Clark's illness with drug therapy. His condition worsened and his doctor sent him to Salt Lake City to undergo treatment with the experimental drug Amrinone in October 1981. But Clark could not tolerate the drug.[86] The progressive deterioration of his heart muscle meant that Clark had developed irreversible heart failure. Because of his age, he was not a candidate for heart transplantation. With no other options to pursue, Clark's doctor, in late 1982, suggested the possibility of a TAH. Barney Clark and his wife Una Loy met with DeVries, Kolff, and other members of the Utah research team to discuss the device implant.[87] According to Una Loy Clark, they "spared us nothing in explaining the highly experimental nature of the implantation."[88] When seeing the calves and sheep with artificial hearts, Barney Clark told Kolff, "These animals cannot speak, but I believe they feel a lot better than I feel at this time."[89] After discussing the experimental procedure with his family, Clark agreed to the operation.

On November 29, 1982, Clark was admitted to the University of Utah Medical Center, where he signed an 11-page consent form—twice, over a 24-hour period—before undergoing the surgery. The consent form outlined the procedure as experimental with no guarantee of a positive outcome and listed many potential complications: device malfunction, infection, machine dependency with limited mobility, and other possibilities, including death.[90] According to Una Loy Clark, her husband "was astutely aware of his critical physical condition and the highly experimental nature of the implantation and DID NOT expect any great personal miracle; he knew FULL WELL that by volunteering, he would be submitting to a totally unpredictable future. . . . There were absolutely no promises made to him."[91] According to his surgeon, Clark agreed to the experimental procedure as a way of furthering medical knowledge about the use of a TAH in a human.[92] At this point, Clark was a very ill man, probably within days or weeks of dying. He was diagnosed with Class IV heart failure, his heart working at one-sixth the capacity of a healthy heart, and he was in "marked decline" with a "very grim" prognosis "without any intervention."[93] It is not unreasonable to assume that many, probably including Clark himself, expected the operation to go one of two ways, either as a failure, in which case he would not survive the surgery or tolerate the device beyond a few hours; or, conversely, a success: the implant would work, delivering a moderately improved quality of life compared to the patient's grave circumstances beforehand. No one, including the medical team, anticipated the extent of complications that resulted or what one bioethicist later referred to as "halfway success."[94]

On December 1, 1982, two days in advance of the scheduled operation, Clark was rushed into surgery owing to the rapid deterioration of his heart. In the operating room, the implant team of surgeons, cardiologists, an anesthetist, a perfusionist, a heart-driver engineer, a heart-driver manager, an artificial heart adviser, and nurses attended to their respective tasks as DeVries removed Clark's diseased heart and

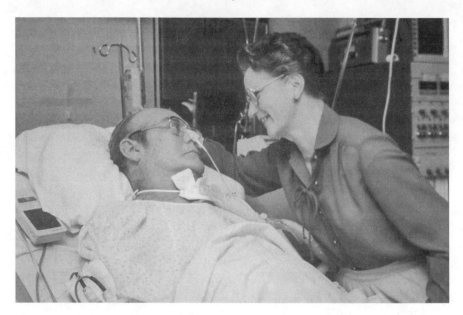

Artificial heart recipient Barney Clark and wife Una Loy, about two weeks after the implant surgery, University of Utah Medical Center, Salt Lake City, Utah, December 1982. Clark lived 112 days with a Jarvik-7 artificial heart but was never discharged from the hospital. Courtesy of Special Collections, J. Willard Marriott Library, University of Utah.

implanted a Jarvik-7 heart.[95] Initially, the implanted left mechanical ventricle failed to pump blood; DeVries disconnected the device, checked the mechanical valve, fiddled with the major blood vessels in Clark's chest to which the artificial heart connected, and repositioned the mechanical ventricle. The device began working properly thereafter. Drive lines penetrated the left side of Clark's body, delivering pulses of compressed air to the implanted device and connecting Clark to a large, 418-pound drive unit on wheels necessary to power and monitor the Jarvik-7 heart. The heart-driver operators monitored the pulse rate, adjusting blood pressure and flow to sustain an adequate cardiac output for the patient, while the surgeons checked for errant bleeding, inserting sutures as needed, before closing the chest. The anesthetist and the perfusionist worked to manage adequate oxygen levels in the patient's blood, attentive to Clark's compromised lung function, caused by suspected emphysema. The surgical team disconnected the heart-lung machine from Clark, who was now being supported by the Utah heart. Clark survived the surgery, opening his eyes and moving his arms and legs within hours after the operation. He was soon able to communicate with his family and the medical team; he let his wife know that he still loved her and that he was not in pain.[96]

DeVries, Kolff, and others on the medical team remained cautious; they had entered uncharted clinical territory. How long would the device continue to work?

Would it alter Clark's physical and mental state for the better? The level of uncertainty was high, and it manifested itself in the range of emotions of the medical team, from the initial sense of accomplishment, happiness, and relief to guarded optimism, concern, and frustration.

It was not long before Clark suffered a series of complications. On day 3 after the operation, DeVries was forced to operate on Clark again to repair ruptured air sacs in his lungs. On post-op day 6, Clark started having seizures. On post-op day 13, Clark experienced heart failure owing to a broken valve in the artificial heart, necessitating replacement of the entire left ventricle of the device in yet another surgery. The team had prepared to react to mechanical problems, anticipating potential device failures with the diaphragm, the connector, or the valves, as well as possible air leaks by the outlets, based on animal implants. In animal testing, investigators could not explain the "sticking" problem of the Bjork-Shiley valve, and they later discovered that in Clark's device, the valve had a defect. Thereafter, they used the Medtronic-Hall valve, which eliminated the sticking and breaking problem.[97] Arguably, this experience bore out Jarvik's and Olsen's earlier hesitation about device readiness for human use.[98] Thereafter, Clark was listed in "extremely critical condition."

Near the end of December, Clark appeared to be recovering—standing for the first time, taking his first few steps, even eating soft food by mouth. Hospital officials released a photo of the patient standing with his physical therapist, and another photo of Clark exercising on a stationary bicycle. The Utah team began to receive congratulations from within and outside the medical community. Feeling uncomfortable with these accolades but still optimistic about Clark's recovery, Kolff wrote, "I will remain very concerned as long as we have not restored Dr Clark to an enjoyable existence. We still have a reasonable chance to accomplish this . . . [and] . . . we fervently hope that we will succeed in getting him well."[99]

But complications returned to plague Clark. In mid-January 1983, Clark underwent surgery to control recurring nosebleeds caused by his aggressive anticoagulant therapy, deemed necessary to prevent blood clotting in the artificial heart. In February 1983, Clark suffered from various kidney and respiratory problems, which were never satisfactorily overcome, and he battled pneumonia, diarrhea, shortness of breath, bloody stool, and fever, among other problems. Una Loy Clark told friends and family, "Barney keeps valiantly trying and we pray we may soon reach the point when things will turn in our favor but the days are hard."[100] Following Clark's recovery closely, NHLBI official John Watson admitted to DeVries and the Utah medical team that "the current clinical results exceeded any of my expectations. The thorough and careful planning for every eventuality has certainly paid off for Dr Clark." The threat of blood clot problems and brain seizures was ever present, however, and Watson suggested the names of two medical experts with whom the Utah group might consult about these issues.[101]

In early March, Clark talked publicly for the first time about living with an artificial heart, calling it a worthwhile experience. In a videotaped interview with

DeVries that was released to the media, a tired and hoarse-voiced Clark commented that the artificial heart is "a thing you get used to. [It] doesn't bother me at all. Yes, it has been hard, but the heart itself has pumped right all along and I think it is doing well. All in all, it has been a pleasure to be able to help people." When DeVries asked what bothered him most, Clark replied his "shortness of breath" and "lack of air" from chronic lung problems, but his symptoms were "getting a little better."[102] During the interview, the sound of the air-driven heart pumping was clearly audible, alongside Clark's labored breathing.[103] The next week, Una Loy wrote, "The days pass and we are still trying to climb a big hill. This last bout with pneumonia was discouraging." Clark was back on the respirator, making communication with friends and family difficult. As Una Loy Clark acknowledged, "he can't talk and it is difficult . . . when all you can do is nod your head and grin."[104]

Clark's care was complicated, and DeVries and his medical team made several therapeutic trade-offs. For example, Clark received antibiotics to prevent infection, but the antibiotics contributed to his renal failure; aggressive anticoagulant therapy was carried out to avoid a stroke, but that therapy caused bleeding that was difficult to control; and the decision to keep device output at high levels was to avoid increasing Clark's pulmonary edema, but doing so was risky for device failure and blood hemolysis reasons.[105] The medical uncertainty surrounding device safety and performance alongside patient care and postoperative management manifested itself openly among the medical team, the patient, and the family, who were thrust into a day-by-day stance. On March 23, 1983, Clark died as a result of severe pseudomembranous colitis and sepsis (infection), which led to multi-organ failure.[106] Barney Clark lived 112 days with his artificial heart.

The Clark case received enormous media attention, with reporters from across the country and the world traveling to Salt Lake City to cover the story. Fearing that inaccurate information would be leaked, University of Utah officials had prepared to deliver accurate, honest, and regular briefings from the beginning, hoping that their statements would not draw criticisms of grandstanding or overhyping the event.[107] Daily press conferences were held in the university cafeteria, presided over by University of Utah vice president Chase Peterson and University of Utah Medical Center Public Affairs director John Dwan. They provided journalists with background information on the Utah artificial heart team, details of the implant procedure, postoperation results, patient updates and schedules, and other data. For example, at the December 15 press conference, Peterson told reporters, "At 9:45 this morning . . . Dr Clark had a sudden drop in his blood pressure. . . . The pressure dropped down to about 80/40, where it had been in the range of 140/80. . . . [The patient went back into surgery, where] a break was found in the wire-housing of the mitral valve. . . . So a new left heart was attached, the same velcro attachment was used, the new drive line was put in, and Dr Clark has now come through the surgery."[108] At times, members of the Utah artificial heart team, usually DeVries and Jarvik, appeared before the press to answer questions.

The university strove to cooperate fully with journalists, attempting to disclose medical information about Barney Clark as it unfolded and to meet the demands of the media. Perhaps this course was chosen because of lessons learned from the high-profile brain operation on the conjoined twins Lisa and Elisa Hansen, in May 1979, also at the University of Utah Medical Center; hospital spokespeople had struggled to meet the media demand for information about that surgery, and two photographers, hidden in laundry hampers, had taken unauthorized pictures in the hospital recovery room.[109] Many of the same reporters who had covered the Hansen surgery had now, in 1982, returned to Salt Lake City, and one journalist commented on the improved university-media relationship.[110] Peterson later admitted that while they had anticipated and prepared for considerable media coverage of the Clark surgery, it had not been enough. They had underestimated the number of journalists and the duration of their stay. Peterson commented, "We expected they would leave several days after the operation. . . . Instead, they stayed, many of them, throughout the long 112 days until Dr Clark's death."[111]

One reporter who criticized Peterson was *New York Times* medical writer Dr. Lawrence K. Altman. He accused Peterson of withholding information from the press, specifically medical details and IRB deliberations, that the public had a right to know. Admitting that they were indeed a "motley crew" of reporters, Altman stated, "There were some of us who wanted the laboratory values and other clinical facts to make our reports more scientific."[112] In responding to such journalist criticisms, Peterson was fully aware of drawing professional disapproval for ignoring the traditional peer review and medical publication process before releasing results to the public. Medical leaders like *New England Journal of Medicine* editor Arnold Relman and American Medical Association president Joseph Boyle argued that case results should be reported in medical science journals, after peer scrutiny, with only limited details offered to journalists before this.[113] Fearing "side-door media probing," Peterson felt that the level of interest and worldwide fascination with the Jarvik-7 heart was simply too great not to engage forthrightly with the mainstream press.[114]

Public interest in the Clark case was due to the novelty of the Jarvik-7 heart as a permanent replacement device and the fact that this patient lived with the device for 112 days. Moreover, unlike the earlier desperate cases in Texas, the Utah patient recounted what it was like to live with an artificial heart. Media reporting of the Clark case was detailed and constant, from the drama of the initial implant procedure through patient recovery highs and lows. Articles tended to be optimistic about the outcome, with technical descriptions of the Jarvik-7 device, glowing descriptions of the surgical team, and praise for Clark, who bravely volunteered to be the first to undergo this experimental procedure. Accompanying the text were many photos— Clark being wheeled into surgery, Clark after the surgery with DeVries at his bedside, sketches of the Jarvik-7 heart and its operation, headshots of DeVries, Jarvik, and Kolff, and even photos of university spokespeople. Headlines included "Artificial Heart Dramatically Improves Condition of Patient," "Artificial Heart Is

Doing the Job," and "Stepping over a Medical Frontier."[115] Setbacks were duly reported, with the much-hoped for recovery described soon thereafter.[116] *Time* and
Newsweek magazines ran similar stories, including "Man Makes a Heart: The Bold
New World of Cardiac Medicine."[117] Focusing on the individual, rather than the
device, *Life* magazine ran a story on Barney Clark in February 1983, entitled "The
Brave Man with the Plastic Heart."[118] When Clark died, the media highlighted his
courage and the "extra" 112 days of his life with the Jarvik-7 heart.[119]

After Clark died, Jarvik's celebrity status rose. Describing Jarvik as "boyishly-
good looking" and "a diminutive Warren Beatty," the medical and popular press ran
stories that depicted him as a talented innovator and a successful entrepreneur as
well as a hip and youthful boy genius, even a visionary. For the *American Medical
News* and *Hospitals* publications, Jarvik answered questions about the benefits, need,
and costs of the technology and posed for photographs, often clad in a suit, sometimes holding the Jarvik-7 heart.[120] At other times, he dressed in jeans and a black
leather motorcycle jacket. He agreed to interviews for *Playboy* and *People* magazines
to speak about the Jarvik-7 heart, but he also talked about his design for a new dildo
and falling in love with his second wife, Marilyn vos Savant, who held the highest
IQ in the world at 228.[121] *Inc.* magazine, a monthly publication tracking the fastest-
growing companies in the United States, profiled Jarvik's achievements as the chief
executive officer of Symbion Inc. under the glib subheading "Has Jarvik Found a
Heart of Gold?"[122] The device inventor and businessman was also photographed
for a Hathaway shirt advertisement, with an eye patch; this photo appeared in magazines and on billboards. "It was a good image for the business," Jarvik said, "[al-
though] admittedly, you're selling shirts."[123] The young, brazen, showy personality
of Jarvik certainly contributed to the public fascination with the artificial heart
and the media attention to it in the 1980s.

This publicity was dismissed as tasteless and indulgent by many in the research
community. However, Jarvik's celebrity profile was hardly out of place in the popular media coverage of the period. In terms of meaningful coverage of artificial hearts,
journalists' accounts were rarely critical, offering only a cursory discussion of such
difficult issues as costs, access, and quality of life. They extolled the patient, marveled
at the device, admired the artificial heart team, and celebrated medical science's attempt to fight heart disease with this technology. Still, media reports both reflected
and shaped public interest in this groundbreaking use of the artificial heart. It was
colorful drama, with constructed heroes and victories, which connected with American hope and faith in medical science and saving lives.

After Clark died, the Jarvik-7 heart was removed from the his body and studied
for signs of device malfunction, deterioration, or blood clotting. None were reported, thus supporting the technological feasibility of mechanically replacing the
heart. For the Utah team, the Barney Clark case was deemed a scientific success—
the Jarvik-7 heart had granted the patient and his family 112 extra days of life. DeVries
stated, "To say to only live an additional 112 days is unsuccessful is ridiculous. His

case was successful because he was going to die that day, and he saw Christmas and his birthday and his anniversary, and even the Brigham Young–University of Utah basketball game on television."[124] Yet success measured as an improvement of patient quality of life had clearly not been achieved.[125] John Bosso, chair of the University of Utah Medical Center IRB, recognized the nuances surrounding the definition of success. When asked by the press if the Utah TAH was successful, he replied, "The TAH showed that it could sustain life for 112 days. But was it successful, well that is a relative thing. We wanted the patient to go home, but the other information that was learned, from that standpoint, it was successful."[126]

Members of the University of Utah Medical Center IRB delayed approval for the next implant, stating that they wanted to evaluate the Clark case more fully and to improve the research protocol before proceeding. Utah's artificial heart program was not being terminated, stated Bosso at a September 1983 press conference.[127] But months passed, with finger-pointing between DeVries and IRB members for who was to blame for the delay in moving forward with the second TAH implant.[128] Further irritating DeVries, university hospital officials asked him to raise funds for future implants, after they tallied the cost of Clark's care. (While the device equipment cost of about $16,000 had been absorbed by Kolff's research program, Clark's hospital bill had escalated to more than $200,000. By signing the consent form, the Clark family had agreed to pay hospital care costs, which had been estimated at $15,000. The actual hospital bill caused considerable anxiety for Una Loy Clark, and in the end, the Clark family was relieved of financial responsibilities.)[129] DeVries stated publicly, "I'm not a money raiser, I'm a doctor."[130] DeVries interpreted the hospital officials' request as wavering institutional support that threatened future clinical cases, and so he left Utah, infuriating Kolff, who was fighting to hold together the Utah artificial heart program.[131]

Four More Implants: William Schroeder, Murray Haydon, Leif Stenberg, and Jack Burcham

On July 31, 1984, DeVries announced that he was shifting his Jarvik-7 heart implant cases from the University of Utah Medical Center to Humana Hospital Audubon in Louisville, Kentucky. The Humana Corporation, one of America's largest investor-owned, for-profit health care companies, offered money, equipment, facilities, and personnel to DeVries to support his artificial heart program and surgical practice through its affiliated Humana Hospital Audubon and Humana Heart Institute private group practice. With deep pockets and plentiful resources, Humana presented DeVries with a commitment to underwrite the financial costs of up to 100 implants. This must have been music to DeVries's ears, when he was frustrated by administrative delays and fund-raising pressures at the University of Utah.[132] The only surgeon authorized by the FDA to implant the Jarvik-7 heart as a permanent device in the United States, DeVries was approved to perform seven implants (subject to IRB case-by-case approval) before he would need further federal consent. He was not tied to the University of Utah Medical Center for the surgery, and Jarvik ran the company that would ensure DeVries had Jarvik-7 hearts to implant wherever such operations took place. In Louisville, DeVries could continue his artificial heart work and build a large cardiovascular practice; the opportunity was irresistible.[133]

How would Humana's for-profit status conflict with or alter the course for artificial heart development? For DeVries, Humana's administrative and financial promises meant that he would perform his second implant case sooner rather than later. It removed him from the institutional inertia and tensions that he felt in Utah, while also expanding Humana's involvement from substantial investor in Symbion and customer of its training programs to primary host as a leading center for this implant surgery. Critics, including Relman and Boyle, remarked that Humana supported the less-than-perfect Jarvik-7 heart for publicity reasons, as a means to establish a reputation as a leading cardiac care facility and attract patients for many kinds of heart surgery.[134] Part of this was true; Humana wanted to be a leading heart disease center. Two years earlier, Humana had proposed setting up an affiliated Center of Excellence at the university hospital in Salt Lake City. Such a cooperative venture would have allowed Humana to share scientific credit and would have provided a place to send Humana physicians for training as well as Humana patients not easily treated elsewhere; Kolff, DeVries, and other University of Utah researchers and clinicians would have secured funding for their heart disease research and treatments. Kolff was open to unconventional ways to finance his artificial heart work, but he was unable to broker the deal. The center never materialized, because it lacked support from Utah officials, queasy over how the direct involvement of Humana and its for-profit mandate would affect their university hospital practices of public teaching, research, and patient care.[135] Now that DeVries would be shifting his work to Louisville, without oversight of university hospital research protocols and standards, similar concerns over clashing institutional goals arose again.

Would a nonteaching, nonacademic hospital, such as Humana-Audubon, be less demanding in its review and approval of protocols for implant procedures, driven by patient demand and economic motives? There was an intuitive bias that public, research-oriented universities like the University of Utah would be more rigorous and were qualified to direct experimental clinical procedures in a way that for-profit hospitals were not; competent cardiac surgical teams are present at both, but not all are suited for clinical investigation.[136] Humana executives openly acknowledged their business orientation, unnerving medical leaders like Relman and Boyle by blurring distinctions between academic centers as traditional sites of research and for-profit hospitals as efficient sites of medical treatments.[137] As Fox and Swazey point out, Humana's increased involvement in artificial hearts ignited concerns about the growth of for-profit medicine in this period and its "presumed negative implications" for health care delivery.[138] The relevance of Humana's for-profit status was how it served to intensify discussions surrounding the clinical use of artificial hearts. For Humana officials, the unspoken reality was that implant success needed to be demonstrated sooner rather than later in an environment concerned with the economic bottom line.

On November 25, 1984 (almost 2 years after the Clark implant), at Humana's Audubon Hospital, DeVries implanted a Jarvik-7 heart in 52-year-old William (Bill) Schroeder, who became the second recipient of a permanent artificial heart. From Jasper, Indiana, Schroeder had been a quality assurance inspector at an army munitions depot, but ill health had forced him to retire. Like Clark, Schroeder was categorized as a Class IV heart failure patient who was not a candidate for heart transplantation. Like Clark, Schroeder had battled heart disease for years, had exhausted all conventional treatments, and had only weeks to live when he decided to undergo the device implant. More emphatic than Clark, Schroeder chose the experimental surgery as a way to live; he wanted more time with his family and wanted to attend his son's upcoming wedding.[139] Agreeing to the implant procedure, Schroeder signed a lengthy consent form, which had been expanded to include graphic details of Clark's medical difficulties with the Jarvik-7 heart. The night before the surgery, a priest read Schroeder his last rites. Prepared for death, Schroeder nonetheless lived, surviving the implant procedure, which was complicated by significant cardiovascular scarring from previous surgery. Schroeder lived 620 days, becoming the

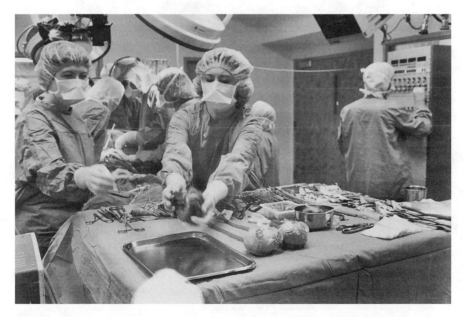

William Schroeder's diseased heart is placed on a tray next to a sterilized Jarvik-7 artificial heart (implanted in halves), Humana's Audubon Hospital, Louisville, Kentucky, November 25, 1984. Photographer: William Strode. Used with permission from Charlotte Strode. Image courtesy of the History of Medicine Division, National Library of Medicine.

longest-living patient with a permanent artificial heart, and for a period he lived outside the hospital in a nearby apartment that had been remodeled for implant patients.[140] His experience was not without setbacks, however. Near the end of Schroeder's life with the artificial heart, his family requested that no extraordinary measures be taken to address the series of infections, strokes, and other impairments.[141]

The Jarvik-7 heart implanted in Schroeder was almost identical to the one implanted in Clark. Schroeder's artificial heart had different valves; the Bjork-Shiley valve in Clark's artificial heart had broken and was replaced by the Medtronic-Hall valve in subsequent device constructions. Perhaps more noticeable to the public was the increased mobility and freedom of Schroeder, as compared to Clark. Schroeder's mechanical heart was powered by a large, bedside drive unit (much the same as Clark's) as well as by a newly available, battery-powered, portable drive unit. Less than 12 pounds in weight and fitting into a large satchel, this portable driver

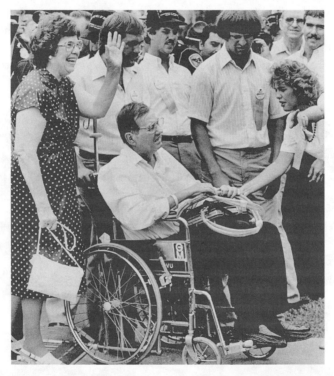

Artificial heart recipient William Schroeder visits his hometown of Jasper, Indiana, where he is greeted by well-wishers before riding in the town's annual German-heritage parade on August 4, 1985. Note the portable drive unit sitting on Schroeder's lap. Cardiac surgeon William DeVries served as the parade's grand marshal. Immediately after the event, Schroeder made the 90-mile trip back to Humana Hospital, Louisville, Kentucky. Schroeder lived 620 days with a Jarvik-7 artificial heart.
(AP Photo/Al Behrman)

could be used by Schroeder for up to three hours, replacing the tethering to the large primary unit. Schroeder was photographed rolling down hospital halls in his wheelchair, going for drives in his modified van with his son as chauffeur, and ultimately moving into a transitional apartment attached to the hospital.

For a brief time, the uncertainty surrounding the Jarvik-7 heart was eclipsed by reports of Schroeder's miraculous recovery and his optimistic outlook. Two weeks after the surgery, an alert and eager-to-talk Schroeder, who was still bedridden in the hospital, told reporters that he felt "super" and that "with this new heart I feel like I've got [another] 10 years." When asked what it felt like to not have a heart, Schroeder said: "It just sits there. I can feel it. It doesn't bother my sleep. It doesn't bother me at all. I've gotten used to it and don't know it's there. There it goes, it's taking off like a horse. Who knows, I may be as well as the bionic man." He asked his interviewers, reporter-physician Lawrence Altman and ABC News correspondent George Strait, to feel his chest, and they described Schroeder's new heartbeat as more prominent and vibrant than a normal human heart. The reporters also commented on the "barely audible" noise of the new portable driver. When asked about his pain and discomfort, Schroeder stated that it was comparable to his previous open-heart surgery experience.[142] These were encouraging early days, during which Schroeder teased the nurses and toasted his recovery with a can of beer, but they did not last. Schroeder's experience with the Jarvik-7 heart soon included seizures, strokes, fevers, short-term memory impairment, and battles with renal failure, among other complications.[143]

The media's coverage of Schroeder's implant was not unlike that of Clark's. Journalists praised the patient, explained the mechanics of the device, and congratulated the medical team. Headlines included "Heart Recipient 'Feeling Good,' Requests a Beer" and "High Spirits on a Plastic Pulse: Schroeder's Joviality and Fast Recovery Astound His Doctors."[144] Photographs contributed to the shaping of this event as a heroic journey, with images of Schroeder going into surgery, the surgical team implanting the device, and family surrounding Schroeder during his recovery. There were pictures of DeVries with his famous patient, of Schroeder on the phone asking President Ronald Reagan about his social security check, of Schroeder in a wheelchair touring the hospital, saying "Feel my heart. Wanna feel my heart? It's beating, it's OK."[145] Most, if not all, of the photographs used in the reporting of Schroeder's case were commissioned by Humana.

Humana played a proactive role in shaping the Schroeder news story. First, Humana contacted the media two days in advance of Schroeder's operation. The 300 or more news people sent to cover the extraordinary surgery found themselves in a well-equipped press center in a downtown convention hall set up by Humana. As one news outlet reported, "Background books, coffee and sandwiches, pictures and videotape, regular bulletins and detailed briefings—all were dispensed with operating room precision as the events unfolded."[146] After studying the cases of Barney Clark and Baby Fae (who only one month previously had been implanted with a baboon's heart in California), the Humana public relations team sought to control the flow of information to minimize errors and prevent animosity with re-porters.[147] For Humana, the costs of cooperating with the media contributed to its goal of building company name recognition. But apparently there were limits. When Schroeder's recovery deteriorated, some journalists accused Humana of intentionally withholding information.

Like Clark, Schroeder experienced setbacks, and the press duly informed the public. On December 13, a week after his upbeat celebratory interview with report-ers, Schroeder suffered a massive stroke, probably resulting from the formation of blood clots in the artificial heart, which then traveled to his brain. When he regained consciousness, he had lost much of his memory, his coordination, his speech, and his jovial personality.[148] Schroeder was paralyzed on the right side of his body and suffered from depression, a common result of stroke. Gloomy headlines announced, "Heart Recipient Suffers a Stroke: Doctor Reports Partial Recovery," and "Heart Recipient Loses Enthusiasm, Doctor Reports."[149] In early February, Schroeder developed a mys-terious fever, which lasted for 60 days, possibly contributing to greater brain damage.[150] Returning to Louisville to cover the story of Murray Haydon (the recently announced third Jarvik-7 heart recipient), journalists were surprised by the extent of Schroeder's decline. Quickly, Humana countered with more positive aspects of Schroeder's experience, such as photos of the patient and his wife eating pizza together. In March, Schroeder did not make the 90-mile trip to Jasper, Indiana, to attend his son's wedding, since doctors deemed it "too stressful for him"; instead, Schroeder, who was reported as being "in really good spirits," attended a dress rehearsal in the hospital lobby, followed by dinner and a reception in the hospital auditorium.[151]

Not long after, Humana officials announced that medical information relating to Schroeder and all future implant cases would no longer be provided to the media; instead it would be guarded for scientific evaluation and publication. According to one publication, DeVries criticized the media for seeking "trivia," such as "whether the patient had strawberries for breakfast."[152] In both the Clark and the Schroeder cases, institutional attempts at full disclosure with the media did not work as advan-tageously as had been hoped by the University of Utah and Humana officials. Nevertheless, those attempts enabled the spotlight to shine as long and as brightly as it did on the people involved.

Within months of Schroeder's implant, DeVries performed more Jarvik-7 heart implant procedures. On February 17, 1985, Murray Haydon, a 58-year-old retired auto assembly plant worker, became the third recipient of a permanent Jarvik-7 heart. Haydon lived 488 days with his artificial heart; however, he never left the hospital and spent a great deal of time attached to a respirator to assist his breathing. In ad-dition to his lung insufficiency problem, Haydon suffered a stroke, bleeding, and a series of infections after the implant.[153] The press dutifully gathered in Louisville to report on the Haydon case, but it did not generate the same coverage as it had for either Clark or Schroeder. Typically, the press celebrates medical firsts more than thirds. As noted by Fox and Swazey, media reports on Haydon were limited to the implant operation, his one-year anniversary with the device, and his death. They stated, "He [Haydon] was a quiet, intensely private man who insisted adamantly that he and his family be shielded from publicity. He was not, as some of his physicians and nurses at first had hoped, destined to be the first permanent artificial heart recipient to make a 'full recovery.'"[154] When Haydon died, his family released a statement expressing their gratitude for the extra 16 months of life afforded Haydon because of the artificial heart. According to them, Haydon "decided to receive the heart because he wanted to live longer, and because he wanted to be a part of something that will someday save many lives. He achieved both of those things."[155]

A full recovery did seem imminent for one patient outside the United States. On April 7, 1985, at the Karolinska Hospital in Stockholm, Sweden, cardiac surgeon Bjarne Semb implanted a Jarvik-7 heart into heart failure patient Leif Stenberg, who had been removed from the heart transplantation list owing to multiple organ failure. Before this, Stenberg had experienced two acute myocardial infarctions (heart attacks) that had damaged his heart, notably compromising its right ventricular function; Stenberg's poor heart function then contributed to increasing kidney and liver problems.[156] Semb had become interested in the artificial heart the previous year after Jarvik had visited the Karolinska Thorax Clinic, part of the prestigious Karolinska Institute, Scandinavia's leading health center. The treatment of heart problems was one of the specialties of the thorax clinic, and Semb, who was already transplanting hearts, keenly signed on to learn more about the Jarvik-7 heart. He and his team traveled to the United States for device implant training, paid for by a Swedish pharmaceutical company, in preparation for the artificial heart's clinical use at the Karolinska Hospital. Semb also visited DeVries in Louisville to see his clinical cases firsthand and to note concerns and challenges for patient recovery. The week before the Swedish surgery, the Jarvik-7 heart and its power supply were shipped to the Karolinska Hospital as a donation by Jarvik's company for Stenberg's surgery (it was a [reported] $15,500 gift that Humana Hospital had not received).[157] As had been the case for DeVries's implant operations, Jarvik was in Semb's operating room as an adviser on the day of Stenberg's procedure.

A glitch occurred in surgery when Semb first attempted to transition his patient from the heart-lung bypass machine to the artificial heart. When activated in Stenberg's chest, the artificial heart provided dangerously low left ventricular cardiac output. Semb detected an impingement of the mitral valve prosthesis by the left atrial catheter, so he had to disconnect the mechanical heart to manipulate the catheter and functioning of the valve. He then reconnected the artificial heart, which proved to work more satisfactorily to support patient circulation, and Stenberg was moved into recovery.[158]

Like the American patients, the Swedish artificial heart case presented an ambiguous experience of postoperative complications and setbacks amid periods of promising improvement and hoped-for recovery. During the first two postoperative days, Semb battled bleeding problems in his efforts to stabilize sufficient blood circulation in his patient, after which Stenberg was finally extubated at 41 hours postsurgery. The medical team tinkered with the anticoagulant treatment and responded to kidney and liver complications experienced by Stenberg. It took several weeks before improved pulmonary perfusion occurred, the patient showed good weight gain, and a general showing of well-being presented.[159] The public was not privy to these medical challenges; instead, they saw the upside of living with an artificial heart: Stenberg leaving the hospital during the day, taking walks through the city, and eating in his favorite restaurants with his portable drive unit powering his artificial heart. At a 90-minute press conference three months after the implant, Stenberg declared that he was "living proof" that this technology could extend a person's life and improve its quality; Jarvik referred to Stenberg as his "best patient."[160] Still, the longer Stenberg remained on the device, the more his medical team worried about the risk of blood clotting and embolic strokes, despite their best efforts at carefully managing his blood-thinning drugs. Semb put Stenberg back on the heart transplant waiting list, even though, at the time of implantation, he had not intended to do so. Stenberg did not receive a heart transplant; he suffered a stroke in September (which then ruled out a transplant), fell into a coma, and died of respiratory and multi-organ failure in November after living with the Jarvik-7 heart for seven and a half months. Semb was ambivalent about the use of the artificial heart as a permanent therapy, and thereafter he implanted only a few more Jarvik-7 hearts as temporary measures before heart transplantation.[161]

On April 14, 1985, DeVries implanted an artificial heart in retired railway engineer Jack Burcham, age 62, who died 10 days afterward. Burcham's death upset DeVries. The oldest patient to undergo the operation, Burcham experienced extensive bleeding, acute renal failure, and cardiac tamponade (fluid accumulation in the sac around the heart). But most disturbing was the poor surgical fit. Despite the standard preoperative CT scan to confirm patient chest dimensions, DeVries struggled to fit the Jarvik-7 heart into Burcham. DeVries acknowledged it as "a tight fit and unusual positioning of the device," which probably contributed to Burcham's demise.[162] Burcham underwent a prolonged operation because of the difficulties in placing the Jarvik-7 heart in his body, and it resulted in only a partial closing of his chest around the device.[163] Unbeknownst to all at the time, this patient turned out to be the last individual to receive a Jarvik-7 heart as a permanent implant.

It is tricky to assess public understanding and sentiment regarding the permanent implantation of artificial hearts. A snapshot of opinions suggests that the public was divided on the issue. In a *USA Today* article, a handful of Americans were asked how they felt about artificial heart implants. Responses ranged from "Artificial hearts tamper too much with human nature" and "Medical technology has finally overstepped its bounds" to "This is a great advancement for medical science" and "If I were in a life-threatening situation, I'd want an artificial heart."[164] In the days after Barney Clark's death, the public empathized with the family's decision to undergo the experimental procedure. One woman who had lost her father prematurely to heart disease said, "What if an artificial heart had been available when we stood helplessly by and watched someone we cared about slip past the physician's skill?"[165] Responding to critics, Una Loy Clark stated, "It is easy for those of us standing here with healthy hearts to criticize and to say what we would or would not do—it is quite another thing to be facing death because our own heart is giving out and have to make a decision about whether to die or to have an artificial heart and prolong our lives and have a chance of survival."[166] It is not surprising that, confronted with death, patients, their families, and doctors struggle with a decision that might offer a chance to live, discounting the experimental nature of the procedure or the rocky clinical courses of past patients. Una Loy Clark's comment may be interpreted several ways. On the one hand, no one likes to be second-guessed about his decisions, particularly after the fact, when many of the "what ifs" are removed. On the other hand, it speaks to the emotionally charged environment in which end-of-life decision making often takes place and the best-case scenarios that families often cling to at those times. It supports the case for advance directives based on timely discussions of medical conditions and end-of-life issues with patients and their families, which might ease such decision-making burdens.

A "Temporary" Spike: A Market for the Jarvik-7 Heart

The mixed results of permanent implant cases did not discourage the use of the Jarvik-7 heart as a temporary device by some surgeons between 1985 and 1991. During this period, a handful of cardiac surgeons implanted TAHs as a bridge to transplantation for deteriorating patients waiting for donor hearts. The intention was for a patient to live temporarily—a matter of days only—with an artificial heart, thus diminishing concerns of limited patient mobility and strokes that had materialized in permanent implant cases. What emerged was a "temporary" spike of TAH cases in the later 1980s that was dominated by the Jarvik-7 device. The spike began in Tucson, Arizona, with a surgeon who championed the technology and became invested in it.

At the University of Arizona Medical Center, cardiac surgeon Jack Copeland was building a world reputation for himself and his institution by performing cutting-edge cardiac surgery with remarkable results. He had completed medical school at Stanford University in the 1960s and, during the 1970s, trained under transplant surgeon pioneer Norman Shumway at one of the top cardiovascular centers in the country. In 1977 Copeland moved to the University of Arizona Medical Center in Tucson to develop a transplant program. According to Copeland, it was a timely opportunity that offered "the freedom to do things that others had not done."[167] Within a short time, Copeland put the University of Arizona Medical Center on the map and saved countless lives. In 1979 Copeland performed Arizona's first heart transplant and, six years later, the state's first heart-lung transplant.[168] In treating patients who suffered from varying degrees of heart failure, Copeland was receptive to the use of mechanical pumps. He approached artificial heart technology as a benefit for heart transplantation.

In March 1985, Copeland performed an emergency implant utilizing the Phoenix TAH in a patient who was in allograft rejection (his body was rejecting a donor heart). The Phoenix heart kept 33-year-old Thomas Creighton alive for 11 hours until a second heart transplant was performed. Like the Jarvik-7 heart, the Phoenix heart was a pulsatile pneumatic device that required tethering to a large drive console. Designed by Phoenix dentist Kevin Cheng, a former employee of the Texas Heart Institute and a co-worker in the construction of Akutsu's artificial hearts, the Phoenix heart had had limited animal testing and had never been used in a human before. Since the Phoenix heart was 25 percent larger than the human heart, Creighton's chest was left open, with the artificial heart pumping, until his transplant procedure. Although the Phoenix heart kept the patient alive until he could undergo another transplant operation, Creighton lived only 39 hours with his second donor heart.[169] Creighton's death was not attributed to the Phoenix heart, but to blood cell and organ damage caused by being maintained on a heart-lung machine longer than the recommended maximum of four hours while his medical team secured his first donor heart.[170]

There was some criticism concerning the use of an untested device that was not FDA approved. Like Cooley, Copeland responded that such emergency implants were legitimately performed by a physician who was exhausting all options to save a patient's life.[171] As a medical practice, the surgeon's decision to implant an experimental device, as Copeland and Cooley had done, did not need FDA approval when surgeons, regulated by their own experience and commitment to their patients, deemed it potentially beneficial. Nonetheless, it created some confusion that was played out in the press: were FDA officials turning a blind eye to bridge implants, in sharp contrast to permanent implants in nontransplant patients?[172] How was it that the Utah group had labored through the regulatory process for the use of their device, while Cooley and Copeland had not? What the public discussion failed to distinguish was that industry, not surgical researchers or clinical surgeons, pursued FDA approval to make and sell their devices. During the 1980s, the Utah group had formed a company to market the Jarvik-7 heart with FDA approval for implantation in specialized cardiac medical centers, hoping to broaden its use and influence the standard of care for heart failure. After the Phoenix heart implant, Copeland traveled to Salt Lake City to learn more about the Jarvik-7 heart and its implantation procedure from the Utah team through its corporate setup. Acknowledging the utility of mechanical support for failing patients waiting for donor hearts, Copeland purchased the Jarvik-7 heart equipment, preparing to use this FDA-approved device instead of another Phoenix heart.[173]

On August 29, 1985, Copeland performed his second artificial heart surgery, implanting a Jarvik-7 heart into a 25-year-old heart failure patient, Michael Drummond. The implant procedure was uneventful, but seven days after the operation, Drummond experienced a series of small strokes. Two days later, on September 7, 1985, Drummond received his donor heart and the Jarvik-7 heart was removed

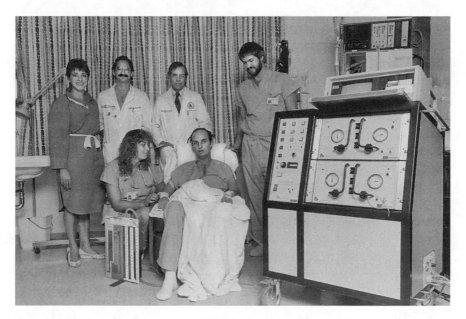

The celebrated first patient case with a Jarvik-7 artificial heart at Tucson's University of Arizona Medical Center, in 1985. Twenty-five-year-old Michael Drummond lived nine days with a Jarvik-7 artificial heart before undergoing a heart transplantation. *Left to right, in back,* Nina Trasoff, information officer; Mark Levinson, cardiac surgeon; Jack Copeland, cardiac surgeon; Richard Smith, biomedical engineer; *left to right, in front,* Debbie Nuetfield, nurse; and Michael Drummond, the artificial heart recipient. Note the drive line connecting the patient's artificial heart to the large drive unit, dubbed "Big Blue," powering and monitoring the implanted device. ©Arizona Board of Regents, University of Arizona Health Sciences. Reprinted with permission. Photographer: Jeb Zirato, FBCA; UAHS BioCommunications.

from his chest. Examination of the device revealed that fibrinous deposits (blood clots) had formed around the valves; the clots probably dislodged to cause the patient's neurological events (strokes).[174] Drummond lived another five years with his donor heart, until infection and other medical complications led to his death in 1990. The case was reported as the first Jarvik-7 heart bridge success, not as a perfect technology, given the stroke event, but for sustaining Drummond well enough to receive his donor heart.[175]

Both the Drummond case and the availability of the smaller, improved Jarvik 7-70 artificial heart contributed to an international wave of artificial heart bridge implants during the late 1980s.[176] The new Jarvik 7-70 heart was 30 percent smaller than the original Jarvik-7 model and designed to fit into smaller patients without compromising performance (or cardiac output). The smaller Jarvik-7 heart of 70 ml capacity was designed for a cardiac output of 7 to 8 liters (around 2 gallons) per minute, compared with the 11 to 12 liters per minute of the original 100 ml Jarvik-7. Jarvik and his team maintained that patients waiting for a donor heart did not demand more than the 8 liters per minute volume output owing to their weakened physical state and limited exercise tolerance. They also acknowledged that the smaller Jarvik heart was a better anatomic fit for more candidates, expanding the candidate pool to include smaller individuals. The team continued to work on improving the device design so as to reduce the risk of blood clot formation around the valves.[177]

According to a registry report produced by the Minneapolis Heart Institute, more than 200 TAH implants took place in roughly 40 specialized heart centers worldwide (including 20 American centers) by 1991; the number of operations peaked in 1986, 1987, and 1988, with 43, 51, and 75 implants, respectively.[178] Of the 11 different device models employed in these operations (not all were American), the Jarvik-7 heart was implanted in roughly 80 percent of the cases.[179] The predominant complications were infection and hemorrhage, but device dysfunction and neurologic events also occurred.[180] The majority of implant patients (65%) subsequently underwent their intended transplant operations, and half (50%) were alive one year later with their donor hearts.[181] Patient survival was related to the nature of the heart disease, not gender, age or indication for implantation, according to the authors of this report. They concluded that the use of artificial hearts as short-term, rather than long-term, devices produced better outcomes, and thus they advocated for the development of less costly, yet technologically superior, devices for treatment of end-stage heart disease. At the time, the more promising devices for short-term support were VADs, which did not require the removal of the native, diseased heart. Would these devices not be a more reasonable option for heart failure patients? TAH researchers remained committed to a device for long-term mechanical circulatory support. But the high development costs and cumbersome government regulation of these devices were real challenges for artificial heart researchers.[182]

The costs of developing the artificial heart from an experimental device to a commercially available product were significant. Initially, Kolff funded research of the Jarvik heart through NIH grants, and he later marketed the device through Kolff Associates Inc. Research on artificial hearts depended on government funding, with the intention that university researchers would partner with industry to transition medical devices from investigative to commercial products. In the United States, the establishment of the Artificial Heart Program at the NIH in 1964 was a catalyst in the development of the artificial heart, through contract funding to both university and industry researchers for targeted research and device development. Through this program, NIH officials organized contractor meetings in an attempt to facilitate knowledge exchange and the dissemination of scientific findings among researchers in the field. Working in a climate of protecting proprietary information, industry researchers were less forthcoming than academic researchers. In many cases, industry-university partnerships had been formed with the intention of commercial development, and thus the partners were reluctant to share promising product details with potential competitors. Kolff's team certainly benefited from NIH funding, securing hundreds of thousands of grant dollars throughout the 1960s and the 1970s that contributed to the improved design, function, and animal testing of the Jarvik heart. Kolff's team did not include an industry partner, and now they grappled with transitioning from device research to commercial development and marketing.

In 1976 Kolff, Olsen, and Jarvik formed Kolff Associates Inc., an independent proprietary company, to manufacture and sell various medical products coming out of Kolff's lab. A board of directors was set up, with Kolff as chair and five other members: son Dr. Jack Kolff and fellow lab colleagues Lee Smith, Clifford Kwan-Gett, Jarvik, and Olsen. At the time, Kolff dismissed any debate of ownership and all objections to his right to market and sell any lab product; it was a lapse of oversight that he refused to double-check intellectual property and licensing agreements.[183] Kolff Associates Inc. advertised its extensive experience in device design, materials processing, device fabrication, and in vivo evaluation. It also offered to fabricate devices designed by other research groups, allowing those laboratories to concentrate on experimentation rather than developing large polymer fabrication groups and manufacturing facilities necessary to produce uniform designs. (It is unknown how many, if any, non-Utah designs Kolff Associates did in fact manufacture.) Through direct marketing to research surgeons, Kolff Associates advertised Jarvik hearts as investigational devices at $2,300 each, LVADs at $800 each, and the Utah Heart Drive at $4,900 each.[184] These were steep prices, and it is unknown exactly how many experimental units were sold at this time. After devices were purchased, Olsen trained the research teams on how to operate the equipment and implant the devices in animals.[185]

At the University of Utah, there were numerous spin-off companies or businesses formed in partnership with university scientists to develop and commercialize new technologies. When Kolff had arrived in Utah, such companies were being organized with the knowledge and permission of the university, with the understanding that patent rights of products created with university support became the property of the university, and researchers sought licenses from the university to manufacture the products. Any federally funded research products were owned by the US government, which was often reluctant to relinquish ownership of patents to universities. In 1980 the Bayh-Dole Act revised US patent and trademark law by transferring discovery ownership and intellectual property made with federal research grants to the universities and small businesses where they were made. It aimed to simplify the "technology transfer" process, encouraged academic institutions to pursue licenses with business, and hoped that institutions would share profits with the inventors. It also made clear that the university owned the rights to such products, much to the chagrin of Kolff. By the mid-1980s at the University of Utah, there existed numerous biomedical university-industry collaborations similar to the artificial heart group, including Motion Control Inc. (the Utah arm prosthesis), Vascular International Inc. (synthetic blood vessels), Life Extenders Corporation (an artificial bladder and artificial sphincter), Deseret Research Inc. (biomedical engineering and testing), and Bonnell Inc. (an infant respirator).[186] Dubbed "academic capitalism," such spin-off firms provided welcome income to university research projects while working toward the commercialization of devices such as the Jarvik heart. It was hoped that successful collaborations would forge a new biotech industry in which profits would fund innovative new research and create high-paying and high-skilled jobs.

Kolff's experience with the commercialization of the Jarvik heart was rocky, partly because of his misunderstanding of device ownership, his lack of business acumen, and his decision to relinquish so much control to Jarvik. No doubt Kolff had some level of faith in the process and the people who were similarly invested in the clinical use of the Jarvik heart. According to Kolff's records, Kolff Associates did adequately well for a new company, making a small profit each year and attracting some investors to purchase company shares.[187] In turn, Kolff Associates contributed some funding to Kolff's research program at the university.[188] But the financial stability of Kolff Associates was far from certain. In 1982 the company was renamed Kolff Medical Inc. and Kolff introduced a board motion to make Jarvik president, a somewhat surprising turn, since their relationship had become one of increasing friction and animosity in recent years.[189] Kolff agreed to be replaced as president because Jarvik had done well to raise the much-needed venture capital to market their device, and Kolff supported Jarvik's high-powered fund-raising style.

After assuming greater control of the company, Jarvik went after big corporate investors and aggressively marketed the device and training programs, promoting implantation beyond Utah in other heart programs nationally and worldwide.[190] It was at this time that it became clear that the artificial hearts were owned by the University of Utah, exposing Kolff's earlier mistaken understanding of device ownership. Kolff Medical secured a technology licensing agreement from the university immediately. Big money rolled in when Jarvik began targeting large investing hospitals; in addition to the cost of the equipment, Jarvik sold high-priced training packages to these hospital groups, which would send surgical staff to the Utah laboratories to practice implanting the device in animals.[191] In 1983 Kolff Medical became a public company, and financial giants such as American Hospital Supply, Humana, Johnson and Johnson, and the Hospital Corporation of America became major stockholders.[192] Jarvik reorganized the company's management structure, began severing ties with Kolff, and soon squeezed Kolff out of the company entirely.

These were harsh actions taken by Jarvik against the man who had forged the Utah artificial heart program and nurtured many careers, including Jarvik's. It undoubtedly hurt Kolff to be removed from the company that bore his name, and colleagues witnessing these events commented privately on the unseemliness of it all. Kolff was angry and bitter about Jarvik's actions. He wrote, "Jarvik wants to stamp out everything that is Kolff. One might think he would have been satisfied after having first reduced the board of directors to a puppet organization when the so-called Management Committee had all the power and after subsequently making life so miserable for me that I resigned as Chairman of the Board of Directors.

That was not enough! Subsequently he has threatened to discontinue payment of the $125,000 per annum to the University of Utah for [artificial heart] research with no strings attached because he felt I was breaking my agreement." Publicly, Kolff refrained from bad-mouthing Jarvik but instead stated that he had resigned from Kolff Medical over the issue of vacuum forming as an alternative to the conventional mould-forming methods for the Jarvik heart. (Kolff argued that vacuum forming was less time-consuming and less expensive without compromising the design and efficacy of the device; however, Jarvik was not convinced.)[193] Kolff later remarked, "If I were a lot younger, I would have resisted it."[194] Kolff returned to the University of Utah full-time, while Jarvik left the university to run the company. In 1984, as Jarvik was ousting Kolff from company management, Kolff Medical changed its name to Symbion Inc.[195]

During this period Jarvik began promoting the Jarvik-7 heart as a temporary device for transplant patients deteriorating on waiting lists. This was in sharp contrast to the Utah team's earlier intent for the Jarvik-7 heart to be a permanent therapy only. In 1986 Jarvik told Judith Swazey that a de facto moratorium on permanent implantation had taken place and the company's focus was on its temporary use. He said, "There is no question that the TAH does work. We always felt it could work, but we weren't sure under what conditions. Now as a bridge we are saving a lot of lives."[196] Promoting the Jarvik-7 heart as a bridge device, Symbion offered implant training programs at the University of Utah Experimental Heart Laboratory that attracted many cardiac transplant surgeons, such as Jack Copeland, who attended before his well-publicized implant in Michael Drummond. Surgical teams from outside of the United States also traveled to Salt Lake City for training after investing in the Jarvik-7 heart technology.[197] Each surgical team's training and equipment added up to a reported $350,000 for Symbion.[198] Symbion also secured contracts with Humana and Hospital Corporation of America, two of the largest for-profit hospital groups in the United States, for approximately $650,000 per year to provide such training to their staff.[199]

Ever the businessman, Jarvik hoped to convert Stanford's Norman Shumway, transplant pioneer and influential leader in the field, to support Symbion's program, which would then persuade other transplant programs to follow suit. But Shumway was no fan of the Jarvik-7 heart, and he never used it. In 1984 he told the *New York Times* that the Jarvik-7 heart was a "crude device with no future" and that the most successful treatment for end-stage heart patients was cardiac transplantation.[200] Two years later, he had not changed his mind. In a rare interview, Shumway bluntly told a *Discover* magazine journalist, "From what I've seen so far, the mechanical heart is nothing more than a marketing or an advertising gimmick."[201] In a *Today Show* segment, Shumway reiterated to host Bryant Gumbel his view: "The [total] artificial heart is really dangerous."[202] Shumway was, however, interested in VADs; these devices attached to the patient's heart, which was left intact and remained partially functional, often improving under its lessened workload. At the time, the Stanford transplant program was collaborating with Peer Portner to refine the Novacor left ventricular assist system to be used as a temporary device for the deteriorating cardiac patient awaiting a donor heart. In 1984 Stanford surgeon Philip Oyer performed the world's first successful VAD implant as a bridge to transplant, with the Novacor device.[203]

In 1987 Symbion announced a modest profit to its shareholders. In large part it was due to the introduction of two new products, an artificial ear and a VAD, as well as the sales and services related to the Jarvik-7 and smaller Jarvik 7-70 hearts.[204] A battery-powered, rather than air-driven, Jarvik-8 heart was under development in the lab, but it was a low priority for Symbion.[205] That same year, the investment firm of E. M. Warburg Pincus and Company mounted a successful takeover bid. Jarvik vehemently opposed it, but the Symbion board overrode his objections to the sale.[206] Reportedly at odds with the board for some time, Jarvik was fired soon after Warburg Pincus took control of the company.[207] The volatility often associated with start-up companies, such as Kolff's, speaks to the strong innovator-research personality and the high-cost, bureaucratic task of bringing a new device into the medical marketplace as standard practice. There was minimal media coverage of Symbion's takeover and Jarvik's dismissal from the company. At the time, press reporting asserted that the artificial heart was "thriving" as a bridge device.[208] In Washington, DC, the Smithsonian Institution celebrated the donation of the Jarvik-7 heart that had been implanted in Michael Drummond as a valuable contribution to the national collection.[209] It was as a temporary measure that the TAH found support, in contrast to the growing disapproval of its use as a permanent therapy.

Criticism of the TAH became more discernible and vociferous with its increased use in the second half of the decade, peaking in 1988 when the device was dubbed "The Dracula of Medical Technology" in a *New York Times* editorial.[210] This piece supported the decision by Dr. Claude Lenfant, director of the National Heart, Lung, and Blood Institute (NHLBI), to cancel federal funding for development of an artificial heart as an implantable, permanent device. (Few people knew that Lenfant actually wrote the unsigned op-ed.)[211] The editorial stated, "During its 24-year life this Dracula of a program sucked $240 million out of the National Heart, Lung and Blood Institute. At long last, the institute has found the resolve to drive a stake through its voracious creation." According to the piece, it took the suffering of five individuals (four in the United States, one in Sweden) to demonstrate that this noisy, burdensome technology offered limited benefits at great cost. Measures of prevention, argued the editorial, are always superior to heroic cures in the fight against disease. Additional newspaper articles echoed the sentiment that government dollars were better spent on heart disease prevention rather than daring replacement technologies.[212] This prevention-treatment dispute was not new, but now it was situated in the broader debate of the 1970s and the 1980s concerning medicine's overall contribution to society's well-being.

Contemporary mistrust and cynicism toward the conventional goals and achievements of medicine fractured the attitudes of optimism and faith in medicine that had prevailed in the 1950s and the 1960s. Thomas McKeown, Ivan Illich, and other commentators contended that medicine placed too much emphasis on cure; some argued that misguided and risky treatments did more harm than good, and others called for a more humanistic, less technology-centered approach in medicine.[213] The clinical use of the artificial heart, with its high costs and questionable returns in quality of life, fueled the debate about the role of curative technologies in medicine. A curative medicine approach foregrounds what has been and can be achieved, and it leads to uncertainty about medical activities when curative technologies, such as artificial hearts, fail to deliver promised outcomes. Still, the hope for medical cure and beneficial treatment will never be completely extinguished, only dampened, with ebbs and flows when it comes to lowering the incidence and prevalence of such deadly diseases as heart failure and cancer. The spectrum of clinical care encompasses disease prevention as well as supportive, curative, rehabilitative, and palliative care. The extent to which medicine and society invest in each is linked to perceptions of related disease management success.

During this period, a new emphasis on individual responsibility for health drew attention to behavioral and lifestyle choices, supporting greater preventive medicine initiatives. Epidemiologists and social scientists studying heart disease, dating from the Framingham Heart Study of 1948 (still ongoing), emphasized the identification of risk factors and related preventive strategies to avoid cardiac problems. For most cardiologists, however, the preventive cardiology movement really emerged in the 1980s with the availability of pharmacological options, notably cholesterol-lowering statin drugs, bolstered by industry and obvious economic incentives therein.[214] Broad-based preventive medicine, not targeted curative interventions (which may or may not work), resonated with many individuals as the more appropriate focus and allocation of medical resources.

The Jarvik-7 clinical experience of near success contributed to the uncertainty surrounding the further development of this imperfect technology. The 1988 editorial emphasized the prevention-treatment debate and gave the artificial heart a contemptuous moniker—"The Dracula of Medical Technology"—that haunted the technology for decades to come. It was a negative spotlight, one that gained public attention and intensified debate and led to more forceful political tactics that ultimately decided program funding. Such criticisms of the device, the perceived lack of federal oversight of the artificial heart program, and the prevention-or-treatment debate were hardly new; throughout the 1980s, bioethicists had queried the various actions of the NHLBI, the FDA, and artificial heart researchers, thereby prompting more agency review and Congressional hearings.

Divergent Opinions and Assessments: Bioethicists and Politicians Weigh In

Bioethics emerged in the 1960s as an interdisciplinary field of academic study in response to advancements in medical science (for example, the availability of new technologies such as in vitro fertilization) and cultural change (including challenges to authority and the rise of patient rights).[215] It was also responding to various research scandals, such as the Tuskegee Syphilis Study and Willowbrook hepatitis experiments, in which patients have unknowingly been subjected to harmful studies.[216] Whereas traditional medical ethics guided doctors in their individual relationships with patients, bioethics sought to provide guidelines relating to broader socioeconomic issues and incorporate greater public involvement and control over medical care and treatment. Central to the new bioethics movement was individual choice, or patient autonomy. Decision making needed to include the research subject or patient to ensure that researchers working with human subjects assessed risks and benefits that were not self-serving and physicians reached critical medical judgments that were not idiosyncratic.[217] Bioethicists study the thorny social, economic, ethical, and political factors associated with medical problems and therapies, such as organ transplantation, reproductive technologies, kidney dialysis, end-of-life care, and health care justice. Their goal is to guide patients, doctors, lawyers, hospitals, government, policymakers, and society in managing many of the dilemmas surrounding medical advancement. The first centers devoted to the study of bioethical questions were the Hastings Center in New York, founded by philosopher Daniel Callahan and psychiatrist Willard Gaylin in 1970, and the Kennedy Institute of Ethics, which opened at Georgetown University in Washington, DC, in 1971. More bioethics centers and academic units emerged thereafter, partly because of such controversial new medical technologies as the artificial heart.

By the late 1970s and the 1980s, the study of bioethics had become institutionalized, and bioethicists were the experts, tasked with addressing the problematic outcomes of the new medical technologies. The notoriety of the Barney Clark case signaled that bioethics had arrived, according to physician-historian Barron Lerner.[218] Bioethicists closely followed Clark's case, homing in on the issue of informed consent and patient autonomy. Did Clark really know what he was getting into before the operation? Did he have the option to say "enough" when recovery appeared elusive? Lerner points to a tension between the bioethicists who seek to "protect" the rights and bodies of patients and the individuals who battle horrific illnesses and assume levels of risk that are perhaps not understandable to outsiders.[219] Bioethicists also weighed in on the larger socioeconomic issues associated with the artificial heart. This narrative countered the more common one of the artificial heart as medical progress. Government agencies such as the NIH sought bioethical guidance; however, excessive criticism was not wanted. Criticism of technology by bioethicists contributed to the perception that bioethicists were antitechnology, or antimedicine, or antiscience, which was not necessarily true. Bioethicists struggled to balance biases while retaining a constructive skepticism as to whether biomedical science and technology contributed to an improved society and to individuals' wellbeing. In the case of the artificial heart implants of the 1980s, the bioethical discourse was less antitechnology in tone than skeptical of the process and benefits of

this experimental therapy. Bioethicists raised many issues, including patient selection criteria (the issue of access), cost (psychological and financial), informed
consent (the issue of autonomy), the criteria for success (patient quality of life), and
patient self-determination (terminating the experiment).[220]

Two of the more interesting lines of the bioethical discussion were the use of
human subjects in medical research and the priorities of public funding in fighting
disease. First, the TAH cases of the 1980s obscured the issues of therapy and experimentation, thus attracting concern regarding the use of human subjects in medical
research and the hot-button issue of informed consent. Was the TAH being implanted as a "life-saving" treatment (so readily reported by newspapers) or to test the
fit and performance of the device as part of the experimental continuum? Was the
intent to treat the patient or to gain data on the device for researchers? Surgeon William DeVries would have responded, "Both."[221]

Bioethicists argued that using human subjects, regardless of intent, required attention to IRB and FDA regulation (protection of the public) and informed consent
(autonomy of the patient). Arthur Caplan of the Hastings Center criticized the regulatory and institutional controls—or lack thereof—in the case of Denton Cooley's
1969 and 1981 artificial heart implants; he was astonished at the silence of the FDA
and the NIH in the aftermath of those well-publicized cases.[222] George Annas, pro-
fessor of health law, bioethics, and human rights at Boston University, criticized the
informed consent form presented to Barney Clark, acknowledging that, though it
was an improvement over consent forms for past implant patients, it did not account
for "halfway success." The form assumed that Clark would either die or survive the
procedure and remain competent; instead, Clark suffered numerous strokes, respiratory complications, bouts of mental confusion, and other difficulties. Annas argued that Utah should have anticipated Clark's "halfway success" and customized
the consent form to allow some measure of self-determination and dignity (such as
asking, When should the experiment end?).[223] The University of Utah IRB committee did contemplate this issue—what if Clark survived the operation but remained
extremely ill? The committee insisted that such a scenario be bluntly presented in the
consent form.[224] The consent form clearly listed all the things that might go wrong,
such as emboli causing a stroke, malfunction of the device, infection of the drive line,
hemorrhaging, and damage to the red blood cells. The procedure as <u>experimental</u>
was underlined. There were "no guarantees concerning the result of the operation"—
Clark would probably require continued hospitalization and medical care and further
surgery and would probably experience considerable postoperative pain and discomfort. And still he agreed to the procedure, signing the consent form twice.[225]

Adding to the debate on patient self-determination was a *New York Times* article
entitled "Artificial Heart Recipients Will Have Choice on Life," which stated that
there was a "key" to "turn off" the machine powering the artificial heart in Barney
Clark's chest. The key was both a physical instrument and a metaphor. Could Barney Clark actually terminate the experiment by using this key to stop the artificial

heart, effectively ending his life by his own hand? The physical key did exist, and it locked the air compressor "on" to prevent accidental shutoff. Initially, DeVries held this key, and then it was unceremoniously taped to the back of the machine, without any discussion of "patient self-determination." According to DeVries, Clark knew the key was there but did not express any desire to use it.[226] It is debatable whether Clark would actually have been strong enough to get out of bed, reach for the key, and turn off the machine, even if he wanted to end his life.

In late 1983, at an "after Barney Clark" conference organized by University of Utah officials, a small group of bioethicists, journalists, and scholars joined the Utah artificial heart team and local participants to reflect on and discuss broader nonmedical issues arising out the Barney Clark case. The conference was designed to offer debate rather than instruction; however, university officials really hoped for some clarity, even a guide, as to how best to navigate the complicated legal, governmental, socioeconomic, bioethical, and media issues surrounding clinical artificial heart cases. Speakers included bioethicists Albert R. Jonsen and Jay Katz, social scientist Renée Fox, medical reporter Lawrence Altman, historian Stanley Reiser, and others. There was debate, with notable tension and disagreement, particularly coming from the Utah medical team as they reacted to the social and bioethical criticism of their program. In the end, the conference did not provide answers for "smoother roads" for university officials and future implant cases. "We have learned that no outside experts or consultants can do our job for us," commented F. Ross Woolley, former chair of the Utah IRB's artificial heart subcommittee.[227] No meaningful consensus emerged out of the conference.

Not surprisingly, one of the key topics raised by bioethicists at the Utah conference was the method of obtaining informed consent from Barney Clark. Unknown outcomes might be anticipated by what bioethicist Albert R. Jonsen suggested, a greater emphasis on negotiation between the patient and the doctor—much like Annas's notion of customizing cases—instead of a static "one-size-fits-all" consent document. Jonsen proposed measures to protect the patient, whereas most medical attendees at the conference viewed informed consent as necessary to protect the hospital and to satisfy university lawyers, the IRB, the FDA, and insurance carriers.[228] Annas argued that the consent form was not well thought out in Arizona either, and he dismantled the Arizona team's justification for implanting the unapproved Phoenix heart.[229] In this instance, lawyer Ellen Flannery implied "regulatory malpractice" by the FDA for failing to protect the public against such devices as the Phoenix heart and suggested that surgeons should be put on notice that such practices of implanting unapproved devices in patients was unethical.[230] Lerner astutely asked, "Should this version thus be considered the definitive story—that Barney Clark [or any other artificial heart recipient], while knowing what he was getting into, nevertheless submitted to an ill-advised and ultimately harmful experiment?"[231] This line of questioning by bioethicists represented only one of many narratives that were occurring.

A second part of the debate questioned the priorities of public funding in fighting disease—prevention or cures? To what extent should public funding support such heroic technologies as the artificial heart? Two days after Barney Clark died, a *New York Times* editorial asked, Was it worthwhile?[232] The issue of quality of life prompted many bioethicists to suggest that many end-of-life technologies only prolonged death, and that public funds would be better spent on prevention programs rather than heroic therapies.[233] Prevention was indeed less glamorous, yet arguably preferable to the costs and limited benefits of the artificial heart in terms of dollars and quality of life.[234] Jonsen argued more forcefully that the high costs of the artificial heart threatened to deprive many people of needed medical care, either in the case of public funds directed away from much needed, more cost-effective prevention programs or in the case of a patient's inability to pay for this expensive device, once perfected. Ironically, Jonsen served on the NIH Working Group in 1985 that reviewed the artificial heart program, and this panel recommended that NIH continue to fund this research. He defended his position by stating that a publicly controlled effort to develop and test the device was preferable to private sector or foreign development of the artificial heart, for reasons of equitable access.[235]

Challenging the endorsement of preventive measures over heroic therapies, according to others, was the technological momentum of the artificial heart. The medical writer Gideon Gil concluded that despite bad patient outcomes, questions of fairness, and informed consent issues, the momentum of the artificial heart was too strong to be stopped, that the results had not been "sour" enough to make profit-seeking manufacturers and alike abandon the device.[236] The momentum of the artificial heart was due, in part, to the lack of an organized opposition to the technology, according to the Seattle cardiologist Thomas Preston. He argued for a public debate on "whether we as a nation want to use it."[237] The historian Barton Bernstein agreed with the need for more public forums, criticizing the persistent closed decision-making practices of the program that were dominated by biomedical experts without much scrutiny by Congress. He also commented on the remarkable technological optimism that had characterized the government-sponsored artificial heart program since its inception.[238] Fox and Swazey identified it as "ritualized optimism" that blended scientific knowledge and clinical judgment with a degree of optimism in the face of uncertainty.[239] Criticizing artificial heart research for taking place in a "largely unquestioning and unquestioned way," Fox and Swazey were clearly disturbed by "the zeal with which the quest for a viable mechanical heart was pursued."[240]

In an attempt to address these concerns, NIH officials commissioned two panel reviews in the 1980s. The NHLBI had maintained a practice of periodic peer review of its artificial heart program from its inception. Arguably a more closed and controlled forum, these review panels attempted to allow for a detached "outsider," albeit medical expert, assessment. They issued recommendations that the NHLBI made public and attempted to follow. In the end, however, these recommendations did not radically challenge or alter the course of the program, despite the inclusion of bioethicists and lay people in the review process.

In 1981 the well-publicized intention of the Utah artificial heart team to implant a Jarvik-7 heart in a human (most notably, their FDA application for IDE status) prompted NHLBI director Dr. Robert I. Levy to form a working group of non-government experts in the field of mechanical circulatory support to evaluate the technical, social, ethical, and economic issues related to the development of an artificial heart. Specifically, this working group was asked to provide two sets of recommendations that addressed issues pertaining to NHLBI's artificial heart program in general and the reported plans for the use of the Jarvik-7 heart at the University of Utah. As in previous program reviews, this nine-person working group (eight of whom were cardiac medical specialists) recommended continuing NHLBI support for artificial heart research, stating that Utah's plans to implant the Jarvik-7 heart in a human was "not a justification for interrupting an orderly development of mechanical circulatory support devices."[241] Other recommendations stated concerns about clinical research conduct and processes, informed consent, quality-of-life issues, and publicity influences, among others. Interestingly, the working group recommended the appointment of a multidisciplinary standing committee to provide greater oversight. The report suggested, "Rather than reviewing the direction and scientific merit of the NHLBI's program at a single point in time, as previous task forces and panels have done, this standing committee would provide *ongoing surveillance* of this important and *potentially controversial* form of therapy."[242] The importance of bioethics and its role in emerging new medical therapies had certainly not been overlooked by NIH officials or experts working in the field. The report neither endorsed nor opposed Utah's plans explicitly, but it did ask researchers to consider VADs that would not require the removal of the patient's heart. Inferred in this document is the expectation that the Utah artificial heart team would proceed with the clinical use of their device, and thus the working group recommended greater involvement of NHLBI and lay participants to address anticipated controversial issues.

After the Barney Clark case, the NIH's artificial heart program was evaluated once again when NHLBI director Dr. Claude Lenfant convened a review panel consisting of nongovernmental medical experts in the field as well as a bioethicist, a social worker, and a lay member. This working group of 13 individuals (of which 7 held MDs and 4 held PhDs) met between September 1983 and February 1985 before submitting their report.[243] The timing is notable, since the group's report is situated within the maelstrom of media attention surrounding the clinical cases of Barney Clark and William Schroeder as well as the robust tide of support for assistive rather than replacement devices. The report's recommendations addressed both of these issues, but it did not refer directly to any specific Jarvik-7 implants. In the end, the working group supported the artificial heart program, their evaluation characterized by one panel member as "a cool and somewhat ambiguous endorsement."[244] They recommended that research on mechanical circulatory support systems should continue, with a return to the original program vision of developing a range of devices; the devices should include partial assistive devices as well as total replacement devices, for both temporary and permanent implantation. Clearly there existed a tension within the research community over the displacement (valid or not) of the TAH device by VADs. The report recommended, "Society should be presented with a balanced view of MCSSs, so that it can anticipate the problems and failures that will be encountered, as well as the hoped-for successes."[245] The members of the working group questioned the public's understanding of the artificial heart and the role played by the media, public relations officials, and others. Society's optimism needed to be kept in check.

The NHLBI review panel's recommendations for increased oversight of the Jarvik-7 implants were addressed more directly by the FDA that year. In 1985 FDA officials, feeling the pressure, took action on two occasions. First, they attempted— then retracted—a serious rebuke of Copeland's decision to implant an unauthorized artificial heart into a dying patient in Arizona. Several bioethicists called for strong FDA action to censure this case of "emergency human experimentation," but in the end, FDA officials simply issued a warning to Copeland to adhere to FDA procedures in the future.[246] This event prompted FDA officials to issue new guidelines covering emergency use of such unapproved devices, offering surgeons a "one-time permit" to use devices without IDE status. The second action taken by FDA officials that year occurred in December, when they convened an advisory panel to assess whether the complications encountered in the first four permanent implants performed by DeVries warranted a withdrawal of FDA approval for any further cases. Several members of the medical and bioethical community had expressed concern about the lack of oversight and scientific reporting regarding DeVries's implant cases after he moved to Louisville, with some critics calling for an official moratorium on further implants. Dr. Charles McIntosh, chairman of the FDA's circulatory system advisory panel, reported that the committee "did not come to any clear-cut conclusion as to whether the problems were device-related"; they recommended that artificial heart implants be allowed to continue, hoping that "the next three patients will provide valuable information."[247] But they also recommended that the FDA take a greater oversight role, specifically, that it increase report requirements, review patient care plans after each case, and adopt a case-by-case FDA approval strategy, with the restriction of no more than one patient every three months. One reporter referred to the FDA inquiry as a "trip to the woodshed" for DeVries and the Humana medical team for lax practices that hereafter would be subject to increased oversight.[248] Jarvik-7 participants denounced the recommendations as bureaucratic overregulation that hampered innovation.[249]

In 1986 a congressional subcommittee held hearings to examine the direction of the government-sponsored artificial heart program. The purpose of the hearings was not to end the program, but to "promote continued progress in an ethically and medically responsible manner."[250] Responding to allegations of human experimentation and negligent oversight by the FDA and the NHLBI, Congress invited both proponents and opponents of the artificial heart to propose how best to proceed. Participants included medical researchers, cardiac surgeons, NHLBI and FDA officials, bioethicists, and family members of implant recipients. Artificial heart insiders Jack Copeland, William DeVries, and Robert Jarvik reported on patient lives saved, scientific knowledge gained, and the therapeutic potential of the device for a nation battling heart disease. Invested in the use of this technology, these device advocates pressed for greater funding for the NHLBI's artificial heart program and opposed increased government regulation. At the other end of the spectrum, Sidney Wolfe, director of the Public Citizen Health Research Group in Washington, DC, called for increased FDA regulation, while bioethicist George Annas proposed a new umbrella advisory group to work alongside the NIH, the FDA, and local IRB officials. Both Wolfe and Annas wanted stronger public oversight of this experimental technology, introducing nonmedical experts to the decision-making process. "Trust in the expertise of those of us who have trained and dedicated ourselves to cardiac surgery and transplantation," urged Copeland, who, like many medical persons, could see little benefit in a nonmedical advisory group.[251]

Strong lines were drawn between artificial heart team members expressing the need to move forward unimpeded, motivated by a mix of altruism and self-interest, and their critics, who warned of zealous, out-of-control use of the device. DeVries stated, "The trend toward bureaucratic overregulation is a real impediment to scientific progress."[252] Annas responded, "The real possibility exists that the tragic 'me too' orgy of heart transplants that followed Dr. Christiaan Barnard's first human heart transplants in 1968 could be repeated."[253] New FDA emergency guidelines for the use of unauthorized artificial hearts constituted an attempt to counter this possibility, yet Annas, Wolfe, and others wanted greater FDA control. McIntosh commented on the delicate balance of the FDA "to act both as an accelerator pedal and as a brake pedal" in their efforts to facilitate access to new, potentially life-saving products while guarding patient safety.[254] Representatives of the NHLBI, the FDA, and the Department of Health and Human Services did not advocate for additional regulatory mechanisms at this time, stating that each agency had intervened appropriately in the past to ensure the proper direction of the NHLBI's artificial heart program. In the end, Congress did not intervene further, thus contributing to the confusion and contestation surrounding the use of the artificial heart.

Throughout the 1980s, there emerged divergent meanings and ambiguous assessments of artificial heart technology. When the NHBLI review panel announced their endorsement of continued support for the artificial heart research program, NHLBI director Claude Lenfant told reporters that he was "surprised," interpreting the decision as "a strong directive for us to continue what we started and to mount new programs to develop fully implantable artificial hearts."[255] The bioethicist Albert R. Jonsen, a member of the review panel, countered by stating that this was inaccurate; the working group recommended only that the present effort continue. In his defense of the panel's recommendation, he alluded to the inevitability of the development of the artificial heart. "A call to cease and desist from any techno-logical development prior to significant demonstrations of its inefficacy, inefficiency, or danger seems bound to fail in our society. The technological imperative, particu-larly when linked to marketability, is powerful. We have, in fact, almost no effective means to bring such developments to a halt. FDA controls on development are limited and specific."[256] Both panels recognized the medical community's shift to the more promising VADs but were hesitant to end funding for TAH research. Perhaps it was too late, as implied by Jonsen; perhaps the technological momentum of the TAH was too great, so it was best to stay involved, mediating its use. But Lenfant's actions in 1988 constituted a challenge to that technological momentum.

In May 1988, Lenfant announced the cancellation of $22.6 million in research contracts (over six years) that had been awarded only four months earlier to four research groups to develop a new, electrically powered, fully implantable TAH.[257] Officially, he defended this decision by citing poor experience with TAHs to date and current funding reallocation needs for the more promising VADs, which were nearing clinical trials. Personally, Lenfant did not support the development of TAHs. It was his view that the Jarvik-7 heart implant cases were a failure and that the technology would not overcome its problems for many years, if ever. He told Fox and Swazey, "I'd rather be put in my grave than have to be five years with such a device."[258] One of Lenfant's management strengths was finding money to support projects that he deemed worthwhile. He favored the development of the less radical VAD, and after encouraging lab results were presented in late 1987, he began maneu-vering financial budgets to ensure funding for clinical testing of these experimental devices. Phasing out all TAH research would provide that funding, but Lenfant later admitted to making a strategic error. Seeking to avoid rumors and misinformation, Lenfant asked Watson to deliver the bad news to the four research groups in advance of the public announcement. Lenfant did not anticipate how quickly and effectively the research groups united to lobby against the withdrawal of their funding, even reaching out to congressional politicians.[259] Lenfant's decision was extremely con-troversial, since it contradicted the 1985 review panel's recommendations and the original goal of the NHLBI's artificial heart program, and it incited strong responses from the contractors and the larger device research community. While some agreed with Lenfant's action based on the fiscal necessity of his decision, others argued that both lines of research were necessary since the devices would serve different patient populations. Moreover, dropping out of the race this way might allow competitors in Japan, Western Europe, and the Soviet Union to forge ahead in developing the artificial heart.[260]

Political pressure bore down on NIH officials to reinstate the funding when out-raged researchers in the field turned to Washington politicians. Led by senators Edward Kennedy (of Massachusetts) and Orrin Hatch (of Utah), Congress threat-ened to block funding for all new NIH programs until all long-term commitments to previous programs—such as the artificial heart research contracts—were honored. (Not coincidentally, the two artificial heart research programs that would be directly affected by this NIH funding decision were Abiomed Inc. of Danvers, Massachusetts, and the University of Utah in Salt Lake City.) NIH director Dr. James B. Wyngaarden conceded, not wanting to jeopardize future budgets. Forced to "eat a little crow," Lenfant reversed his decision, realizing that he had been outmaneuvered, but he resented the congressional intrusion of "a handful of senators [working] in private negotiations with the institutes."[261] The editorial page of the *New York Times* agreed, stating, under the headline "Senators Doctors Kennedy and Hatch"—with a slash crossing out the word *Senators*—that Kennedy and Hatch had "second-guessed Dr Lenfant in a way that lards their own pork barrels."[262] In the end, funding for TAH development continued, and Lenfant redirected money from other NHLBI programs to fund the VAD work.

Then in 1990, the FDA recalled the Jarvik-7 heart, withdrawing its earlier IDE approval, citing record-keeping and quality control problems by Symbion Inc.[263] By the next year, the FDA instructed Symbion that use of its mechanical hearts must cease immediately. In compliance with this ruling, Symbion asked that hospitals destroy the devices or render them unusable.[264] The Jarvik-7 heart was no longer available for implantation. Overall, hospital demand for the device had fallen. In comparison with the TAH, VADs offered surgeons more flexible patient management as bridge-to-transplantation support. There had been no more permanent implantation of the device since Jack Burcham in 1985. Furthermore, members of the earlier Jarvik-7 team were not interested in fighting Symbion's battle with the FDA. In 1988 Robert Jarvik moved to New York to focus on the development of the Jarvik 2000 VAD and his new company, Jarvik Research Inc. That same year, William DeVries left Humana to concentrate on building his surgical practice; he expressed no further interest in implanting artificial hearts.[265] NHLBI-funded researchers at the Cleveland Clinic, Pennsylvania State University, and the Texas Heart Institute were working on the next-generation TAH—one that was fully implantable and was electrically, rather than pneumatically, driven. As stated by Jack Copeland, "the heyday of the Jarvik-7 [had] passed," its clinical use apparently over, with the knowledge gained to be encapsulated in a better, technologically superior device.[266]

Resiliency and Adjustment

Three significant things emerged out of the Jarvik-7 clinical cases of the 1980s that influenced the development of artificial hearts over the next two decades. First, it was clear that the technology was flawed, most critically its blood-biomaterial interaction and risk of embolism; future devices would have to be better. Building a clinically useful artificial heart remained a challenge, because the body's systems are innately opposed to implanted objects of metal and plastic. "We thought the problem wasn't going to be as complicated as it turned out to be," admitted William S. Pierce, inventor of the Penn State TAH. "As we've solved some problems, we've uncovered others."²⁶⁷ Some researchers in the field suggested that the Jarvik-7 heart might play a role as a temporary device for bridge-to-transplantation use, but others called for its outright abandonment, arguing that the patient risk of embolism and strokes, as well as its tethering to power drives, undermined its efficacy and reliability. In 1988 Lenfant told reporters, "While the device itself seemed to work well, the biology didn't work. The human body just couldn't seem to tolerate it. . . . We were left wondering whether the idea of a permanent replacement will ever work. . . . but it may also help us develop a device that works better."²⁶⁸ There was clearly an ambivalence about the meaning of the poor clinical results with the imperfect technology. Should artificial heart research stop because of the "failed promises" of the Jarvik-7 heart? Or, conversely, had researchers now gained a valuable understanding of the operation and function of mechanical pumps in humans that could be applied to improving the technology?

In hindsight, it is clear that this experimental device was not ready for clinical use as a permanent heart replacement. When poor patient results were reported, the implants were widely criticized as premature. Calves were not people, and more harm than good had been experienced by patients Barney Clark, William Schroeder, and others. Artificial heart researchers countered that valuable knowledge had been gained from these clinical cases that could not have been produced in the lab. According to cardiothoracic surgeon Robert Bartlett, the case of Barney Clark sent a wave of excitement through the field. It embodied decades of research in dozens of laboratories, demonstrating that normal organ function could be sustained with a mechanical heart, although thrombotic complications needed to be addressed.²⁶⁹ Nuclear physicist Peer Portner, inventor of the Novacor left ventricular assist system, stated that Barney Clark's 112-day experience with the Jarvik-7 heart provided more complete information about the placement and function of an artificial heart than had been possible with the earlier short-term Houston experiences with the Liotta and Akutsu artificial hearts.²⁷⁰ Researchers in the field of mechanical circulatory support systems all agreed that the Jarvik-7 cases were milestone cases, not for being the first clinical implants or for delivering improved patient health, but for boldly demonstrating that artificial hearts could replace human hearts in people. Texas Heart Institute surgeon O. H. Frazier applauded the Utah artificial heart team, saying, "We certainly are indebted in this field to the Utah Group for getting us off the farm, if you will, and into the clinical area with the artificial heart. No matter what the outcome of this, their place will never be among those timid and cold souls that know neither victory nor defeat."²⁷¹

For the public, it was a case of hope and fear, the hope that experimental devices would work along with the fear that the use of the devices might make patients worse off in the end. They hoped that the artificial heart would deliver additional time to dying cardiac patients to attend family weddings, to welcome new grandchildren, and more. This happened for some artificial heart patients, although their postoperative experiences included many complications. The negative outcomes of the Jarvik-7 permanent implant cases realized much of the fear surrounding experimental devices, and the hideous moniker "The Dracula of Medical Technology" stalked future artificial hearts, courtesy of the media. Clinical uptake and acceptance of artificial hearts was now slower as a result, with hospitals, practitioners, and patients all wary of repeating the poor experiences. It was going to be an uphill battle for artificial heart researchers in many ways, including convincing the public that the technology had improved and that it was worth paying for and living with.

Second, bioethicists were now firmly entrenched in artificial heart matters. They found many clinical events and patient experiences in the 1980s to comment on, such as the surrogacy case of Baby M; Baby Fae's chimpanzee heart implant; the case of Libby Zion, whose death raised questions about the long working hours of medical residents in relation to patient safety; and the social and ethical issues surrounding HIV-AIDS. When it came to the Jarvik-7 implants, bioethicists raised many issues regarding aspects of human experimentation that predominantly focused on patient autonomy and patients' rights to receive and discontinue new clinical therapies. Who has the authority to say "enough" when complications arise? They explored the role of the FDA and hospital IRBs as "guardians" in policing enthusiastic clinical cases. They impressed upon the NIH that publicly funded projects needed to include social scientists, bioethicists, and other nonspecialists in their deliberations of continued support for research projects. By this time, artificial heart research programs—any medical research programs—hardly had the luxury not to include bioethicists, as a result of FDA regulations, new medical device legislation, hospital management structures, and the demands of the device industry. These were good measures, intending to protect the public good without stifling research innovation, although there was much grumbling from scientists unaccustomed to engaging with nonmedical outsiders. Yet, in situating these cases within the longer historical trajectory, one notes that many of the issues raised in the 1980s were not new. In the 1960s, issues of informed consent and the use of experimental treatments were monitored by institutional IRBs, such as the case at Baylor College of Medicine during Michael DeBakey's early artificial heart research. In the 1970s, concerns regarding the public good and the allocation of government funding were voiced surrounding the development of atomic hearts. What was different in the 1980s was that the role and opinion of bioethicists assumed a higher profile during the Jarvik-7 implants owing to the timing of this nascent movement. As a result, their involvement in future artificial heart patient trials was now assured.

Third, the clinical cases of the 1980s revealed the involvement of additional stakeholders in the development of artificial hearts by this time. The sandbox had become crowded with different groups engaged for different reasons, with varying degrees of power and influence. The traditional stakeholders were the researchers, medical practitioners, patients, and NHLBI officials who were motivated by the scientific challenge, by being involved in a new clinical therapy, by stalling death, and by the national investment in cutting-edge American research. The clinical introduction of artificial hearts brought industry, for-profit hospitals, bioethicists, and politicians into the mix in a more prominent way than in the past. The commercialization of devices was too costly and time-consuming for academic researchers, who welcomed (and often invested their own money in) device companies for the purpose of developing their prototypes. Through its artificial heart program, NHLBI officials promoted academic-industry research collaborations through their contract funding mechanism, which was expected to lead to industry commercial development. By the 1980s, Symbion Inc. and its vigorous marketing of the Jarvik-7 heart exemplified such development. For-profit hospitals, like Humana, latched onto the artificial heart to seek publicity as a leading technology health care facility. Bioethicists raised numerous issues surrounding the business of medical devices as well as the experimental nature of these early clinical cases. Politicians weighed in at various times; sometimes they held hearings to shed light on the state of the field, with questionable impact, and other times they championed the research work being done in their constituencies. They wanted to maintain a public perception of research support for solutions to the nationwide problem of heart disease.

In 1988 the fate of the TAH was precarious. Given the disconcerting outcomes of DeVries's implants, public disillusionment propagated by the media, the business troubles of Symbion Inc., and the desire by some NHLBI officials to stop funding for the device, this was the moment when the limits of the TAH seemed apparent. Surely this was the time when most stakeholders would acknowledge the infeasibility of artificial hearts over their desirability. At this moment, the contentious debate surrounding the Jarvik-7 cases seemed strong enough to break, or at least retract, the momentum behind the development of artificial hearts as a technological fix for heart failure. But it did not. The majority of stakeholders endorsed more than countered the scientific enthusiasm to build artificial hearts. Some critics such as social scientists Fox and Swazey had become alienated by the drive to "rebuild people." They called it a "hubris-ridden" endeavor of "overzealous" researchers that was diverting attention and resources away from other basic health care needs.[272] The Jarvik-7 cases did not quash the pursuit of TAHs, from the perspective of artificial heart researchers, some clinicians, industry, and politicians. Yet these cases did affect Humana's position: Humana executives withdrew institutional support of an artificial heart program when they recognized that Jarvik-7 permanent implants no longer garnered positive publicity and that the program appeared to be nowhere near an acceptable therapeutic course for heart failure anytime soon. However, these negative reactions were not enough to turn the tide entirely.

Extensive media coverage, characterized as "a sustained orgy of media excess" by Portner, significantly contributed to the contested 1980s period of artificial heart development and use.[273] Whereas the 1970s had been a decade of more critical and suspicious medical reporting, the 1980s resembled the 1960s in their celebration of innovation in science and technology. Dorothy Nelkin states that this 1980s style of reporting reflected press perceptions of what people wanted to read; thus, journalists shaped their stories to fit with prevailing hopes and beliefs in medical advances.[274] Contributing to such perceptions, institutions, researchers, and clinicians affiliated with the artificial heart promoted the technology with authority and enthusiasm. But by the mid to late 1980s, a more ambivalent, often negative, tone pervaded media reporting as a result of the turbulent medical courses of Barney Clark, William Schroeder, and other artificial heart recipients. DeVries told Louisville *Courier-Journal* reporter Gideon Gil that the negative news reports had a great impact on patient referrals; in 1985 more than 100 artificial heart requests a week had come into his office, but by 1988 that number had been reduced to an inquiry every other week.[275] Jarvik seriously wondered whether public criticism would indeed kill the entire artificial heart program.[276] The media provided a forum for political and bioethical debate of the artificial heart, bluntly challenging the earlier enthusiasm, even naïveté, surrounding this device as a potential technological fix for individuals in end-stage heart failure. Bioethicists and nonmedical commentators raised issues of patient autonomy, quality of life, cost, and genuine worry that perhaps medical technology had run amok. They expressed open misgivings about the use of this experimental device in humans, concerned that the Jarvik-7 heart was more harmful than beneficial. The Utah team bore the brunt of the criticism owing to their device-readiness stage, their open regulatory and business proceedings, and their commitment to using the Jarvik-7 heart as a permanent therapy.

The Utah team involved with the Jarvik-7 heart chose specific regulatory and business courses that contributed to the rise and fall of the device in the 1980s. By complying with FDA and IRB regulations, the Jarvik-7 team worked toward their goal of unencumbered (approved) marketability of the device, once perfected. They secured Investigational Device Exemption status for the Jarvik-7 heart in 1982 (this approval was later withdrawn by the FDA in 1990) as a step toward collecting clinical data to support a future premarket approval application to the FDA. The university-industry collaborations to develop new medical devices may be effective in bringing together key expertise, but they present a muddied setting for objective evaluations of the clinical use of these devices. Surgeons worked with for-profit device companies, together selling the experimental devices, such as the Jarvik-7 heart, and offering training sessions (at a cost) for hospital customers. For-profit hospitals clamored to acquire the latest technology, to raise their profile in a competitive medical marketplace.[277]

The formation of Kolff's start-up companies, which morphed into Symbion Inc., marked the transition of the Jarvik-7 heart from an investigational research device to an emerging commercial product, with the subsequent manufacturing and marketing challenges therein. The competition and financial demands of the medical device industry contribute to its volatility, and companies are absorbed by others in the health sector as they are in other sectors. Symbion worked to remain financially stable, changing from a privately owned to a publicly owned company that eventually ousted its two principal founders, Willem Kolff and Robert Jarvik. Ironically, it was the regulatory process, so duly followed through the years, that ended the distribution of the Jarvik-7 heart in the United States.

During the 1980s, other artificial heart research teams worked to devise better TAH devices than the Jarvik-7 heart. Cardiac surgeon William S. Pierce implanted the air-driven Penn State TAH, the only other TAH licensed for implant in the United States, in three different patients as a bridge device, but he reported no transplant survivors.[278] Developed by Pierce's research team, the Penn State TAH had a slightly different pump design, but arguably it was not any safer than the Jarvik-7 TAH. It represented more than a decade of research and had been tested in more than 60 calves before its implantation in a patient. It was not a competition, according to Penn State bioengineer Gerson Rosenberg and Utah researcher Don B. Olsen, who respected each other's work, discussed shared problems, and only sought to find the better approach.[279] In Germany and Austria, surgeons Emil S. Büecherl and Felix Unger implanted the experimental Berlin heart and Unger heart, respectively, to bridge several transplant patients. The European devices were air-driven and conceptually similar to the American TAHs but were no more successful.[280] By the late 1980s, early clinical data on the use of VADs reported that this technology worked as well as TAHs to bridge transplant patients. These were early days in which to declare the better device, but attaching a VAD to the heart, with the device resting outside the body, seemed intuitively to be the safer route. The increased clinical adoption of VADs translated into a declining use of the TAH overall.

By the end of the 1980s, the lack of public consensus regarding the success and meaning of the Jarvik-7 implants created an ambiguous environment for the artificial heart's development as compared to previous decades. But many artificial heart researchers were not put off and embraced the clinical experiences of the 1980s to improve the technology, surgical procedure, and postoperative patient care. Jack Copeland refused to abandon the Jarvik-7 technology, convinced of its necessity to provide biventricular support for many end-stage heart patients. Promising results with mechanical assist pumps suggested that the new LVADs would be safer, but what about the patient who needed mechanical support to off-load both failing ventricles? LVADs were not an option for patients with compromised right ventricle function. Copeland and his colleagues acknowledged the diversity of the heart failure patient population and supported research for many mechanical circulatory support devices, harking back to the Artificial Heart Program's original goal of building a family of cardiac devices. The challenges of bleeding, infection, and the need for a better implantable power source exposed through work with TAHs were also being studied by VAD researchers. VAD research gains with better biomaterials, device designs, or power sources might then transfer back to TAHs. Researchers had identified the problems, and they set out to resolve them; for Copeland, that meant improving the Jarvik-7 heart.

Jack Copeland and Don B. Olsen "saved" the Jarvik-7 technology by negotiating its transfer from Symbion Inc. to CardioWest Technologies Inc., a newly formed, nonprofit organization that was a joint venture of the University of Arizona Medical Center and the MedForte Research Foundation.[281] The device was re-named the CardioWest temporary TAH, and in 1992 Copeland received Investiga-tional Device Exemption approval from the FDA to use the device in six American medical centers as part of a clinical study; ultimately, four sites provided patient implant data. The research team reported a list of adverse patient events, from bleeding problems to drive line kinks, but positioned the artificial heart as a "suc-cess" since it had bridged the majority of the patients to cardiac transplantation. Minimal fanfare accompanied the implants; the technology still had flaws. Cope-land spent the next decade refining and implanting the CardioWest heart as a bridge to transplantation in dozens of patients, intending to commercialize the device for others to use.[282]

Elsewhere, artificial heart researchers also continued with their work, having just won a political battle with NHLBI officials to reinstate program funds. During the late 1980s and early 1990s, there were three major research programs with NHLBI contracts to develop implantable TAHs. Unlike the air-driven Jarvik-CardioWest technology, these were electrically powered artificial hearts under development in col-laborative academic-industry teams: the AbioCor heart at Abiomed Inc. in Massachu-setts, working with the Texas Heart Institute; the Penn State heart at the Pennsylvania State University Hershey Medical Center, working with Sarns 3M, in Michigan; and the Cleveland Clinic heart at the Cleveland Clinic Foundation, in collaboration with Nimbus Inc., of California. Research work on TAHs also continued at the University of Utah, the Baylor College of Medicine, the Milwaukee Heart Institute, and outside the United States, including Japan, Germany, and Austria.

In many of these labs, researchers also worked on VADs. TAH researchers were well aware of the state of VAD research and did not see VADs as competing devices, since they were limited to single ventricular support. In the lab, at meetings, and in publications, there was a natural crossover of VAD and TAH research concerning compatible biomaterials, drive systems, power sources, and other matters. With prom-ising clinical results starting to emerge, VADs gained more attention in both medical and nonmedical communities. The NHLBI awarded more funding for this line of research, contributing to a noticeable shift to partial artificial hearts that was happen-ing concurrently with the events surrounding the Jarvik-7 heart. NHLBI director Claude Lenfant had wanted to allocate greater funding to VADs in 1988, hedging his bets that this was the more promising technology. Less dramatic than the implant of a TAH, the VAD implants received moderate, more subdued media coverage. No doubt, they were orchestrated this way by academic and industry researchers ne-gotiating the FDA approval system with their respective VADs. In the aftermath of Barney Clark, the artificial heart research community was going to be tentative about any more pronouncements to the public of success or promising new devices.

Nonetheless, hopes for a technological fix for end-stage heart disease remained, despite the 1980s contentious experience with the Jarvik-7 heart. As suggested by

David Rothman in his analysis of the iron lung and the kidney dialysis machine, it was the "resurrectionist capacity" of such technologies that appealed to society and, most certainly, the media.[283] The bait was the promissory nature of artificial hearts as a life-sustaining treatment, a medical technology that might alter the usual course of events that when a person's heart failed, the person died. Artificial hearts teased society with a notion of immortality, but at best, any resurrection was certainly limited. With resiliency and determination, artificial heart researchers and their industry partners continued their research and development work, from which some stakeholders soon received clinical and commercial rewards—not with TAHs, but with VADs.

CHAPTER FIVE

Clinical and Commercial Rewards

Ventricular Assist Devices

Although some members of this [surgical meeting] audience may feel that such [VAD] devices are either impossibly expensive or ethically unrealistic, it is clear that they are rapidly emerging from the realm of science fiction to clinical application.

Dr. Eugene F. Bernstein, cardiovascular surgeon (1980)

A ventricular assist device is a type of mechanical heart that helps the weakened ventricles of the native heart to maintain blood circulation in the body. Conceptually, VADs, which do not replace the native heart, represented a less radical approach than total artificial hearts in mechanical circulatory support. In the majority of heart failure cases, patients suffered left ventricular malfunction, so arguably they needed mechanical pump support for only one side of the heart. By implanting this device, surgeons could provide cardiac assistance without removing the patient's biological heart. A VAD serves as a partial artificial heart; it unloads the pumping work of the heart and supports the pulmonary or systemic circulation. The standard device used for augmenting cardiac function in this period was the intraaortic balloon pump, developed in the previous decade by Adrian Kantrowitz. But balloon pumps worked only for limited and temporary assistance, and not in all heart failure cases. Extracorporeal membrane oxygenation (ECMO), delivered by a modified heart-lung bypass machine, provides temporary support for patients with reversible heart or lung failure and serves as a bridge to recovery or sometimes a bridge to a more robust support device.[1] During the 1980s, ECMO gained use as a mechanical circulatory support system for acute heart failure in roughly 50 specialized cardiac centers in the United States.[2] For about three decades, this technology provided the only cardiac support system for children, until the introduction of the Berlin Heart Pediatric VAD.[3] In comparison to balloon pumps and ECMO, VADs offered short-term assistance and more, filling an important niche for those patients requiring longer-term cardiac assistance.[4] VADs met the temporary circulatory support needs of the postoperative heart patient as a bridge-to-recovery (BTR) device as well as providing extended cardiac assistance for patients battling chronic heart failure.

There are numerous mechanical blood pumps classified as VADs. Some VADs are used singly to assist the function of the right ventricle (to pump unoxygenated blood through the pulmonary artery and into the lungs) or the left ventricle (to pump oxygenated blood to the ascending aorta and to the body). In some cases, a patient's condition may require biventricular support, and two VADs are used to assist the work of both ventricles. More often than not, heart failure presents first in the left ventricle, the heart's main pumping chamber. In this case, the left ventricle dilates or expands, holding more blood and ejecting less blood with every heartbeat. Less common is right ventricular failure, which usually occurs with left-side failure. VAD investigators experimented with both short- and long-term use of this device, as well as with its position outside (paracorporeal or external) and within the body (intracorporeal or implantable). In light of the ambiguous results of the Jarvik-7 TAH cases of the 1980s, many end-stage heart patients and medical practitioners opted for VADs as temporary assist devices for patient recovery after heart surgery or as bridge-to-transplant (BTT) devices to bolster deteriorating cardiac conditions while patients waited for donor hearts. Later, the Food and Drug Administration approved the permanent implant of some VADs, referred to as destination (or final) therapy for patients with end-stage heart failure who were poor candidates for heart transplantation.

It would be misleading to frame the history of this technology in binary terms, such as whether to develop a partial or total mechanical heart, whether to assist or replace a damaged heart, or whether to provide short- or long-term support. Since the beginning, the goal of the NIH's artificial heart program has been to develop a family of cardiac devices for MCSSs, for temporary and permanent use, in which assist pumps and TAH research programs would share basic science, bioengineering, and clinical knowledge, with the aim of serving a diverse and sizable cardiac patient population. Over the past 50 years, federal research grants and contracts have supported both lines of device research, focusing on component research and later device integration. Beginning in the 1970s, targeted federal funding for assist devices, from design concepts to prototype testing in clinical trials, stimulated new research and greater interest in VADs, laying the foundation for the development of this particular device.[5] The media, however, favored the more glamorous sibling—the TAH—despite FDA approval and commercialization of several promising VAD models during the 1980s and 1990s.

VADs are both similar to and different from TAHs in the ways they contribute to the MCSS family. VADs may be implanted inside the chest or situated outside the body, may be used for short or long durations, and may be used as a bridge to recovery, a bridge to transplantation, or a destination (permanent) therapy. Like TAH researchers, VAD investigators faced technological challenges of finding suitable biomaterials and power sources for their devices and reported operational difficulties of blood clotting, thrombus, and infection in animal models and patients. These shared device problems stimulated research crossover and exchange among the different artificial heart teams at various professional conferences. Not surprisingly, device projects overlapped in laboratories and among investigators. At the

University of Utah, Willem Kolff's laboratory developed both TAHs and VADs for several decades. Robert Jarvik lent his name to a TAH, the Jarvik-7 heart, and later to an assist pump, the Jarvik 2000 FlowMaker. At Baylor College of Medicine, Michael DeBakey's well-funded research program conducted TAH work, boasted the first cardiac assist devices implanted in humans in the 1960s, and, for decades thereafter, collaborated with the National Aeronautics and Space Administration and MicroMed Technology Inc. to develop the DeBakey VAD. Like TAH researchers, VAD investigators needed to navigate the FDA regulatory system to conduct clinical trials and to market their devices. With government funding and industry partnerships, VAD researchers moved their devices through clinical testing and product positioning in the marketplace more successfully than TAH investigators in the 1980s and 1990s. One key characteristic of VAD development was that academic researchers worked more collaboratively with experienced medical device companies, such as the Baxter Healthcare Corporation and the Thoratec Laboratories Corporation, to develop VAD technology. Not all devices transitioned from research prototypes to viable commercial products, however, and some companies spun off, sold off, or took over competing device product lines for a variety of reasons.

This chapter argues that VADs, not TAHs, made the greater gains toward clinical adoption, owing to their less complex nature, both technologically and conceptually, which facilitated industry collaboration and eased the formidable task of shepherding these devices through regulation, clinical trial, and commercialization stages. Industry buy-in and clinical uptake were linked to what this simpler device technology offered: the potential for fewer device problems and a wider patient population that might benefit from cardiac assistance rather than replacement. Intuitively, it seemed more doable and less drastic to all stakeholders to develop a viable device that would not require removal of the native heart. A VAD or partial artificial heart, not needing to compensate completely for the biological heart, left the patient's organ in place as a somewhat reassuring backup. Implanting a VAD—at a time when artificial heart valves and cardiac pacemakers were considered standard treatments—was much less radical than implanting a TAH. In addition, VAD recipients tended to be less-sick patients, with some ventricular function and less severe heart failure, and they often fared better than TAH recipients. Clinicians asserted that the hearts of many patients were not damaged enough to warrant complete removal and replacement with an imperfect TAH. In the 1970s and 1980s, VAD researchers addressed many of the technical bioengineering and patient care issues that beset TAHs and worked to develop smaller assist devices that would sustain a wider heart failure patient population.

Key funding for VAD research, such as the testing of biocompatible blood materials, power sources, and percutaneous (through the skin) or transcutaneous (across the skin) energy transmission mechanisms, as well as funding for integrated systems readiness trials and other matters, flowed through the circulatory support program at the National Heart, Lung, and Blood Institute. Investment by industry, such as by Thermo Cardiosystems Inc. and Thoratec Laboratories Corporation, significantly contributed to the marshaling of several VADs through product development, testing, and launching, positioning them within a marketplace already receptive to cardiovascular devices. In comparison to the TAH, more VAD prototypes were under development by industry groups in this period. This chapter foregrounds the science and business that shaped VAD technology as the more rewarding venture, technologically, conceptually, and commercially. The timing, the context, and the stakeholders involved—researchers, heart specialists, industry, government, and patients—shaped VAD development in a more incremental, less contentious, and lower-profile way, compared to TAH development.

The First-Generation Devices: The Pulsatile VADs of the 1980s

During the 1970s, the NHLBI prioritized the development of VADs over TAHs as a more manageable approach to address the significant technological and biocompatibility problems associated with mechanical circulatory support at this time. Designing a partial artificial heart that assisted rather than replaced the native heart appeared to be a less daunting task with a shorter development timeline, one that would bring a quicker return on investment. As recommended by the NHLBI Cardiology Advisory Committee, long-time NHLBI deputy director Peter Frommer initiated sizable funding for extramural research on the device materials, energy systems, blood pump, and associated mechanics needed to build a reliable short-term cardiac assist system. NHLBI officials insisted that the research and development undertaken for VADs would be directly applicable to TAHs thereafter (and much of it did transfer). Frommer also contributed to reorienting the mechanical heart program from nuclear-powered systems to electrically energized devices in this period.[6]

In 1976 John Watson, a mechanical engineer and physiologist, joined the NHLBI to oversee the artificial heart program. He shaped program goals, advocated new research areas, managed program finances, and nurtured investigator relationships to realize improved mechanical circulatory support systems. Watson instilled a "progressive style" of targeted, component research and deliverables that necessitated stronger academic-industry collaboration. This focus on components rather than system design was initially controversial, and some investigators balked at it. These artificial heart researchers argued that there would be significant problems with the system when it came time to integrate the components; they anticipated difficulties such as component mismatch, interface complexity, and compromised performance.[7] But the money was too good not to accept it and adapt, and the artificial heart community complied with NHLBI's approach. Watson was committed to developing the best devices with the best expertise within reasonable time lines, and he enjoyed a respected and congenial relationship with device researchers and industry executives in the field. Government funding in the form of one-year industry contracts gave way to multiyear development contracts, coupled with the standard investigator-initiated research grants, to address the significant engineering and basic science work needed. During his 27-year tenure at NHLBI, Watson provided sizable VAD research contracts to numerous collaborative academic-industry teams, sustaining their research programs when they might otherwise have been abandoned. He also facilitated NHLBI support of clinical testing, often working with researchers and industry leaders in the design of clinical trials. Driven to accelerate the development process to bring cardiac devices more quickly to market, Watson worked to assist VAD research teams with funding and regulatory guidance. During the 1970s the NHLBI, through the artificial heart program, doled out roughly $10 million a year, the majority of which supported VAD contracts rather than basic research grants.[8]

Greatly assisted by this NHLBI contract funding, four VAD research teams produced promising cardiac assist systems:

- Aerospace engineer David Lederman at Avco-Everett Research Labs led the development of a sac-type assist device (a multisegment balloon pump) called the AVCO LVAD, which later became the ABIOMED BVS 5000 manufactured by Abiomed Inc.
- Cardiac surgeon William S. Pierce led a team at Pennsylvania State University College of Medicine that devised a pusher-plate diaphragm type pump, the Pierce-Donachy pump, which was further developed and manufactured by the Thoratec Laboratories Corporation and renamed the Thoratec PVAD system.
- Physicist-turned-bioengineer Peer Portner at Andros Inc. built a dual pusher-plate diaphragm type pump referred to as the Andros solenoid-actuated LVAS system, later the Novacor LVAS distributed by Baxter HealthCare Corporation, Edwards Lifesciences LLC, and eventually the WorldHeart Corporation.
- Texas Heart Institute cardiac surgeon John C. Norman teamed up with Thermo Electron Engineering Corporation's engineer Victor Poirier to develop a pusher-plate diaphragm type pump, which evolved into the HeartMate assist device, manufactured by Thermo Cardiosystems Inc.[9]

With the acceptance of NHLBI contracts came mandatory attendance at NHLBI-organized contractors' meetings to present and exchange research information, intended to facilitate better and timely device development. While sharing research knowledge was familiar practice among academic researchers, industry partners were sometimes more guarded, cautious about giving out too much proprietary information. Nonetheless, Poirier remembers these meetings as beneficial and productive in the overall development of the technology.[10] Individuals from the FDA and other government regulatory agencies often participated in these contractors' meetings to help industry navigate necessary device-approval stages for clinical trials. In the end, the NHLBI's focus on partial artificial hearts and the agency's novel development approach paid off.

The NHLBI's contract-supported, component research and integrated systems approach that forged academic-industry partnerships resulted in the resolution of many of the technological challenges of mechanical circulatory support for VAD development in advance of TAH work. The AVCO LVAD, operating on the counter-pulsation principle, evolved into a reliable external biventricular cardiac assist system; it is catheter-mounted for short-term use in predominantly postoperative patients. In 1992 it became the first cardiac assist device approved by the FDA for sale in the United States for patients after open-heart surgery as a BTR system.[11] The success-ful development of this device by aerospace engineer David Lederman, through his company Abiomed Inc., formed in 1981 with the cardiac device patents and tech-nology purchased from Avco, turned out to bankroll Lederman's research on a TAH. This chapter focuses on three other NHLBI-supported cardiac assist device prototypes—the Thoratec, Novacor, and HeartMate systems—which played larger roles in the overall development of VADs. Based on a different technology platform than the AVCO LVAD, the development of these three longer-term car-diac assist devices came to characterize the era of the first-generation VADs, which consisted of large pulsatile devices that mimicked the function of the natural heart.

The Thoratec PVAD

Soon after arriving at the Pennsylvania State University College of Medicine in 1970, cardiac surgeon William S. Pierce formed the multidisciplinary Artificial Heart and Circulatory Support Group to develop practical MCSSs. A collaborative effort between the colleges of medicine and engineering, this research team consisted of Pierce; mechanical engineers John Brighton, Winfred Phillips, and Gerson Rosen-berg; fabrication specialist and machinist James Donachy; several veterinarians and animal care technicians; and later other faculty and graduate students from mechanical, aerospace, and chemical engineering and materials science.[12] Pierce's formation of a multidisciplinary team was key and his timing was ideal. Over the next several decades, the Penn State group benefited significantly from NHLBI's grants and targeted contracts approach for component research, which delivered crucial funding for this group to develop its research prototype and later transition it into a successful commercial device.

Like Michael DeBakey's research team at Baylor College of Medicine, the Penn State group aimed to develop a paracorporeal (external), pneumatically powered device to pump blood from the left ventricle to the aorta. Over the next few years, this group developed several prototypes of a left ventricular assist pump system. Early models of this device mechanically functioned satisfactorily, but there were problems of blood damage and clotting that needed to be resolved. The Penn State group experimented with different blood-interface materials and modified device construction, from sac tethering to the use of a separate diaphragm. In 1974 the research team reported that its latest model—the paracorporeal Pierce-Donachy device—functioned better in both bench testing and animal testing and provided longer-term cardiac support in calves than had been achieved by DeBakey's pump of the 1960s.[13] This was a substantial research development, since DeBakey's pump had been used only for very short-term use—days rather than weeks—for the cardiac patient unable to be weaned from cardiopulmonary mechanical support after surgery. At this point, DeBakey's device was still experimental and not available beyond Baylor College of Medicine. Concerns over the formation of thrombus in this device had made DeBakey hesitate to use it again until his research team improved its construction and function.

The paracorporeal Pierce-Donachy VAD was a pneumatically driven, single-chamber device, consisting of four main components: a pump, an inflow cannula (tube), an outflow cannula, and a drive console. The pump sat exterior to the body, alongside the abdomen, with the cannulas piercing the skin to connect to the heart and the great vessels. Blood flowed from the heart through the implanted tube into the VAD located outside the body and was pumped back into the body through another implanted tube. The pump connected to a drive console that monitored and powered the pump. It worked by alternating positive and

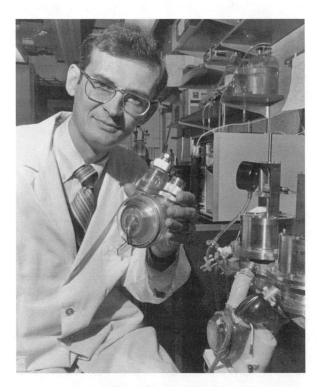

Cardiac surgeon and researcher William S. Pierce holds a paracorporeal ventricular assist device, developed at the Pennsylvania State University College of Medicine and marketed commercially as the Thoratec PVAD system. Used with permission from the Eberly Family Special Collections Library, Penn State University Libraries.

negative air pressures or pulses of air, transmitted through a hose, which compressed and emptied a flexible, polyurethane blood sac. A sensor detected when the pump was full of blood, triggering the ejection of blood from the pump. Tilting prosthetic valves positioned in the inflow and outflow ports ensured that the blood flowed only in one direction. The pump mechanism itself was encased in a hard outer shell.[14]

One of the debatable areas of technological development of these devices at this time concerned the lining of the device, which came into contact with the blood. How best to avoid potentially fatal thrombus (clot) formation when blood came into contact with this foreign surface? The Penn State researchers chose a smooth lining, whereas the opposing approach was a textured or flocked lining to anchor clots and let them construct a smooth lining. In their research, Penn State researchers provided data demonstrating the superiority of a smooth lining and its reduction of incidences of thrombosis. They also defended the external positioning of the device, arguing that its placement was less invasive to the critically ill heart patient and allowed for easier monitoring and removal. Moreover, in this position, their VAD could be used for either left ventricular support or right ventricular support, or two VADs could be used simultaneously for biventricular support. In 1974 research colleagues praised the Penn State team for their device achievement and research contributions surrounding blood interactions and longer-term mechanical circulatory support.[15]

It appeared that the Penn State team had overcome some, but not all, of the previous decade's technological obstacles. Pierce's group conducted more mock circulation testing to challenge mechanical failure and more animal studies to study device biocompatibility; and within months, their confidence in the device led them to seek permission to implant their experimental VAD in humans. In 1976 the Penn State team received approval from the Clinical Investigation Committee of the Milton S. Hershey Medical Center to use the experimental pump as a left ventricular assist device on critically ill patients facing heart failure (and death) after surgery. The hospital review board granted permission to implant the VAD in patients unable to be weaned from cardiopulmonary bypass or who developed profound cardiac failure shortly after being removed from bypass (known as postcardiotomy recovery).[16]

Between December 1976 and August 1977, Pierce and his surgical team implanted the Pierce-Donachy pump as an LVAD in four patients. In three of the four cases, the pump sustained blood circulation for several days; after attaching the device, patients were taken off bypass, left the operating room, and fully recovered. One patient, a 39-year-old woman, utilized the VAD for eight days postoperatively, a record length of "prolonged use" for such a device in this period. Diagnosed as a Class III heart failure patient, she underwent mitral valve replacement on July 28, 1977, but was unable to be weaned from the cardiopulmonary bypass support. Surgeons tried a variety of drugs and inserted an intraaortic balloon pump in their unsuccessful effort to stabilize her blood pressure. Having now exhausted all standard modes of therapy, Pierce used his experimental cardiac assist device, which was assembled, connected, de-aired, and pneumatically actuated for left ventricular support. The VAD stabilized the patient's blood pressure, and the woman was taken off cardiopulmonary bypass. The medical team monitored the patient, and on the eighth day surgeons assessed her heart to be strong enough to function without the aid of the mechanical pump. She returned to the operating room for removal of the VAD and remained stable thereafter. Improvement was slow but steady, and the patient eventually left the hospital after four months.[17]

Pierce's group argued that the Pierce-Donachy VAD managed the two greatest problems that had plagued left ventricular assist pumps at the time: thrombus (blood clotting as a result of poor blood-contact surface materials) and infection (from problematic percutaneous lines). Their device minimized thromboembolic complications by its smooth inner surface and reduced the threat of infection by improved tissue fixation at the site of the cannula insertion. Problems did exist, however, such as excessive bleeding, renal difficulties, and preoperative conditions, that complicated or prevented patient recovery. Still, Pierce reported that more than 50 percent of his VAD patients survived, supporting its use as a short-term (less than 10 days) assist device. In 1980, based on data collected from additional mock circulation bench testing, animal studies, and those early clinical cases, FDA administrators awarded Investigational Device Exemption status to the paracorporeal Pierce-Donachy VAD as an experimental device for postcardiotomy recovery.[18] Commenting on its recent clinical use, Pierce stated in 1981, "Engineering developments have made implantable motor-driven left ventricular assist pumps a reality. These units . . . will surely compete, in about five years, with cardiac transplantation for patients with end-stage left ventricular dysfunction."[19] This IDE status was an important step in the clinical use of the Pierce-Donachy VAD, and it marked the point for greater industry involvement, toward its commercial realization.

During this period, federal funding offered some support to transition VAD technology from experimental devices to commercial products, though such support is atypical in the medical device industry. Public moneys tended to support basic and applied research in academic settings; private funding typically brought a prototype into the marketplace and reaped any economic benefits. Before investing in an experimental device, companies sought a safe and cost-effective product, a reasonable time line to bring a sound device to market, a receptive and sizable consumer market, and, of course, a good margin of profit. But artificial hearts were expensive, complex devices, and there were multiple ways in which a business time line could become delayed and much costlier than originally planned. Artificial hearts—VADs or TAHs—were a high-risk endeavor for industry, owing to the prolonged development and significant regulatory, reimbursement, and acceptance barriers faced by these new devices.[20]

Recent federal regulations raised the cost and time involved in bringing a new device to market. The Medical Device Amendments of 1976 (in effect as of 1978) enacted greater premarket and new postmarket requirements, especially in the case of such high-risk Class III devices as artificial hearts. As a result, industry needed to support clinical trials (with IDE-approved devices) and collect data toward meeting FDA regulations for premarket approval and widespread distribution. Industry needed to demonstrate "proof" to FDA administrators, the medical profession, and the public that the device worked safely and effectively in order to garner greater clinical acceptance and thereafter reimbursement by various insurance and health management organizations.

The typical three-year return on investment expected by traditional venture capitalists was practically impossible for these devices. The financing and marketing of artificial hearts as viable commercial products, with the many attendant uncertainties, was a steep challenge. It was too heavy a financial burden for industry to assume alone. To mediate in the process, the government-sponsored artificial heart program took an instrumental economic role in transitioning promising VAD technology into the marketplace.[21] Contract money from the government lured industry into partnerships with academic-based research groups by subsidizing the high costs and lengthy time period associated with the commercial development of artificial hearts. In the case of the Pierce-Donachy VAD, Thoratec Laboratories Corporation of Pleasanton, California, became an industry partner with the Penn State group to manufacture, market, and distribute the IDE-approved device. Thoratec executives committed to further development of this device, and the Pierce-Donachy pump became the Thoratec paracorporeal ventricular assist device (PVAD).[22]

In 1976 biomedical engineer–entrepreneur Robert Harvey and cardiovascular surgeon Donald Hill purchased the Research and Development division of Searle Cardiopulmonary Systems to cofound Thoratec Laboratories Corporation (named to reflect "thoracic technology"), intending to make the firm "a leader in circulatory support devices, that is, the artificial heart and related products."[23] During the mid-1960s, Harvey had worked for Thermo Electron, conducting research on artificial hearts, but he left in 1968 to complete his doctoral degree in biomedical engineering at Worcester Polytechnic Institute in Massachusetts. As CEO of a new medical device company, Harvey encouraged development of new biomaterials for circulatory support and vascular graft products, specifically a polymer material with a high flex life for durability, plus good blood compatibility to eliminate any need for anticoagulants.[24] Harvey worked to bring the Pierce-Donachy pump to market as a technological solution for heart failure patients, servicing the postcardiotomy BTR patient population as well as the new and growing BTT market of patients. The slow pace of device development tested the perseverance and financial solvency of many companies, but Thoratec Laboratories hoped to survive by developing a solid product line to dominate the VAD market.[25]

With the introduction of the immunosuppressant drug cyclosporine in 1980, heart transplantation surgery shifted from an experimental procedure to a viable operation for some heart failure patients. Most cardiac surgeons had abandoned heart transplantation after the dreadful results of the late 1960s, a greater than

75 percent mortality rate because of organ rejection.[26] With improved immunosuppressive drugs, such as cyclosporine, to combat organ rejection, one-year survival rates of cardiac transplant patients increased to 80 percent by the mid-1980s. Increased acceptance of heart transplant surgery supported the increased use of artificial hearts as "bridges," or short-term devices, to keep failing heart patients alive while they waited for a donor heart. Whereas the Utah group intended the Jarvik-7 artificial heart to serve as a permanent device for heart failure patients who were not viable transplant patients, they also supported its expanded use as a BTT device for critical patients awaiting donor hearts. But in comparison to TAHs, VADs presented a less radical, more effective technology for short-term mechanical circulatory support for many individuals in this patient population. VAD researchers and industry investors embraced the BTT market for their assist pump systems.

In 1984, at San Francisco's Pacific Presbyterian Medical Center, Hill implanted the Thoratec PVAD in a 47-year-old heart failure patient as a bridge to transplantation.[27] The device provided two days of effective cardiac support, after which the patient underwent a successful cardiac transplantation. This case bolstered the use of the Thoratec PVAD by other heart transplant programs across the United States. Reporting from eight other medical centers, those surgeons commented positively on the mechanical pump's function and dependability, its support of single- or biventricular assist, and the ease of attaching it for short-term support, either as a BTR or a BTT device.[28] For those patients who needed biventricular support, the Thoratec PVAD competed with the Jarvik-7 TAH and the Symbion Acute Ventricular Assist Device as a bridge device until Symbion lost its FDA approval status for these two products in 1990.[29]

But there were shortcomings of the Thoratec and Symbion assist devices. Both VADs contained mechanical valves, were powered by air, and battled problems with patient infection and thromboembolism after too many days of device support.[30] One of the main drawbacks was the need to have the patient tethered to large air consoles as the device's main power source. The ideal device would have to be implantable to provide greater patient mobility. For decades, researchers experimented with various power sources, including nuclear power, in their quest to develop a nontethered, implantable device. During the 1980s, the clinical introduction of electrically driven, implantable VADs suggested that the ideal had possibly been attained.

The Novacor LVAS

In 1969–70, Peer Portner demonstrated the feasibility of an implantable ventricular assist system—to be known as the Novacor LVAS—while working at Arkon Scientific Labs, renamed Andros Inc., in Berkeley, California. This company was broadly involved in instrument and device development; it received primary support for its VAD initiative from federal funding and venture capital.[31] Portner's aim was to develop a totally implantable system for long-term support of end-stage chronic heart failure patients. He designed a unique, high-efficiency, pulsed solenoid energy converter as the driving mechanism to be integrated with a pusher-plate sac pump. He also experimented with implantable compensating mechanisms as an alternative to the vent tube for solving the problems of displaced pump volume.[32] For years, Portner and his team worked to develop an energy transmission system whereby electrical energy could be transmitted with high efficiency across intact skin to power the pump unit. This system would eliminate problems of infection from the drive lines that penetrated the skin. Portner's group envisioned an electrical transformer that consisted of a single-turn secondary coil designed for implantation beneath the skin around the waist, where it would be connected via a wire to the implanted electric control and pump units. A multiturn primary coil, resembling a conventional belt, would be worn outside the body and would overlie the implanted secondary coil. The primary coil would be powered from either portable, rechargeable batteries (worn by the patient during the day) or by conventional 120 volt sources (using a wall plug during the night).[33]

The Novacor LVAS revived earlier visions of the utility of MCSSs—imagine the patient freedom with such a wearable implantable VAD! The Novacor device was substantially different from the Thoratec PVAD in its design, actuation, and connection to the patient, illustrating the variety in device research and development pursued by clinicians and bioengineers. Most notably, the Novacor LVAS was an electrically driven and implantable device that promised to offer greater patient mobility, and presumptively a better quality of life, challenging the tethering requirement of the Thoratec PVAD. Patients would no longer need large abdominal punctures for percutaneous energy transmission lines (as required by the Thoratec devices). Yet the Novacor LVAS development team had to wait for improved miniaturization of the electronic control and power circuitry before realizing their design concept.

In 1980 Peer Portner founded Novacor Medical Corporation out of Andros Inc., to more aggressively pursue development of the device system and market it to a larger patient population.[34] Certainly patients recovering from heart surgery may benefit from short-term use of a VAD. Certainly unstable heart failure patients awaiting transplantation could be sustained with longer-term use of a VAD. What about cardiac patients whose heart dysfunction may be reversible if their heart is allowed to "rest" while on a VAD? And could a VAD be used for permanent assistance for those patients with irreversible disease not treatable by transplantation?[35] Both Novacor Medical and Thoratec Laboratories executives embraced such possible cases, wishing to market their respective VAD products to a broader patient population.

In 1984 the Novacor LVAS consisted of three components: an implantable electrical energy converter, a blood pump, and an external control console. The energy converter and the blood pump were assembled in a single unit. The energy converter or actuator transformed electrical to mechanical energy by means of a highly efficient solenoid. This pulsed-solenoid energy converter transferred energy via a spring mechanism to drive two symmetrical pusher plates within the blood pump. The blood pump was a sac type, with a smooth blood-contacting surface (like the

Thoratec PVAD to resist clotting), through which blood collected and then was pushed through by the pusher plates. A regulated pumping cycle maintained optimal flow. Whereas the Thoratec pump rested outside the body (paracorporeal), the Novacor pump was placed inside the body in a subcutaneous pocket (slightly under the skin) created in the upper abdomen. The superficial location of this pocket allowed for easy access to remove the device. The pump unit was implanted, but the electrical power source was not. An external console provided energy to the pump and also monitored device function and patient adaptability. The control mechanism in the drive console allowed the medical team to document device performance as well as physiological changes in the patient. The implanted device needed to be connected to the console, which required a cannula (tube) to pierce the skin in the abdomen of the patient, providing a power line and air vent. As with any percutaneous line, the medical team needed to be vigilant against infection.[36]

In September 1984, Stanford cardiothoracic surgeon Philip Oyer implanted a Novacor console-based LVAS in a 51-year-old man diagnosed with ischemic cardiomyopathy. For eight and a half days, the device supported the patient, who then underwent a cardiac transplant operation and lived for years thereafter. This BTT case led to more Novacor LVAS implants at Stanford, as well as in the transplant centers at St. Louis University, Johns Hopkins University, Vanderbilt University, and the University of Pittsburgh over the next four years. During this period, a total of 20 patients, ranging in age from 25 to 63, received cardiac support from a Novacor device, ranging in duration from one hour to 90 days; however, only 10 implant patients (50% of the group) survived to undergo heart transplant operations. The most common patient complication was bleeding, which necessitated reoperation in some cases and caused death in others. While implanted with the Novacor LVAS, 6 patients battled infections, 5 patients went into severe right heart failure, 4 patients died of kidney problems, 2 others died of multi-organ failure, and 2 patients experienced fatal cerebrovascular events.[37] Of the 10 patients who received a heart transplantation, 8 individuals left the hospital and lived for months, even years, thereafter. The Novacor LVAS research team reported that during the weeks of device support, 10 patients were ambulatory, walking with some assistance, and several patients exercised on a stationary bicycle. Commenting on his experience with the Novacor pump, 42-year-old James O'Brien said, "I was so comfortable with that device. . . . I felt 100 percent stronger. I was on that device for a week and during that time I was able to clear my lungs, clear my kidneys, improve the liver function. I got stronger . . . and I'd been flat on my back for over a month. It gave me a much better chance (in the transplant operation)."[38] Individual patient results varied, and there were device and patient management problems to be resolved.

Still, the Novacor LVAS researchers drew mostly positive, but cautious, meaning from these clinical cases. The group stated that, first, the Novacor LVAS proved to be mechanically reliable (not perfect) as both a bridge to recovery after surgery and as a bridge to transplantation. Second, the Novacor LVAS team reported no clotting

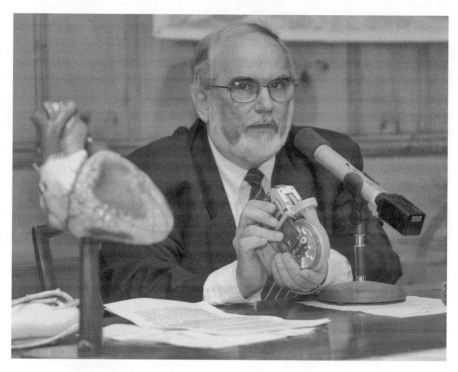

Device inventor Peer Portner talks to the press about the Novacor left ventricular assist system at the three-year survival mark, a long-term VAD support record at that time, of Novacor implant patient Robert "Pete" Kenyon on August 9, 2001. Five months later, in January 2002, Kenyon received a donor heart at the Yale–New Haven Hospital, New Haven, Connecticut. (AP Photo/Bob Child)

or evidence of thrombotic material in the pump, the conduits, or the valves of their explanted devices. Yet two patients had experienced embolic events, the dreaded complication of these devices. In the end, thromboembolic complications became the major weakness of this device.[39] Third, they described removal of the Novacor LVAS as straightforward and not problematic for the subsequent cardiac transplant procedure. The obvious limitation for the Novacor LVAS was that it was not useful for the patient in right ventricular failure.[40]

Overall, the results of the Novacor LVAS and the Thoratec PVAD clinical cases as BTT devices in this period were presented as validating the use of mechanical circulatory support beyond only postoperative recovery. With these results, the device teams pushed onward. Thoratec executives concentrated on meeting FDA standards for premarket approval (PMA) and commercialization of their system.[41] The Thoratec PVAD became the "workhorse" device and remained more or less the same device for the next 30 years, contributing significantly to the company's cardiovascular product line. But the Novacor device's implantability marked a key moment in the field; the goal of an implantable artificial heart, partial or otherwise, seemed closer to realization. This factor prompted its competitor, Thoratec, to pursue research into an implantable device version. And the Novacor LVAS evolved, as had always been the intention. In 1984 the Stanford team viewed the Novacor console-based LVAD as representing only an intermediate stage of development.[42] Stanford's cardiac transplant pioneer Norman Shumway supported the Novacor LVAS for its future goal of longer-term support for the transplant-ineligible patient. He certainly favored VADs over the use of TAHs. And he reminded the field that VAD use as bridge devices for transplant patients did not resolve the donor heart shortage and that they unfairly prioritized the implant patient on long waiting lists.[43]

The HeartMate LVAD

In the mid-1980s, a third serious contender for the VAD market emerged—the implantable HeartMate LVAD—which threatened to edge out both its competitors. Like the Novacor LVAS, the HeartMate LVAD was a pulsatile pusher-plate blood pump, implanted in the abdomen of the patient, and required tethering to a power console. While the Novacor LVAS was electrically driven, the HeartMate LVAD used compressed air as its power source (as did the Thoratec PVAD). A unique feature of the HeartMate LVAD was its use of a textured blood-contacting surface, in contrast to the smooth lining employed in both the Novacor and the Thoratec devices. Artificial heart researchers experimented with various blood-compatible surfaces in their devices to combat clot formation and thromboembolism. Whereas a smooth lining discouraged a buildup, a textured surface promoted the growth of a living lining of endothelial cells that resembled the inner surfaces of arteries and veins. HeartMate LVAD patients would then require less anticoagulant drug therapy (to reduce the formation of blood clots) than was necessary with competing devices. (Next-generation VAD technology made the smooth-or-textured surface debate moot.) In 1986, at the Texas Heart Institute, cardiac surgeon O. H. Frazier successfully used an experimental HeartMate LVAD in an end-stage heart patient awaiting transplant surgery, and he continued to report positive results with additional HeartMate LVAD cases thereafter.[44]

Trained by Michael DeBakey and Denton Cooley in the 1960s and 1970s, Frazier played an "instrumental role in the design, development, testing and subsequent clinical introduction" of VADs, implanting more LVADs than most likely anyone else in the world.[45] Under DeBakey's mentorship, Frazier became involved in the field of mechanical circulatory support in 1965 as a second-year medical student at Baylor College of Medicine, working on DeBakey's assist pumps as well as Liotta's TAH. Frazier completed his general surgery residency under DeBakey, then shifted to THI to train in cardiac surgery under Cooley in 1974. The high volume of cardiac surgical patients, as well as a robust mechanical device research program, allowed Frazier to meld clinical insights with experimental laboratory work. During the 1970s, he worked with John C. Norman on the development of an abdominally implanted, pulsatile assist device—the Model-7 ALVAD. Cardiac surgeons at THI implanted the experimental ALVAD in 22 patients between 1975 and 1980 and reported their first positive patient experience with this device as a bridge to transplantation in 1978.[46] In 1981 Frazier succeeded Norman as director of the Surgical Research Laboratory at THI. His leadership contributed to further achievements with mechanical pumps through THI cardiac device development projects and various collaborative partnerships with other device innovators and industry, all of them supported with significant NHLBI funding. His program offered the full package: excellent research facilities, laboratory testing capabilities, and animal implants, as well as patient cases at nearby St. Luke's Episcopal Hospital. In this way, Frazier was instrumental in the development of the HeartMate LVAD.

Engineer Victor Poirier designed the HeartMate LVAD for Thermedics Inc., later spun out as Thermo Cardiosystems Inc. with Poirier as president and chief executive officer; the two firms were subsidiaries of the Thermo Electron Corporation of Waltham, Massachusetts.[47] Thermo Electron, a supplier of various scientific instruments and equipment, had been developing mechanical circulatory support devices for decades, since its first government contract from the Artificial Heart Program in 1966. For a time, the company pursued development of both a TAH and an assist device, but by the mid-1970s it focused more on the development of an LVAD. It was at this time that Poirier joined Thermo Electron full-time and redirected his efforts from the company's main project—thermionic energy conversion to develop new power sources for space problems funded by NASA—to the development of cardiac assist devices. In 1975 Poirier shifted research efforts away from the older axisymmetric pump (the principle of pressure from hydraulic fluid in a pumping chamber to move blood through) to a pusher-plate pump (a two-chamber pump with a pusher plate in the lower chamber to exert pressure to move blood in the upper chamber). This marked the conception of the HeartMate device. Its new design was smaller in size and better in mechanical function and, hopefully, reliability. Also at this time, Thermo Electron developed the textured surface for the interior of blood pumps and explored pneumatic, electric, and nuclear power sources in various development projects. Poirier did not incorporate nuclear power in any of his various HeartMate LVAD prototypes. He explored two different power sources—pneumatic and electric—and tested both in a transcutaneous energy transfer system and in a system with a direct percutaneous lead to carry either the electrical energy or the pneumatic pulse from the external console to the blood pump.[48] A battery pack would offer some mobility for patients using either the HeartMate IP (implantable pneumatic) LVAD or the HeartMate VE (vented electric) LVAD.[49]

Dating from the 1970s, Poirier and his Thermedics team worked collaboratively with leading surgeons at busy heart centers to improve the HeartMate device. The effort included cardiac surgeons William Bernard of Boston Children's Hospital and John C. Norman and O. H. Frazier of THI, who refined surgical implant techniques, developed patient management protocol, and suggested device improvements.[50]

Thermo Electron, the parent company of Thermedics, had a history with THI when Norman collaborated with Thermo engineers to design and test possible nuclear-powered VADs. At the same time, THI was conducting a complementary VAD research program with some success in the late 1970s. Given the volume of heart patients and the profile of heart surgeons at the THI, it was the ideal setting for testing the HeartMate LVAD. Most notable was cardiac surgeon Denton Cooley, who was unapologetic in his willingness to use experimental devices to save his patients if he judged that such an option was available. For the HeartMate LVAD, it was Frazier's insight into the problems of poor compliance-chamber performance (volume displacement) and inflow-graft occlusion (blood clotting) that led to two key design changes. To resolve these problems, which had emerged repeatedly in his animal implants, Frazier suggested percutaneous venting (to replace the compliance chamber) and a shorter inflow graft (to reduce blood pooling and clotting).[51] Frazier reported more positive clinical outcomes with the improved HeartMate LVAD as a BTT device, and this experience contributed to the launch of Poirier's device.

Companies like Thermedics now looked toward larger clinical case studies—multicentered, controlled clinical trials—that would produce the patient data required to obtain PMA status for their medical device from the FDA. For device manufacturers, the FDA process to secure PMA status was time-consuming, costly, and fraught with agency delays, but it was absolutely necessary for the commercialization of devices in the United States. It was a pivotal stage that buttressed the additional efforts

TABLE 5.1
Selected pulsatile VADs and FDA regulatory status

Device	Description	FDA status
HeartMate IP LVAS, by Thermo Cardiosystems Inc.	An implantable, pneumatic LVAD	1994 PMA granted
Thoratec PVAD, by Thoratec Laboratories Corp.	A paracorporeal, pneumatic BiVAD	1995 PMA granted 2003 PMA granted for home use with TLC-II Portable VAD Driver
Novacor LVAS, by Novacor Medical Corp.	An electrically powered, wearable assist system, with portable battery pack	1998 PMA granted
HeartMate VE LVAD, by Thermo Cardiosystems Inc.	An electrically powered, wearable assist system, with portable battery pack	1998 PMA granted
Thoratec IVAD, by Thoratec Corp.	An implantable version of the Thoratec PVAD	2004 PMA granted

Note: FDA = Food and Drug Administration; LVAS = left ventricular assist system; LVAD = left ventricular assist device; PMA = premarket approval (to distribute device commercially in the United States); PVAD = paracorporeal ventricular assist device; BiVAD = biventricular assist device.

of industry to secure device reimbursement and buy-in for the use of their new devices from medical practitioners and patients. Different stakeholders collaborated in designing, organizing, and participating in VAD clinical trials for different reasons, united in their goal of delivering a new medical device as an acceptable standard of care for heart failure patients.

Getting to the Commercial Market: FDA Regulation and Clinical Trials

The Medical Device Amendments of 1976 greatly shaped VAD testing and the VAD's pathway into the medical marketplace during the last quarter of the twentieth century. In early experience with mechanical pumps, clinicians attached laboratory prototypes to patients who were near death, with hopes that industry would ultimately make and sell the devices. After 1976, the FDA regulated the manufacture and clinical use of medical devices more strictly in the United States. Industries now needed to secure FDA approval, which would be based on clinical trial data satisfying the FDA that the device was safe and effective, before producing and selling it. The cost of testing and collecting data for FDA evaluation was significant, and industries would be paying these costs. The regulatory and financial aspects of device development were enough to threaten any promising innovation. In the case of VADs, several large device companies successfully navigated this new regulatory pathway, thereby shaping the recipient pool and clinical indication for the use of these devices.

Artificial heart research is an example of practical biomedical research, or translational medicine, which emphasizes a collaborative, multidisciplinary approach to advance therapeutic innovations from the bench to the bedside more quickly and effectively. In the case of artificial hearts, the clinical problem was heart failure, which initiated laboratory study and device innovation. Early clinical trials were conducted with experimental pumps, and then it was back to the laboratory for device improvement and study. More clinical trials followed, and eventually an acceptable device was produced, with patient care guidelines to treat the clinical problem. This process of developing a device from concept to clinical use may be viewed as passing through three distinct phases: innovation, regulation and clinical trials, and commercialization and marketing. In the first phase, innovation occurred with the emergence of artificial hearts as a concept (anyone can think up a concept); next came early bench and lab studies (involving surgical researchers, bioengineers, and research scientists) and then the clinical introduction of device prototypes (by a surgeon). A surgeon's decision to use an experimental artificial heart clinically is guided by the surgeon's judgment regarding its potential benefit compared with its risk. Compelled to offer the best care for their patients, surgeons proceed based on their sense of competency. Mechanical heart implants are complicated procedures performed in hospitals, regulated to some extent by internal policies related to credentialing, certification, privileges, and institutional review boards, as well as by state policies on hospital licensure. Surgeon-researchers Michael DeBakey, Adrian Kantrowitz, Denton Cooley, Robert Bartlett, William S.

Pierce, O. H. Frazier, and others operated within this innovation phase of device development, steered by their research work, clinical experience, hospital environment, and commitment to their patients.

In the regulation and clinical trials phase, industry and the FDA become involved to fund and to grant approval for new devices to be marketed to a wider audience. An expectation of commercial success will entice industry to support this development phase, working with research teams to navigate FDA regulation. The regulatory process deals with evidence of innovative therapies before offering new treatments to patients and influencing the standard of medical care. In the United States, companies, not individuals, submit data and specific claims for any new device in the attempt to gain FDA approval for its widespread use and commercialization. The FDA judges the quality of the data and ultimately decides whether to approve the sale of the device by the company. For FDA approval to market devices, data demonstrating device safety and efficacy, from definitive controlled clinical trials, must be submitted. These trials can cost millions of dollars, whether they are successful or not. Industry assumes much of this cost with expectations of reaping device profits later.[52] Clinical trials allow investigators to test whether a particular device or intervention potentially will improve the health outcomes of participants. Such trials produce essential data for evaluation by different groups with different aims regarding new medical treatments. In the case of VADs, clinical trials test the performance of the new technology: does such a device function appropriately in the human body, and does it contribute to improved health for the end-stage heart failure patient? Hospital officials, doctors, and patients have to be convinced of its viability as a treatment option. Regulatory agencies, charged with public oversight, seek to ensure the safety and efficacy of new products for patients. Accordingly, FDA officials approve the clinical use of new devices in stages: first, as investigational devices (with IDE status) for specific clinical trials held in specific medical centers with specific patient indications or a targeted population; if satisfactory patient outcomes result, then, second, as a commercial product (PMA status) for wider distribution for specific patient populations.

Commercialization and marketing is the third phase of device development, when commercial sales, device reimbursement, and clinical acceptance take place. Market reimbursement is crucial to the survival of any new technology and its incorporation into standard practice. In the United States, health care reimbursement is predicated on the concept that any new medical procedure or product must be "reasonable and necessary."[53] FDA approval of any new device is essential to secure Medicare and commercial, or third-party, payers to cover the cost of the technology, the surgical procedure, and any patient supplies or accessories related to the treatment.

In Europe, device manufacturers go through a less stringent approval system to receive Conformité Européene (CE) marking. For device certification or CE approval by the European Commission, industry submits data from European clinical trials to demonstrate that the device is safe and functions as marketed by the company. In the United States, industry must provide safety data and efficacy details. That is, for a VAD, industry must provide reliable information related to its safety for human implantation, its function without mechanical fault, its operational performance as advertised, and its use as beneficial for some patients. Because European approval lacks the efficacy component, new devices tend to be introduced into European medical markets more quickly. Although some type of US clinical trial is required for FDA approval applications, industry will add data from European clinical trials as supporting documentation. Europe's more permissive environment for the testing of new devices by industry is perhaps related to cultural and political differences. Few European countries have matched American enthusiasm for new unproven medical technologies, and public demand for greater government oversight did not materialize there as it did in the United States.

Whether American or European clinical trials are conducted, industry needs favorable data to apply for device reimbursement in different countries. Unlike medical device approval, the process for medical device reimbursement in Europe is not uniform; it differs from country to country based on state government health care policy.[54] In Canada, new medical devices are regulated and reimbursed in ways similar to the US policies. Health Canada approves new technology in stages, with postmarket surveillance, and reimbursement is secured through public and private health insurance providers.[55] For industry, penetrating the American market is most important to reach device profitability, owing to its sheer size and lucrativeness. In the United States, device reimbursement approval from the Centers for Medicare and Medicaid Services (CMS), sanctioning financial coverage of specific medical treatments, is key in transitioning new devices into wider acceptance and standards of care. Thus, clinical trials are essential to demonstrate to clinicians, patients, hospital ethics boards, device regulatory bodies, and government and commercial health insurance payers that VAD technology warrant use and payment.

Pre-1976 clinical studies in the United States were quite straightforward and involved temporary extracorporeal (outside the body) devices. These early clinical cases focused on the ability of the experimental VAD to sustain life until the heart recovered. Typically, the patient had undergone heart surgery and had been unable to be weaned from cardiopulmonary bypass. The patient was in postcardiotomy shock, and death was imminent if the patient could not be rescued with a temporary VAD. All standard therapies had been exhausted—such as drug regimens or the insertion of an intraaortic balloon pump—and surgeons resorted to an experimental VAD as a last-ditch effort. Michael DeBakey at Baylor College of Medicine was using experimental VADs in this way in the 1960s, and John C. Norman at THI and a handful of other surgeons did so in 1970s. Not all of these early cases were successful, but the data gathered contributed to ongoing bench and animal testing to improve device prototypes, to reduce mechanical failure, and to refine surgical and patient care procedures. The significance of the early cases is that they established the concept of MCSSs for short-term use, with potential for longer-term use. As a result, some cardiac surgeons were encouraged to expand VAD use for other heart failure patients, such as cases of cardiogenic shock caused by myocardial infarction or acute myocarditis. Several researchers sought to push VAD use beyond temporary measures if a better device could be developed.

In the 1970s, academic and private research teams introduced more durable and implantable VADs, intended for longer-term use than the earlier temporary, postoperative devices. Innovators like Peer Portner and Victor Poirier envisioned their devices as a permanent support technology and a viable alternative to heart transplantation. At this time cardiac transplant surgery was considered a "reasonable and therapeutic treatment to extend life" in selected individuals only. This standard was hardly a ringing endorsement for heart transplantation, and understandably so, given the low patient survival rates. At five years after transplant, only about one-third of patients were still alive, the most common causes of death following the surgery being infection and organ rejection.[56] Research teams developing MCSSs offered another therapeutic option—artificial hearts (total or partial)—but poor biomaterial and performance outcomes needed to be overcome. Things changed during the 1980s with the introduction of effective immunosuppressant drugs, and cardiac transplantation became the established therapy for end-stage heart failure. There were 10-year survival rates after transplantation for about 50 percent of patients over the next two decades.[57]

The establishment of heart transplantation as the better treatment course for some heart failure patients solidified a role for VADs not as an alternative to transplantation but as a bridge to transplantation for patients on donor organ waiting lists. FDA administrators played a role in this process by limiting the eligible patient population for the VAD from all heart failure patients to transplant patients only. When device companies approached the FDA administrators about their aim for VADs as an alternative to transplantation, FDA administrators expressed justifiable concerns about long-term VAD performance and safety. They restricted clinical testing of VADs as longer-term devices to only patients eligible for heart transplantation. FDA administrators insisted upon this limitation as a safety measure; in the case of failure of these implantable devices, heart transplantation could provide a potential backup for such very sick patients. According to cardiac surgeons Lyle Joyce, George Noon, David Joyce, and Michael DeBakey, this FDA course of action marked "a paradigm shift" for artificial hearts as a BTT device rather than as a destination therapy device.[58] Arguably, since the intent of the Artificial Heart Program had always been to develop a range of devices for both short- and long-term use, the FDA course of action was less a paradigm shift than a prioritizing of VAD use, nonetheless still directing the course of development (and commercialization) of this technology at this time.

For economic reasons, industry pushed for additional clinical indications for long-term VAD use beyond bridge to transplantation. Thoratec CEO Robert Harvey always envisioned a varied line of cardiac pump products to serve a broad heart failure patient population. During the company's first six years, Harvey spent more than $5 million, a major corporate investment and financial risk, to develop a "family" of devices. "Our corporate goal is to make VADs available on a mass basis," stated Harvey, to serve "different degrees" of heart failure and patient need.[59] As argued by Peer Portner, mechanical hearts were high-risk devices for manufacturers, given the substantial research and development investment; in terms of profit prospects, industry needed to navigate stiff regulatory, reimbursement, and acceptance hurdles to secure any kind of return on their investment.[60] Industry was not alone; many device innovators remained committed to developing mechanical hearts as a permanent treatment course for non-transplant-eligible heart failure patients.[61] Device designers and industry thus had to comply with FDA requirements in order to enter the American medical marketplace in a meaningful way. In collaboration with device innovators and clinical researchers, industry took a step-wise approach to expanding the patient pool, moving from short-term to long-term use of VADs based on good device performance and patient outcome results. Objective data supporting safety and efficacy would contribute to greater clinician buy-in, expanded indications, and better reimbursement for mechanical hearts.[62] In their effort to secure this data, VAD stakeholders grappled with the complexity of the randomized controlled trial (RCT) to evaluate surgical interventions, and how best to move their device testing beyond the traditional case series with historical controls to generate rigorous, convincing data for FDA administrators.

The RCT became the gold standard in evidence-based medicine for evaluating new therapies, although its adoption for innovative surgical interventions met with logical resistance.[63] An RCT is an experimental study conducted on clinical patients, in which the investigator controls an intervention through random assignment while blinding the physician and the patient to the assigned treatment to eliminate biased measurement. This experimental design is meant to offer clinically meaningful results; that is, to result in strong cause and effect conclusions about the safety and efficacy of new therapies, often in direct comparison with older treatments. Dating from antibiotic research during World War II, RCTs aimed to replace traditional methods of evaluation, such as retrospective case studies, by producing objective, rigorous data on the therapeutic efficacy of new drugs, devices, and procedures in medicine. Was a new treatment better than an older one? Could RCT evidence change conventional knowledge and improve clinical practice with the adoption of new therapies? The RCT sought to remove uncertainty surrounding novel treatments. However, as medical historian Harry Marks and others have demonstrated, RCTs did not always provide convincing data or resolve therapeutic controversy.[64]

But is the use of RCTs to evaluate surgical interventions even feasible or arguably better than other experimental and observational studies? According to medical historian Christopher Crenner, postwar use of controlled clinical trials in surgery emerged out of the field's interest in evaluating new procedures and their therapeutic effects beyond the traditional case series study. Focusing on the controversial use of sham surgery, Crenner shows how placebo-controlled studies exposed subjective patient experiences and the flawed value of two popular surgical procedures: internal mammary artery ligation and gastric freezing. Measuring surgical success beyond the conventional case series to the broader-sanctioned clinical trial in medical research suggested progress, less bias, and more accurate evidence of therapeutic value, according to RCT proponents. But as Crenner states, there was no "straightforward history" of clinical trial data supplanting traditional case series evidence in surgery; the use of RCTs in surgery was "contested and slow."[65]

Many surgical researchers resisted RCTs for good reasons.[66] RCTs were expensive and difficult to conduct, and as some surgeons argued, there are fundamental differences between testing drugs and evaluating new surgical procedures or technology. In surgery, there are simply too many variables to control in order to offer objective results. Surgeons possessed varying skills and different levels of competency, operated in various institutional centers, and faced unique patient cases despite similar diagnoses. Double-blinding the surgeon and the patient was not always feasible, and any random assignment might possibly be unethical when experimental treatments were assigned to life-threatening illnesses. Unlike drug trials, surgical procedures and technologies tend to undergo refinement during the course of a study, resulting in improved outcomes in the later operations, compared with early operations. When a surgical intervention is being compared with a nonsurgical treatment, both surgeon and patient will likely know the treatment assignment, and this in turn may shape outcome expectations and perhaps bias results. When it comes to heart surgery specifically, the life-threatening and urgent situations of cardiac patients may challenge cooperation, since very ill patients may not wish their treatment to be decided by chance or may not be comfortable with the irreversibility of some surgical options.

Debates about the best cardiac therapies—both surgical and medical treatments—abounded in the 1970s and 1980s. Medical historian David Jones describes the fierce controversy among physicians over the efficacy of coronary artery bypass grafting, which was not settled by RCTs in those decades.[67] Still, RCTs in surgery need not be dismissed, according to Jones; he acknowledges the entrenchment of the traditional surgical research methods of animal experiments, case reports, and case series to evaluate new procedures.[68] Yet because regulatory bodies tasked with granting market approval and reimbursement of new medical devices, such as the FDA and the CMS, required rigorous evidence of therapeutic benefits over risks for patients, surgical researchers needed to reconcile the technical and ethical complexities of using RCTs in surgery to fit within the evidence-based medicine model.[69] Large RCTs of VADs eventually were conducted, but not before multicenter observational studies of VAD cases generated positive data for the viability of such devices to provide long-term support.

Once academic and industrial device teams produced a workable VAD—with mechanical and functional kinks worked out through bench and animal testing—they moved from contained clinical cases, with one surgeon or one medical center trying out their device, to more sophisticated multicenter clinical trials to collect data for their commercial approval submissions to the FDA. The 1980s clinical trials with VADs focused on primary and secondary outcomes, specifically device function and patient experience. These multicenter clinical trials sought to measure such things as device performance, efficacy, frequency of serious adverse events, patient neurocognitive levels, and general quality-of-life issues. Obviously these clinical trials sought to demonstrate that the devices worked well, but for whom and to what extent? Industry wanted to satisfy FDA administrators to commercialize their respective VADs, whereas clinicians and inventors sought to establish these cardiac devices as a standard, if not preferred, treatment course for end-stage heart failure patients. As more data was collected, FDA administrators were able to set benchmarks (or performance measures) for experimental VADs—how long should the device function to be safe and effective? What adverse events would negate its safety for patients? FDA administrators established these benchmarks based on the use of the device as an implantable BTT device, with expectations that a longer-term device would work safely and effectively for weeks and months (from data suggesting that the average wait was six months for a donor heart), as opposed to the short-term support (measured in days) of temporary, external devices. Also, threats of infection and thromboembolic events needed to be minimized.

Between August 1985 and September 1993, there was a multicenter clinical trial to evaluate the pneumatically driven HeartMate LVAD that involved 108 nonrandomized patients in 17 clinical centers in the United States.[70] Competing with Thoratec and Novacor devices, Thermo Cardiosystems Inc. (TCI), formerly Thermedics Inc., executives supported the HeartMate LVAD and set up the trial to gather data to support FDA applications for device commercialization. Participating institutions included THI, the Cleveland Clinic, Temple University Hospital, Columbia Presbyterian Medical Center, and others. All medical teams obtained informed consent and patient data from all participating individuals, in compliance with their respective institutional review boards. All 108 patients had been approved for heart transplantation, and 75 of them received a HeartMate LVAD while waiting for a donor heart. The other 33 patients, who became the control group, met the criteria for implantation of the device but did not undergo the implantation owing to either unavailability of the device or patient refusal of the treatment. These patients received intraaortic balloon pump support and/or drugs to increase myocardial contractility. The participating medical teams collected data related to device performance, patient experience, and any adverse effects such as bleeding, hemolysis (blood damage), infection, right ventricular failure, embolic (blood clot) events, and renal (kidney) dysfunction. Cardiac surgeon O. H. Frazier reported the first successful HeartMate LVAD implant, as a bridge to transplantation, in 1986.[71] Eight years of data from this clinical trial provided encouraging and positive findings for long-term use of the HeartMate LVAD as a BTT device.

In addition to providing safety and efficacy data on the HeartMate device, this multicenter clinical study demonstrated that heart failure patients with this implanted device fared better than the heart failure patients who were not treated with the mechanical system. For TCI, this finding would hopefully influence broader clinical acceptance of mechanical support as treatment and also position the HeartMate device as the best LVAD available. The study reported a significant (55%) reduction in mortality for the LVAD patients in comparison with the non-LVAD patients awaiting a donor heart. Moreover, LVAD patients experienced renal and hepatic (liver) function improvement as well as greater general physical wellness; these results suggested that LVAD support rehabilitated them to be stronger before undergoing the heart transplantation. Better patient condition at the time of transplant surgery contributed to a higher survival rate for LVAD patients compared to non-LVAD patients one year after transplantation. The trial was neither blinded nor randomized, but still an effort to avoid bias was made through identical entrance criteria for both control patients and LVAD patients, which worked satisfactorily to make the trial results meaningful. The fact that there were no reported mechanical failures or performance-related problems with the HeartMate LVAD was a positive finding to support FDA applications.[72] But these were not unique results. These HeartMate LVAD results reinforced similar findings in comparable clinical trials of the Novacor LVAS and the Thoratec assist systems, bolstering the case for the effectiveness of ventricular assistance.[73]

What was unique in the clinical trial experience of the HeartMate LVAD was its performance of acceptable cardiac output and low incidence of embolism. Clinicians reported that thromboembolism, a serious complication in the use of mechanical pumps, had not been a problem with this device. The number of strokes related to embolic events was quite low (4%) in HeartMate LVAD patients, in comparison to the higher rates in Thoratec PVAD patients (8%) and Jarvik-7 TAH patients (57%) at that time.[74] This low rate was attributed to the HeartMate LVAD's use of textured surfaces, which promoted the formation of a natural biologic lining, or pseudo-endothelium. With this device, patients did not need to take the anticoagulant warfarin, but instead took aspirin as the only antiplatelet therapy. Whereas the Thoratec PVAD drew criticisms of patient tethering to a pneumatic drive console, the HeartMate LVAD soon offered patients a portable driver, which increased their mobility and allowed them to leave the hospital. In addition, the strong pump flow of the HeartMate LVAD, characterized by a complete fill-to-empty pumping action, provided a complete washout of blood with each stroke and reduced the opportunity for clot formation.[75] Frazier remarked that the HeartMate LVAD was "the only device that works well and will be the device of the future."[76] Participating clinicians in this study received the medical community's praise, and overall confidence in the device swelled. TCI officials submitted these results as part of the PMA application to the FDA, and as they had hoped, FDA administrators in 1994 approved the HeartMate LVAD (pneumatic) for commercial use in the United States as a safe and effective BTT therapy for heart failure patients.[77]

TCI's HeartMate LVAD was the first but not the only VAD to receive FDA approval for sale in the American market during the 1990s. Both Thoratec Laboratories and Novacor Medical (acquired by Baxter Health Corporation in 1988) supported multicenter trials in the United States and Europe to generate clinical data attesting to the safety and effectiveness of their respective devices. These trials with the pneumatic Thoratec PVAD and the electric Novacor LVAS produced device performance and patient experience results comparable to those of the earlier-approved HeartMate LVAD, and it was this data that supported their respective FDA-approval submissions.[78] For example, successful cases of VAD-supported heart failure patients who underwent cardiac surgery were 69 percent of Thoratec PVAD patients and 78 percent of Novacor LVAS patients, compared with 71 percent of HeartMate LVAD patients.[79] The Thoratec PVAD received FDA approval for sale in December 1995, thereafter competing with, and expanding beyond, the potential HeartMate LVAD patient population. The Thoratec PVAD was a paracorporeal (not implantable) device, and it was the only biventricular assist system available.[80] (The company later received commercial approval for a smaller, implantable version—the Thoratec IVAD—which competed more directly with the implantable, pneumatic HeartMate IP LVAS.)[81]

In 1998 the FDA approved two wearable LVAD products for commercial use— the electric Novacor LVAS and the electric HeartMate LVAD. Fourteen years after its first clinical implant, the Novacor LVAS evolved from a console-based to a wearable system that was supported by a small electronic controller and batteries worn on a belt, thus boasting much greater mobility (and untethering) for patients.[82] Novacor Medical supported European multicenter clinical trials in the mid-1990s, gaining European commercial rights before FDA approval. The trial results demonstrated that, in comparison with other VADs, the Novacor LVAS had similar survival and complications rates, with a greater number of at-home supported patients before transplant surgery. There was a low incidence of device malfunction, and confidence in the reliability of the system was bolstered. This data supported results generated from Novacor LVAS implants in the United States.[83] Almost simultaneously, TCI introduced an electrically actuated, wearable HeartMate LVAD that consisted of two external batteries worn on a belt or a vest or in a shoulder bag. This model resolved the patient mobility issues of the earlier FDA-approved, pneumatically actuated Heart-Mate device. By the late 1990s, American medical centers had their choice of multiple commercial VADs. TCI, Thoratec Laboratories, and Novacor Medical responded by pushing to enlarge the possible VAD patient population in the increasingly crowded cardiac device market.

Emerging Rewards

Whether for reasons of profit or improved patient care (or both), VADs in this period contributed to the momentum of cardiac devices as technological fixes to the problem of heart failure. VADs, not TAHs, dominated the field of MCSSs by the 1990s. Scientists, engineers and practitioners had succeeded in resolving many of the technical and biocompatibility problems to reach safety and efficacy standards, and NHLBI officials and device industry executives had funded and marshaled the transition of select VADs from prototype to market product by demonstrating the VAD's health benefits. VADs, not TAHs, emerged as the more rewarding MCSS device technologically, conceptually, and commercially.

In this period, VAD technology worked better than TAH technology for more patients for many reasons. To start with, a TAH is a much more complex device that necessitates removal of the native heart, whereas VADs are designed to augment the work of the weakened, but still functioning, biological heart. TAHs must provide twice the workload of VADs, so they contain more valves and moving parts and a greater blood-contact surface area; they also require more power to operate than assist pumps. Many practitioners continue to question whether a mechanical heart could truly replace the human heart for any extended period, and they point out that the challenges of size and durability are significant hurdles. But many VAD researchers, such as William S. Pierce, Peer Portner, and Victor Poirier, have stated that these technological limitations were surmountable in the case of assist devices, a less daunting task than building a TAH.[84] During the 1980s and 1990s, a period of miniaturization of device components and the introduction of better blood-contact surface materials allowed VAD researchers to build smaller, implantable, and more durable devices. The improvement in batteries as power sources was significant, along with better pre- and postoperative care of VAD patients based on accumulated clinical experience. There existed a cross-fertilization of ideas among researchers as they addressed the problems of thrombosis and infection that plagued the body's acceptance of mechanical hearts. At conference meetings and through medical publications, device teams shared their research on biomaterials, energy transfer systems, cardiac output functioning with prototype devices, and other issues, thereby contributing to steady and incremental advances in the field of MCSSs.

The business of medical device innovation is costly and precarious. In particular, the development of mechanical circulatory support devices is very capital-intensive and risky because of the regulatory, reimbursement, and clinical uptake challenges that come with this technology.[85] Typically it takes 25 years to bring a medical device prototype from proof of concept to clinical adoption—much too long, according to NHLBI official John Watson.[86] After initial design work, scientists tested their devices in vitro (bench testing) for function and durability, then in vivo (in animals) to study further the safety and efficacy of the device. Both stages were necessary steps to refine the prototype and compile data for FDA approval before proceeding to clinical trials. Next there are the staggering costs of clinical trials. Raising money for the trials was no easy task, and the negative media coverage of the Jarvik-7 patient cases had scared a lot of potential investors away. Poirier remembers, "I'd get up at investor meetings and hear comments in the back like, 'Goddammit, not another artificial heart.'" He slowly convinced them with "straight talk" and "promising data" that implantable VADs were better technology with tremendous therapeutic potential for the growing heart failure patient population.[87] In many cases, researchers formed their own startup companies, raised venture capital for ongoing development, and then their companies might be taken over by larger established corporations with deeper pockets, more business expertise, and expanded product lines to further commercialize new innovations.[88] Development costs were staggering, according to Poirier: "In the case of the HeartMate blood-pump system, we initiated the design in 1975. It took 10 years to complete the development and testing needed to obtain an investigational device exemption from the FDA. Our clinical trial took 9 years to complete, from 1985 to 1994. The cost of this trial was $41.6 million. Coupled with development costs, our total investment was $62 million."[89] The financial strain of development weighed heavily, and it was not uncommon for device companies to change ownership regularly, as was the case with the Novacor device.

Portner makes clear that the development of the Novacor LVAS system started with NHLBI funding and some venture capital at Arkon Scientific Laboratories, later renamed Andros Inc.[90] Portner became president and chief executive officer of Novacor Medical, formed to complete VAD development, to manufacture the device as well as to market the product. In 1988 the Baxter Healthcare Corporation acquired Novacor Medical, retaining Portner's involvement, and took steps to enhance and broaden the clinical use of the Novacor LVAS. Baxter's cardiovascular products division was later spun off to Edwards Lifesciences LLC. In 2000 Edwards Lifesciences sold the Novacor technology to the WorldHeart Corporation, a Canadian company set up to commercialize the HeartSaver VAD that was under development at the University of Ottawa Heart Institute. Facing serious financial difficulties by 2004, the WorldHeart Board of Directors made several major changes: CEO Rod Bryden was replaced by Jal Jassawalla, the majority of device development work was moved to Oakland, California, from Ottawa, and the technologies of the Novacor LVAS and the HeartSaver VAD were amalgamated to develop a smaller, improved, fully implantable Novacor II LVAS.[91] In 2006 the company reported animal testing of the new Novacor II device, but its development stopped there. In 2008 WorldHeart stopped manufacturing the original Novacor LVAS and sales were discontinued worldwide. Three years earlier, WorldHeart had acquired the assets of MedQuest Products Inc., a spin-off company of the University of Utah, which added advanced rotary pump and MagLev technology to WorldHeart's VAD technology platform.[92] WorldHeart then focused on its Levacor VAD technology, banking on that device's promise as a next-generation bridge device as well as a permanent implant. However, by 2011, WorldHeart felt that this device would not be commercially competitive, so the firm abandoned its development in favor of the newer, miniature MiFlow VAD technology.[93] In 2012 the WorldHeart Corporation was acquired by Heart Ware International Inc. Bear in mind that this all started with the NHLBI, under a targeted research contact framework that supported researcher-industry collaboration and the provision of the initial funding critically needed in the early development of VADs. Full industry development (or abandonment) of these devices occurred thereafter.[94]

For those companies that could weather the prolonged development course of this technology, the payout promised to be lucrative. Congestive heart failure is a major health care problem, affecting 5.8 million people in the United States and more than 26 million worldwide, with limited treatment options available; roughly half of all heart failure patients die within five years of diagnosis.[95] The market potential appeals to industry, especially with the aging population demographics and the expanding clinical application of VADs from BTT devices to lifetime therapy. After FDA approval of Thoratec's PVAD system in December 1995, Thoratec Laboratories reported revenues of $7.5 million in 1996, which then tripled to $22.5 million by the end of the decade.[96] Between January 1996 and March 2000, a total of 1,200 patients worldwide were implanted with a Thoratec PVAD, still hardly a ripple in the potential pool of 26 million heart failure sufferers.[97] Thoratec executives proposed generating future device revenues and profitability in several ways, most notably by increasing the VAD market with expanded clinical indications, by securing greater buy-in by cardiac surgeons and heart failure cardiologists to use VADs, and by continuing to develop improved pump devices, which may involve the acquisition of companies with complementary products or technologies.[98] Thoratec executives were well aware that their main competitors in the VAD market—TCI and Novacor Medical—would vigorously defend their market positions. The projected size of the VAD market was exaggerated, given the need for specialized cardiac centers and trained implant surgeons; in the end it would be difficult to support many competing devices. The economics of "staying in the game" was rough, necessitating company mergers, spinoffs, and aborted device development, and it favored those companies that had a viable device, secured market placement of their products first, and successfully staved off the competition.

Realizing that market adoption of new devices was critical, industry spent time and money educating medical professionals and society in general about the potential of VAD therapy. Device companies also supported working relationships with cardiovascular surgeons and cardiologists to influence medical device selection and purchase decisions at medical centers. Large multicenter clinical trials introduced new devices into several leading cardiac centers; industry hoped for positive outcomes to capture professional buy-in for VAD therapy and for specific products. Companies such as Thoratec expanded their reach through advertisements in medical and popular media. One such ad downplayed the device in lieu of a much larger image of a VAD-supported mother sitting under a tree playing with her baby, with the title "Thoratec PVAD: 30 Years at the Heart of BiVAD support."[99] Patient testimony and images describing an improved quality of life are intended to dispel any lingering images of moribund patients tethered to large consoles, reminiscent of the 1980s Jarvik-7 heart cases. Deliberately moving the spotlight from the device to the improved patient, active outside of the hospital, industry focuses, in almost all commercial literature, on patients living with, but not dominated by, this life-extending technology. Patient testimony, an age-old standby in the history of medicine, remains a marketing gem for selling medical products.

In the United States, VAD therapy became more commonplace because of the increased positive reporting of clinical cases, patient-centered industry marketing, improved physician awareness and training, expanded indications for VAD use, and VAD reimbursement by both private health insurance providers and the CMS. Medicare payment for an item or a service is dependent on a national coverage determination (NCD), issued by the CMS, which can be requested by beneficiaries, manufacturers, providers, suppliers, medical professional associations, or health plans. An NCD grants, limits, or excludes Medicare coverage and is binding on all Medicare carriers, fiscal intermediaries, quality improvement organizations, health maintenance organizations, competitive medical plans, and health care prepayment plans. From industry's viewpoint, reimbursement of costly cardiac assist technology was key to the financial viability of VADs. It was not a simple process, and in the past decade, new devices had typically taken between two and five years to secure national medical coverage.[100]

As industries successfully secured widening application of VADs for more patient populations, they also diligently worked to obtain device reimbursement at each stage. Targeting payers, industry labored to influence Health Technology Assessments for commercial payer coverage and to push the CMS to issue an NCD for VAD use. Its lobby efforts succeeded on both fronts. During the 1990s and the early 2000s, both Medicare and third-party payers paid for VADs in stages as patient indication and sites for implantation broadened. For example, in 1993 VADs as postcardiotomy treatment were approved for reimbursement; in 1996 VADs as BTT therapy were added; in 2001 the CMS covered VAD implantation at sites other than Medicare-approved heart transplant centers; and in 2003 VADs as destination therapy were approved for reimbursement.[101] So VAD reimbursement in the United States came incrementally, following FDA-approval stages. In Europe, there were some profits in VADs but with restrictions. For example, in France, not all CE mark–approved VADs received reimbursement, and in the United Kingdom, VAD implant reimbursements were restricted to patients eligible for and awaiting a heart transplant.[102] Still, this reimbursement in American and European markets contributed to entrenching VAD therapy as a viable treatment for heart failure patients.

In comparison to the TAH, the VAD gained greater clinical use for several reasons: its technological characteristics as a simpler, less radical device; its demonstration of safety and efficacy through positive trial results and improved clinical lives; and its attainment of FDA approval and CMS reimbursement to make it available in the American market—all of which contributed to a greater buy-in by the medical community and patients. Intuitively, one thinks that building half a heart would be easier than building a full heart, but it was more than that. VAD designs incorporated improved technology, in comparison to earlier artificial heart devices with their tremendous problems of clotting, hemolysis, biocompatibility, and energy sources. The better technology of VADs contributed to better patient outcomes, which led to greater buy-in and clinical uptake of VADs by medical and nonmedical groups.

The assistive, rather than replacement, nature of this pump appealed to physicians and patients; it was the less risky device that would meet the needs of the majority of heart failure patients who suffered left ventricular failure only. Leaving the native heart in the patient also meant that a mechanical failure of the device was not necessarily fatal. Its commercial success owed much to being a workable product as well as to industry partnerships and government advocates who labored to bring the technology to the market. Stakeholders in this technology repeatedly stated that the assist devices would continue to improve, their high cost would be reduced, and their availability would be extended beyond specialized cardiac centers. Much of this prophecy came true when a change in technology platforms shifted the design of VADs from pulsatile to nonpulsatile devices, introducing new, second-generation, continuous-flow assist pumps in the early years of the 2000s.

CHAPTER SIX

Securing a Place

Therapeutic Clout and Second-Generation VADs

I'm wired now [implanted]. . . . It's a great piece of equipment [HeartMate II LVAD]. . . . I was in bad shape 14 months ago. Now I'm back to leading a relatively normal life.

Former US vice president Dick Cheney, *USA Today,* 31 Aug 2011

In 2010 former US vice president Dick Cheney, age 69, received a mechanical heart pump implant after battling heart disease for more than 30 years. Cheney suffered his first heart attack at age 37 during his first congressional race in 1978. Thereafter he agreed to exercise, to eat better, and to quit smoking, but those lifestyle changes did not prevent additional heart attacks in 1984 and 1988. After his third heart attack, he underwent a quadruple bypass surgery and, for the next 12 years, managed his heart disease with medication. Two weeks after the stressful election of 2000, in which Cheney became the US vice president, he suffered a fourth heart attack. There were compromised, blocked arteries surrounding his heart, one of which required a stent, and later Cheney underwent angioplasty to open up other narrowed vessels. A year later, doctors implanted a cardioverter defibrillator in the vice president to detect and treat life-threatening arrhythmias. Cheney's fifth heart attack occurred after he left office in 2010. Subsequent tests and several months of increased discomfort confirmed that Cheney was in end-stage heart failure.[1]

In July 2010, surgeons at the Inova Fairfax Hospital and Vascular Institute in Virginia, outside of Washington, DC, implanted the Food and Drug Administration–approved HeartMate II left ventricular assist device in Cheney to compensate for his severely damaged heart. It would extend his life beyond the expectations of many individuals. According to his long-time cardiologist Jonathan Reiner, the implanted LVAD "provided a cardiac output that Cheney had not experienced since the 1980s."[2] A statement was released to the press, informing them about the LVAD operation and the status of Cheney's progressive heart failure. Based on comparative patient experiences, journalists gave Cheney a 50-50 chance of surviving for two years.[3]

The next year, Cheney was back in the public eye, commenting on national politics and promoting his memoir, *In My Time.* He was thinner after his surgery and quite willing to talk about his recent LVAD operation, praising modern medical

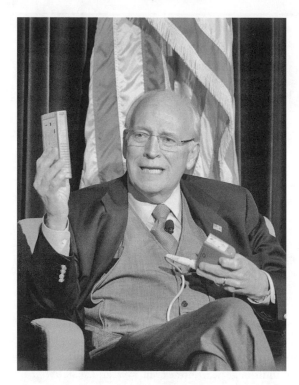

Former vice president Dick Cheney holds up the battery and control unit of his implanted HeartMate II left ventricular assist device. Cheney lived 20 months with the HeartMate II pump before undergoing a heart transplant. Photo taken on September 20, 2011, roughly 15 months after Cheney's surgery. (AP Photo/David McNew, File)

technology for resurrecting him after suffering his latest heart attack.[4] On national television, Cheney showed off his equipment, holding up the battery pack that connected via wires through his chest to the implanted mechanical pump. Sometimes Cheney disconnected the battery, setting off alarms (and unnerving some journalists), and then reconnected it and repositioned the components in his customized vest.[5] "It's brought me back from end-stage heart failure," Cheney told reporters. "I was in bad shape 14 months ago. Now I'm back to leading a relatively normal life. I fish, hunt a little bit, write books, [am] able to travel."[6] Reporters asked if a heart transplant was next, but Cheney was noncommittal at the time. Reiner answered questions about Cheney's health and activity level with the HeartMate II LVAD but commented that Cheney's recovery had certainly not been "event free."[7]

In fact, Cheney spent 35 days in the hospital after the LVAD implant, predominantly in the ICU, battling problems of bleeding, a kidney injury, pneumonia, respiratory failure, and a pneumothorax (an air leak from the lung). Cheney wrote that the LVAD surgery was "by far the toughest" in comparison to his previous heart procedures; in the past Cheney had never been this weak physically, with a severely failing heart and declining liver and kidney functions.[8] It took months of adjusting to the device and extensive rehabilitation for Cheney to start feeling well again after the implant. The device tethering was an issue for him, as it had been for past patients. Cheney found that it required "a lot of effort to adjust to always having to be plugged into a power source. . . . It was mandatory that I *never* be without power for the LVAD."[9] At a six-month follow-up appointment at the ventricular assist device clinic, Dr. Shashank Desai, director of the heart failure program at Inova Fairfax Hospital, examined Cheney and later wrote Reiner, "He [Cheney] had truly turned a corner. . . . His VAD continues to perform well. . . . I am happy to see that he has returned to a near normal quality of life."[10] It was at that point that Cheney made the decision to proceed with a heart transplant. Reiner supported the choice, stating, "I viewed the VAD as a life raft for Cheney, not a destination."[11] In March 2012, Cheney underwent a successful cardiac transplantation after living 20 months with the HeartMate II LVAD. Political cartoonists and comedians had great fun with Cheney's heart operations, for example, depicting Cheney waking up in his hospital bed as a Democrat after surgeons mistakenly transplanted a "bleeding heart."[12] Jokes aside, Cheney's "change of heart" raised the profile of VADs and further endorsed technological fixes for end-stage heart failure patients.

Cheney benefited from second-generation VAD technology. His successful outcome is linked to two previous but pivotal and overlapping events in the recent development of artificial hearts that launched this second-generation technology. First, the landmark REMATCH study, a large-scale randomized clinical trial that compared the permanent implant of first-generation VAD technology (not leading to cardiac transplantation) to conventional medical care, produced noteworthy results that forced practicing heart specialists and their patients to consider mechanical pumps more seriously. This was the first study to compare VAD technology to medical therapy as a definitive therapy, and its results compelled people to reevaluate the clinical use of this technology. According to the 2001 REMATCH study results, VAD patients lived more than twice as long as heart failure patients who were treated with medications only. The medical community debated the significance of these results: had VAD technology reached a meaningful juncture of fruition? For some medical practitioners, the results did not negate major practical and economic concerns surrounding these devices.

Second, a key change in technology platforms shifted the design of VADs from volume-displacement, pulsatile devices to continuous-flow, nonpulsatile pumps, resulting in second-generation VADs. These devices were smaller, quieter, safer, and more effective than the clunky first-generation VADs. The new continuous-flow VADs significantly reduced the problems of thromboembolism, infection, patient mobility, and device breakdowns, but the physiological implications of pulseless flow presented new, difficult clinical issues, such as dangerous gastrointestinal bleeding. Many researchers involved in first-generation devices transitioned into developing continuous-flow pumps, including Robert Jarvik, O. H. Frazier, Michael DeBakey, George Noon, and others, who wanted smaller, simpler, implantable devices to assist in ejecting blood out of damaged heart ventricles. This second-generation VAD technology built on the "bridge" use of older assist pumps and increased support for VADs as destination therapy. Not without problems, the newer VADs nonetheless worked better for select patients, swaying many in the cardiac medical field and in society to consider mechanical assist pumps as a viable option, maybe even a course that was preferable to traditional pharmacological treatments and heart transplantation in the treatment of heart failure. The story of Cheney's VAD experience, as well as other accounts publicized in the media and posted online, matched the crafted message of the device industry that VADs were a valid treatment choice and offered an extended quality of life. How society understood and approached heart failure was changing as a result of improved technology, better patient outcomes, committed researchers and surgeons, and the profit-seeking device industry.

"Proof of Concept" for Prolonged VAD Support: The REMATCH Study

During the 1990s, the clinical promise of first-generation VADs and the limited treatment options available for transplant-ineligible heart failure patients encouraged a group of cardiac surgeon-researchers to expand the use of VADs beyond a temporary therapy. First-generation VADs had already demonstrated success as a bridge-to-transplantation device, but it was uncertain whether the use of these devices could be broadened further. What was the "life expectancy" of the device, and was it safe to implant in people for a longer period? For patients in severe heart failure, would permanent VAD implants provide better outcomes than conventional drug therapy? The high cost of the technology made it more expensive than drug therapy, but would this cost be offset by the long-term benefits?[13] There was genuine uncertainty among clinicians about the relative value of these two different treatments, and thus the stage was set for an active comparison trial. It was not clear whether VADs represented better treatment than optimal drug therapy; the uncertainty inferred clinical equipoise and bolstered the case for a randomized controlled trial. As medical historian Christopher Crenner points out, a "high bar in testing" might serve to legitimate a technology for a wary audience, should outcomes favor the use of the device. While Crenner acknowledges a grand "quest for exact knowledge about therapeutic effects" in clinical research overall, device companies bound by increasing regulation in the American medical marketplace had economic motives to gather RCT data in order to secure commercial approval for their products.[14] The REMATCH clinical trial sought to generate data to resolve the uncertainty surrounding the permanent use of VADs in heart failure patients.

The first phase of clinical testing was a pilot study, dubbed the PREMATCH trial, which yielded valuable information that was needed before a large-scale clinical trial was conducted. Between April 1996 and April 1998, 21 patients in five medical centers were randomized to receive either a pulsatile HeartMate VE LVAD implant or conventional drug therapy. The value of this trial was the collection of preliminary data on patient outcomes and device reliability. Could this older, sicker, and transplant-ineligible group of patients withstand the LVAD implant surgery? Yes. Did LVAD patients fare significantly better or worse than those treated with medications? It remained uncertain. At three months, each treatment group had an almost 30 percent mortality rate, which substantiated clinical equipoise for a definitive, larger clinical trial.[15] Was the LVAD technology reliable? Yes. The HeartMate VE LVAD was a vented electric pump, which Thoratec researchers were still modifying, but the pilot study provided sufficient safety and efficacy data to secure premarket approval of this device from the FDA's Circulatory System Devices Panel in 1998. It also offered the opportunity for surgeons to gain further experience with the device before the main clinical trial.[16]

In addition, the pilot study prompted investigators to refine certain aspects of the study. Most significantly, researchers tightened the comparative focus in their study. Instead of comparing LVAD technology with standard community heart failure care, investigators chose to test device implant outcomes against optimal drug therapy for severe heart failure. What would the "optimal" protocol look like? Answering this question necessitated the development of standards for both the medical treatment and the surgical treatment of patients in the absence of explicit guidelines for optimal medical management and long-term LVAD implants. As a result of the pilot study, investigators finalized the REMATCH protocol design and consolidated support for the second phase of clinical testing—a definitive multicenter RCT.[17]

The REMATCH clinical trial, conducted from May 1998 to July 2001, remains the only RCT that has compared the permanent implantation of an LVAD with conventional drug therapy in transplant-incligible heart failure patients. It was an investigator-initiated study collaboratively conducted between Columbia University, the National Institutes of Health, and Thoratec Laboratories. The trial was led by cardiac surgeon Eric Rose, who was chair of surgery at Columbia University and surgeon-in-chief at Columbia Presbyterian Medical Center. The NIH provided financial support for the costs of data collection and analysis as well as operation costs, as did Thoratec Laboratories, which also donated the LVADs and related equipment for the trial.[18] The Centers for Medicare and Medicaid Services paid for all treatment costs, except for the implant hospitalization, which was covered by participating hospitals. Some medical centers chose not to participate in the trial because of the financial burden of the implant hospitalization. No RCT patients were charged for any study costs, since it would be unethical to financially exploit vulnerable patients with a life-threatening condition. The REMATCH trial took place in 20 US cardiac transplantation centers with expertise in the treatment of severe heart failure. The clinical trial was supervised by a steering committee and carried out by an operations committee with an independent coordinating center. Institutional review boards at all of the participating medical centers approved the study protocol, and all patients signed written informed consent forms.[19]

The REMATCH study enrolled a total of 129 patients in severe heart failure, and none were eligible for cardiac transplantation. Various clinical conditions made a patient ineligible for cardiac transplantation, including peripheral vascular disease, pulmonary hypertension, obesity, substance abuse, psychosocial factors, renal problems, and pulmonary dysfunction. Most commonly, a patient's age kept him or her from organ donor waiting lists. Given these contraindications for transplantation, patients in the REMATCH study were older individuals (the average age was 66) with severe left ventricular dysfunction as well as other medical problems. These were very sick people, with complex medical issues, looking to extend their lives. Through random assignment, 68 patients received an LVAD—Thoratec's HeartMate XVE LVAD (an improved, modified version of the HeartMate VE model)—and 61 patients followed a drug treatment regimen, including angiotension-converting-enzyme inhibitors, which focused on optimizing organ perfusion and minimizing symptoms of congestive heart failure.[20] Individual investigators at each medical site determined the eligibility of patients for the study, and a gatekeeper at the coordinating center ensured that all candidates met strict trial patient criteria. The REMATCH study was not a double-blind trial because of the surgical risk associated with the LVAD operation and the obvious nature of its implantation. The patients, surgeons, and other investigators were not blinded to the treatment assignment, but most were blinded to interim outcomes. Statisticians recorded interim outcomes for both groups. Also, Thoratec investigators monitored LVAD patient data for device safety reasons, but they were blinded to all outcomes from the medical-therapy patient group. After the death of the 92nd patient, a predetermined study endpoint, no more patients were enrolled in the clinical trial.[21]

Given the uncertainty surrounding LVAD technology as a long-term therapy in an older, sicker population, the results of the study surprised many in the medical community. REMATCH investigators reported that LVAD patients lived significantly longer than medical-therapy patients. After one year of treatment, 52 percent of LVAD patients were still alive, compared with 25 percent of medical-therapy patients; after two years, the survival rate was 23 percent for LVAD patients compared with 8 percent of medical-therapy patients.[22] LVAD patients stayed in the hospital longer (median number of days: 88) than did the drug therapy group (median number of days: 24). For those who died during the study, medical-therapy patients succumbed to heart failure, while LVAD patients tended to die of infection or mechanical failure of the device.[23] The REMATCH study confirmed conventional knowledge that available cardiac drugs managed mild-to-moderate heart failure much more successfully than end-stage heart failure.

Nevertheless, the REMATCH results pointed to significant LVAD complications and adverse events for LVAD patients, including problems of bleeding, neurological dysfunction, infections, thromboembolic complications, and renal failure.[24] The percutaneous (through the skin) line that connected the implanted LVAD with external power and controller units became infected in many cases, and as a result, sepsis was the most common cause of death in the device group. Device reliability continued to be an issue. During the course of the trial, 17 devices in 52 patients needed replacement, usually owing to mechanical pump failure or inflow valve incompetence, prompting LVAD modifications by Thoratec device researchers and the implementation of infection management guidelines by REMATCH investigators.[25] The number of adverse events experienced by LVAD patients reportedly declined thereafter.[26]

Even with these occurrences, LVAD patients reported a better quality of life and functionality than the medical-therapy patients, according to the REMATCH study. Did this represent an acceptable tradeoff for LVAD patients, given the natural history of advanced heart failure? REMATCH trial investigators stated that it did.[27] It was clear that the survival rate for heart failure patients with medical therapy was poor and that LVAD implantations improved upon that survival rate. When the trial ended in June 2001, three out of the five surviving patients in the medical-therapy arm of the study crossed over for an LVAD implant.[28] Still, the overall two-year LVAD patient survival rate of 23 percent was hardly cause to rejoice, and reported LVAD-related complications strongly called for device improvement.[29] The study results did not fully erase the uncertainty surrounding these devices, and there were varied responses from the medical community.

To what degree were the REMATCH trial results significant? The study demonstrated that long-term support with an LVAD was feasible and that it provided higher survival rates than optimal drug therapy for severe heart failure patients who were not candidates for cardiac transplantation. Yet the device was not a cure for heart failure. As REMATCH investigators admitted, cardiac transplantation far exceeded the survival rate of LVAD-implanted patients in their study.[30] Still, the REMATCH results suggested a promising role for LVADs for some heart failure patients as a life-extending device, indeed as a "lifeboat," commented cardiac surgeon Stephen Westaby at a medical meeting of thoracic surgeons in 2003. Westaby stated, "The clear survival advantage for patients receiving LVADs now justifies the use of circulatory support well beyond the transplant setting."[31] In the medical literature, including standard medical reference texts like *Braunwald's Heart Disease,* the REMATCH trial was increasingly being described as a "remarkable," "unprecedented," and "landmark" study for moving the potential clinical use of LVAD technology forward in a way that past case studies had not.[32]

Yet there were undeniable practical and economic concerns with this technology, which several members of the medical community raised in response to the REMATCH study. Cardiologist Lynne Stevenson, a nationally renowned leader in heart failure and director of the Cardiomyopathy and Heart Failure Program at the Brigham and Women's Hospital in Boston, acknowledged the "exciting new option" of LVADs but promoted a cautious view of its use.[33] For clinicians, end-stage heart failure management emphasizes individual care; physicians seek to relieve patient symptoms and to decrease disease progression in mild-to-moderate stages, and in advanced heart failure cases, they concentrate on prolonging function and quality of life for their patients. As a therapy for end-stage heart failure patients, Stevenson stated that device durability was the predominant limiting factor against the widespread clinical use of LVADs.[34] The most obvious issue was that these devices were far from perfect.

Stevenson and other cardiologists worked in a rapidly changing medical landscape and acknowledged that the field of heart failure management was progressing quickly in this period.[35] Cardiologists did not sound an anti-LVAD technology horn, but they were restrained in its clinical uptake. The complexity of therapeutic options was increasing, and, as pointed out by Stevenson and her colleagues at the American Heart Association, this fact made shared decision-making more crucial and challenging in the management of advanced heart failure.[36] For the most part, cardiologists acknowledged the LVAD as an evolving technology and advocated for better devices and patient care practices to improve outcomes. Arguably, these steps would help lower the high rate of complications associated with LVAD implants, a necessary factor if this technology had any hope of widespread adoption. Clinical information about device implantation and performance and patient care management had been built on knowledge gained in the laboratory through bench testing and animal experiments with the devices. As investigators continue to engage in these "learn-by-using" experiences, any clinical shortcomings or potential new applications of the technology will necessarily lead to more bench research and design modifications, which will in turn loop back to improved patient outcomes.[37]

REMATCH investigators anticipated and adjusted for such a learning curve scenario with implantation of the Heartmate XVE LVAD. In the early stages of the REMATCH trial, surgeons reported an inflow valve incompetence problem with the LVAD that negatively affected blood flow through the device. During the second half of the study, several device modifications were made, specifically, the screw ring connectors on the inflow and outflow grafts were now locking to avert disconnection, and the outflow graft had added "bend relief" to prevent kinking.[38] Similar "learn-by-using" changes occurred with patient care after implantation. The problem of sepsis in LVAD patients declined after specific infection management guidelines, which defined the choice of antimicrobial prophylaxis, were written and post-op patients wore abdominal binders, which immobilized the exiting drive line, reducing trauma and deterring infection.[39] LVAD patients who enrolled later in the study benefited from these changes, an improved-outcome trend that continued after the REMATCH trial.[40] REMATCH investigators monitored device performance carefully to ensure that any redesign made to address one problem did not introduce the possibility of another problem. Nevertheless, cardiac surgeon Matthias Loebe stated, "If we want to consider mechanical assist devices as a real alternative . . . we definitely have to improve their technical performance."[41] Understandably, persistent reports of device malfunctions made clinicians wary.

Would the introduction of LVADs as destination therapy lead to an indication "creep," with pressure to implant these devices in less ill patients? University of California cardiologist Barry Massie warned that "this is a treacherous path to follow."[42] Granted, the patients enrolled in the REMATCH study were extremely ill. As Massie points out, many of these patients were "too far gone" at the start of the trial to realistically recover from any operation or device complications. As Stevenson indicated, the field was learning to identify those patients who were "sick enough" to warrant an LVAD implant and yet "well enough" to survive the surgery.[43] Arguably, a less ill group of heart failure patients would have responded better to an LVAD implant in the REMATCH study. But then this same group might have also improved considerably with optimal drug therapy, without device and implantation risks. Massie reminded others that individual cases of patients delisted from transplant lists after responding well to drug treatment were known in the field. Given the present state of LVAD technology, he argued that the complications associated with the device outweighed the potential benefit for less-ill heart failure patients.[44]

Wrapped up in the discussion of device durability and patient outcomes was the issue of cost. University of Pennsylvania cardiologist Mariell Jessup stated the obvious: "We now know that ventricular assist devices prolong life; we do not yet know for how long and at what cost."[45] LVAD technology and its management were very expensive and labor intensive. REMATCH investigators reported that the mean total cost for the LVAD patient in the study was $210,187, which included the $60,000 cost of the device and other direct medical costs related to surgery and recovery. (At approximately $200,000, the average cost of cardiac transplantation is roughly the same as the first-year cost of LVAD therapy.)[46] This cost was significantly greater than the expense of treating the patient in the drug therapy group, the difference directly related to the lengthy hospital stay for the LVAD patient. On average, LVAD patients stayed 88 days in the hospital, and patients in the drug-therapy group stayed only 24 days. The cost of taking care of the LVAD patients, roughly $4,000 a day, elicited considerable negative reactions from hospital administrators.[47] The pressure for cost containment was evident if adoption of LVADs as destination therapy was to occur.

The REMATCH study results prompted other device clinical trials, initiated by other device companies seeking entry into the medical marketplace.[48] Between 2000 and 2003, the Investigation of Nontransplant-Eligible Patients Who Are Inotrope Dependent (INTrEPID) clinical trial took place in 13 medical centers in the United States and Canada that had experience implanting the Novacor Left Ventricular Assist System (LVAS) as a bridge to transplantation. Like the REMATCH trial, the INTrEPID study sought to demonstrate mechanical device superiority over optimal medical management (OMM) of non-transplant-eligible patients, but this time the device to be implanted permanently was the Novacor pump. The INTrEPID study was a prospective, nonrandomized clinical trial with fewer patients, who were younger but otherwise had characteristics similar to those of the patients in the REMATCH trial. The results of the INTrEPID study reinforced the REMATCH data by demonstrating that LVAD patients survived longer, with improved functional capacity and quality of life, than OMM patients.[49] Together, these two studies provided a "proof of concept" that prolonged LVAD support for heart failure patients was promising.[50]

But LVAD patients still had the ghastly mortality rate of almost 75 percent at one year, hardly enough for the "fledgling field" of mechanical circulatory support systems to trounce competing heart failure treatments, according to Stevenson.[51] While the trials demonstrated that LVADs could provide longer-term support for a critically ill patient population (Class IV heart failure was the criterion for inclusion), issues of device durability and function remained. No one disputed that incidences of device failure and adverse medical events needed to be lowered. In addition, patient selection was important—could patients not so critically ill benefit more from this technology? As Stevenson admitted, the REMATCH study included "the sickest group of heart-failure patients ever to enter a clinical trial."[52] In addition, improved postoperative and longer-term patient management strategies needed to be defined. In any case, the results of the INTrEPID trial prompted another clinical trial with the Novacor LVAS, this time comparing it with its prime competitor.

The Randomized Evaluation of Novacor LVAS in a Non-Transplant Population (RELIANT) trial, which began in 2004, was a randomized patient study to compare morbidity and mortality outcomes in patients implanted with the Novacor LVAS compared with patients implanted with the HeartMate XVE LVAD. Both devices were electrically actuated, wearable pulsatile pumps with comparable patient results from single-device studies. The Novacor device was larger and heavier than the HeartMate pump. Although the Novacor LVAS had comparable mechanical reliability and durability, Novacor device patients experienced a higher rate of thromboembolic events leading to stroke, and subsequently, clinicians tended to favor the HeartMate XVE LVAD. But the researchers behind the Novacor system argued that their device was the better LVAD and wanted RCT results to prove this. Corporate bidding trumped biomedical research wishes to answer this question. The Novacor LVAS was phased out of investigational use before the completion of the RELIANT study, and no reports of the study were ever published.[53] The manufacturer, World-Heart Corporation, discontinued its support of the study in late 2006 to redirect funding to the development of a different technology platform.[54] While the industry-academic alliances were necessary to develop this technology, their relationship was not always smooth and noncontroversial; corporate bottom lines tended to dominate loftier research pursuits.

Like the WorldHeart Corporation, other industrial-academic teams also pursued multiple technology platforms, prompting the emergence of next-generation VADs. New biomaterials, miniaturization, and improved pump designs promised to resolve problems of thromboembolism, infection, and patient mobility that had challenged the older pulsatile LVADs. A clear enthusiasm for nonpulsatile devices emerged, specifically the axial-design, continuous-flow rotary pump technology of the HeartMate II device, the Jarvik 2000 pump, and a handful of other competing devices. Development of these next-generation devices clearly benefited from the clinical trials of the older technology, notably the influential REMATCH study for its data supporting longer-term device use in patients and extended clinical indication.

The distinction between temporary and permanent use of these devices became blurred. Back in the 1980s, bioethicists first raised this issue after numerous "temporary" Jarvik-7 TAH implant patients experienced complications that removed them from transplant lists. These cases of temporary-turned-permanent bridges meant that patients unintentionally found themselves spending their remaining days tethered to a machine.[55] Would LVAD-implant patients be more willing to accept these risks? Because of long waiting lists, LVAD-supported patients waiting for a heart transplant might well continue to be implanted with their device for a year or longer, and during that period their transplant status might be altered if their health deteriorated.[56] Were LVADs better than TAH technology, making this only a remote risk? Conversely, patients initially ineligible for transplantation might improve on LVAD support enough to resolve their previous contraindications and thereafter become eligible candidates. The categories for use of LVADs were merging clinically as the distinction between temporary and permanent therapy became less relevant for patients and clinicians. As cardiac surgeon James Kirklin said, "the clinical reality is that few therapies are exclusively 'either/or' for the duration of the heart failure patient's life."[57] The ambiguous nature of transplant status for many patients led surgeons to employ a strategy of "bridge to candidacy" or "bridge to decision," an emerging grey zone between "bridge to transplantation" and "destination therapy" indications for the clinical use of LVAD technology.

The Second-Generation Devices: The Continuous-Flow VADs of the 1990s

During the 1980s and 1990s, the majority of cardiac surgeons in the United States and Canada were not implanting the sophisticated and expensive pulsatile VAD pumps—the Thoratec PVAD, the Novacor LVAS, and the HeartMate LVAD.[58] Instead, surgeons used intraaortic balloon pumps, centrifugal pumps, or roller pumps to provide short-term support for the patient unable to be weaned from the heart-lung machine after surgery.[59] Developed back in the 1960s, these devices constituted the primary method of mechanical circulatory support because they were commercially available, simple to use, and inexpensive. Balloon pumps are counterpulsation devices, inserted into the aorta, that assist with moving blood to the coronary arteries, thereby increasing oxygen delivery to the heart, but with only minimal cardiac output support of blood flow to the body. Centrifugal and roller pumps are external mechanical devices with slightly greater cardiac output support than balloon pumps. Adrian

Kantrowitz invented the intraaortic balloon pump from a modified LVAD design to provide temporary assistance for patients in cardiogenic shock.[60] The drawbacks of the balloon pumps, centrifugal pumps, and roller pumps were that all had a relatively low flow rate, insufficient for large patients or patients with severe cardiac malfunction, and patient mobility was greatly reduced because of the cannulation and tethering of the patient to a drive console. More limiting was the fact that these pumps could be used only for short-term support, about one week or less.

Many cardiac patients required stronger and longer mechanical circulatory support, but it was not clear that the pulsatile VAD pumps under development would meet this need sufficiently, owing to their technological limitations.[61] The pulsatile design of first-generation VADs was biomimicry; the technology attempted to imitate the form and action of the heart. Two major drawbacks of this design were its large size and issues of durability; smaller patients needed smaller devices that would function for longer than two years. A major shift in design approaches ensued, from pulsatile to nonpulsatile flow of blood in assist pumps, marking a key turning point in the development of VADs.

In the early 1980s, physician Richard Wampler and the Nimbus Corporation in Rancho Cordova, California, presented a different VAD design based on continuous-flow (nonpulsatile) technology—the Hemopump. The Hemopump is a miniature axial flow pump (about the size of a pencil eraser) that is inserted into the aorta, just above the aortic valve, and powered electrically by an external motor. This VAD uses pulsing electromagnetic fields to rotate a permanent magnet, spinning the pump blades rapidly to draw oxygenated blood from the left ventricle out to the body. Intended as a short-term device, the Hemopump sought to assume up to 80 percent of the left ventricle's pumping action, allowing the heart to rest and ultimately recover from heart failure within a matter of days.[62] Compared with other VADs, the Hemopump was much easier to implant—no need for major surgery—since it was catheter-inserted through the femoral artery. Wampler, working with mechanical engineers Ken Butler and John Moise, intentionally copied this feature of the balloon pump while making the Hemopump more effective in its flow capacity.[63] The Hemopump was a simple and inexpensive device that produced sufficiently promising animal and bench testing results to warrant FDA approval for clinical trial in 1988. But good clinical results did not materialize; issues of device reliability emerged, with reports of improper device placement and dislodgement, kinking of the tube, blocked inflow openings, and other problems.[64] Some clinicians reported some success with the device, but it was not enough for the FDA's Circulatory System Devices Panel to approve the device for commercial sale in the United States. Wampler's Hemopump did gain approval in Europe, but it failed to penetrate the lucrative American market in its existing form at this time.

The significance of the Hemopump is that it demonstrated the promise of continuous-flow technology. Its smaller and simpler design suggested greater mechanical durability, quieter operation, and fewer medical complications than the

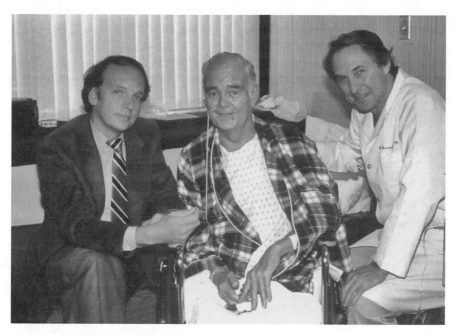

Hemopump inventor Richard Wampler (*left*), patient Herb Kranich (*center*), and cardiac surgeon O. H. Frazier, after the first clinical implant of the Hemopump on April 17, 1988. Kranich recovered and later received a heart transplant. Courtesy of the Texas Heart Institute.

pulsatile VADs.[65] There was only one moving part—the internal rotor—and the device required no valves, thus reducing clotting risks and mechanical malfunctions. Its small size permitted the use of a smaller implantation pocket, reducing infection risks and allowing its implantation in smaller patients. It required less power to operate and a thinner drive line connection to its power console. But would the body tolerate the nonpulsatile movement of blood? What about the physiological importance of pulsatile blood flow in the body?[66] The first-generation VADs had been built based on a working principle parallel to the action of the human heart, with filling (diastole) and ejection (systole) phases, mimicking blood movement and ventricle emptying to augment decreased native organ function. For many clinicians, it was intuitive that mechanical simulation should replicate natural heart function as closely as possible, and it was the dominant view that the arterial pulse played an important physiological and metabolic role in the body. Intermittent, pulsatile blood flow maintained and regulated vascular tone, blood pressure, capillary circulation, organ perfusion, kidney and liver function, and cellular metabolism.[67] In 1974 surgeon-researcher Eugene Bernstein published a key research paper addressing contemporary concerns on the harmful effects of decreased pulsatile blood flow; he demonstrated that dogs lived months, sometimes years, with nonpulsatile blood flow without experiencing bleeding problems, compromised organ perfusion, or other harmful effects.[68] This evidence should have settled the physiological question, but it remained controversial, and an uncertainty surrounding the body's need for pulsatile blood flow remained.

The physiological, metabolic, and hematologic effects of continuous-flow, constant-high-speed, nonpulsatile pumps continued to be debated. Surgical researchers, clinicians, and physiologists reviewed reports of blood trauma, increased bleeding in the gastrointestinal tract, limited cardiac unloading, vascular malformations, end-organ function, and aortic valve insufficiency with the use of continuous-flow VADs.[69] When first approached by Wampler in the late 1980s, cardiac surgeon O. H. Frazier told him that a continuous-flow pump would not work—calling it a "potential blender for blood" (too harmful for fragile blood cells)—and then recanted after animal studies and patient experiences with the device at the Texas Heart Institute proved otherwise.[70] Clinical cases with the Hemopump showed that, despite the high speed of the blades, there was minimal blood damage or hemolysis and the body did appear to tolerate the nonpulsatile movement of blood. Studies reported that blood circulation and organ perfusion were in no way compromised. Still, was it the non-pulsatile characteristic of the Hemopump that explained the promising results in some of the heart failure patients implanted with this device? Or was it something else? The operating mechanism clearly offered a smaller, more durable, quieter device that might lessen the larger adverse effects of the older VADs, but it did not provide complete ventricular unloading or remove all risk of embolism or infection.[71] Nevertheless, it prompted various VAD research teams to pay greater attention to pump miniaturization, device placement, and continuous-flow technology.

The HeartMate II LVAD

In 1991 the Nimbus Corporation formed a partnership with the University of Pittsburgh's McGowan Center for Organ Engineering (later incorporated as the McGowan Institute for Regenerative Medicine) to develop an improved continuous-flow pump for longer-term use, altering the Hemopump device in several ways. This collaboration of the Hemopump team of Wampler, Butler, and Moise with the Pittsburgh group of cardiac surgeons Bartley P. Griffith and Robert Kormos and bioengineer Harvey Borovetz produced a device with a different bearing design, which, in calves and sheep, generated better cardiac flow with minimal trauma detected. But the Nimbus-Pittsburgh project was underfunded for many years, and research and development limped along slowly.[72] In 1996 Nimbus was acquired by Thermo Cardiosystems Inc., which in turn was acquired in 2001 by Thoratec Laboratories, and this brought TCI's broad-based engineering capabilities and its Heart-Mate (pulsatile) device experience under engineer Victor Poirier to the Nimbus-Pittsburgh project.[73] In 1997 the National Heart, Lung, and Blood Institute's circulatory support program awarded multiyear funding to this group to test their device, which became known as the HeartMate II (continuous-flow) LVAD.

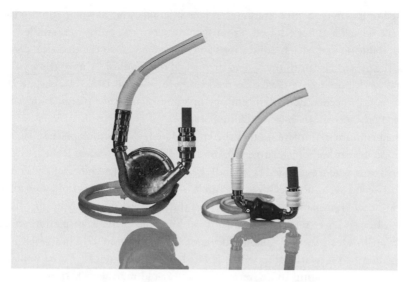

The HeartMate XVE Left Ventricular Assist System (LVAS), a first-generation, pulsatile pump (*left*), and the HeartMate II Left Ventricular Assist Device (LVAD), a second-generation, continuous-flow technology. HeartMate II and St. Jude Medical are trademarks of St. Jude Medical Inc. or its related companies. Reproduced with permission of St. Jude Medical, ©2016. All rights reserved.

The HeartMate II is an axial-flow rotary VAD that consists of a blood pump, a percutaneous lead, an external power source, and a system driver. The pump has only one moving part, a cylindrical impeller or rotor with blades that propels blood along its axis from the left ventricle through the pump and into the circulation system. A magnetic field spins the rotor on its blood lubricated bearings, and all inner surfaces of the device are covered with a textured, blood-coating system (also used in the older, pulsatile HeartMate device) to resist clot formation. The operating speed of the HeartMate II device is generally 8,000 and 10,000 rpm, to generate an impressive flow rate of 10 liters (more than 2.6 gallons) per minute (stronger than pulsatile pumps' rate). Cardiac surgeons implant the HeartMate II device in approximately the same location as the older pulsatile VADs, using similar methods. As in first-generation VADs, a system driver operates the HeartMate II pump, sending power to the device and receiving information from the device, through the power base unit that tethers to the patient. For greater mobility, patients may use a battery pack to provide power to the pump for two to four hours.[74] (Over the next 10 years, improved battery power liberated patients from the stationary drive unit for up to 12 hours.) Smaller and lighter than the earlier model, the HeartMate II pump was one-seventh the size and one-fourth the weight of the older HeartMate pulsatile LVAD; it was also quieter and had only one moving part, a 40 percent smaller lead, and greater long-term durability.[75] But did it work better? Animal and bench testing attested to its safety, demonstrating that blood damage and biocompatibility issues with the device had been solved. From 1997 to 2000, the pump was studied in 51 calves, resulting in device modifications and improvements to the electrical connections, the power base unit, the system driver, and the monitor. Almost three years of animal work produced a device deemed ready for clinical trial. HeartMate II researchers now needed data on its efficacy in humans, and they planned for clinical testing first overseas, then in the United States.[76]

The first human implantation of the HeartMate II device took place in Israel, in July 2000, by cardiothoracic surgeon Jacob Lavee, a previous trainee at the University of Pittsburgh, who was assisted by attending McGowan team members. (The connection between Lavee and McGowan researchers dated back 10 years to Lavee's fellowship in heart transplantation and VADs at the University of Pittsburgh Medical Center. In 1991 Lavee returned to Israel to establish the Heart Transplantation Unit at the Leviev Heart Center, Chaim Sheba Medical Center, in Tel Hashomer, Israel, and maintained a relationship with his Pittsburgh colleagues.)[77] Lavee implanted the HeartMate II pump in a severely ill, 64-year-old man who had exhausted all other treatment options. At the time of the operation, it was reported that the patient had only 10 percent working heart capacity and that he would have died within six hours. The implant procedure took 12 hours, and the patient lived another five days before succumbing to multiple organ failure. Lavee told reporters that the device "functioned perfectly" and that it had "not been responsible" for the patient's death.[78] It encouraged the McGowan team and its TCI industry partner to plan for more implantations in Israel and for a four-center European study to document the safety and feasibility of the HeartMate II.

The goal of the European study was to measure the device's performance to keep heart failure patients alive for six months and to present this data to the FDA's Circulatory System Devices Panel for approval for American implants.[79] But few patients survived that long. The study was stopped early, after fewer than 10 patients, when the HeartMate II team discovered a device design problem that caused a high incidence of pump thrombosis.[80] In this case, an effective device design that worked in the older, pulsatile HeartMate LVAD caused a problem for the newer HeartMate II device. In the pulsatile HeartMate LVAD, the use of textured inner blood-contact surfaces created crucial biocompatible tissue lining in the pump, promoting and anchoring blood clots, facilitating smooth blood flow, and avoiding thromboembolism events (strokes) in patients. But in the HeartMate II device, the textured surface of the stators (or stationary parts of the rotor) created anchored clots too near the pump openings, narrowing the blood flow path, allowing clots to form, and compromising cardiac output.[81] The HeartMate II team redesigned the device by replacing the textured surface with a smooth, polished titanium surface, and this move virtually eliminated the thrombus problem. Specifically, the HeartMate II pump motor and blood tube have smooth titanium surfaces, while the inlet and outlet elbows and the intraventricular cannulas have textured linings.[82] In 2003 HeartMate II clinical studies resumed in Europe, and thereafter in the United States, with the redesigned device. At THI, Frazier reported excellent results with the redesigned HeartMate II, in comparison to his experience with other VADs; 80 percent of his HeartMate II patients on transplant waiting lists met one-year survival rates, and his permanently implanted HeartMate II patients reported improved heart function, general health, and quality of life.[83]

In 2005 and 2006, a large, prospective clinical trial of the HeartMate II as a BTT device, sponsored by Thoratec in consultation with FDA administrators, took place at 26 US medical centers with notable results. In this study, 133 heart failure patients, who were on heart transplantation waiting lists but declining in heart function, received HeartMate II implants. As a result of the HeartMate II device, the study reported that the majority of VAD patients experienced significantly improved hemodynamic status, with recovered heart function and better quality of life. Seventy-five percent of the patients reached the six-month survival mark with their HeartMate II implant, at which time they underwent heart transplantation, had the device explanted because their heart function had sufficiently recovered, or continued with their VAD support.[84] Two years later, a follow-up study of this cohort as well as new heart failure patients reported similar positive results with their HeartMate II implantation.[85] At about the same time, between 2005 and 2007, there was a randomized trial of 200 patients to compare the efficacy of the older, pulsatile HeartMate LVAD with the newer, continuous-flow HeartMate II device as a permanent therapy for heart failure patients ineligible for heart transplantation. After two years, the study recorded that the HeartMate II patients had a significantly better rate of survival, improved heart function, and good quality of life.[86]

Not all patients who participated in the HeartMate II clinical trials enjoyed successful outcomes. This result was not surprising, since these were very ill patients, often in the last stages of congestive heart failure. In every HeartMate II trial, there were reports of adverse events related to the device and the management of care. The more common problems included VAD-related infections from the percutaneous drive line or the pump pocket, clotting or thrombosis incidents with the device, and gastrointestinal bleeding. Some patients died, as a result of strokes, device malfunctions, and coexisting medical conditions. The continuous-flow pumps supported left ventricular function only, and in some cases, patients also required right VAD support to pump blood to the lungs; thus their overall heart operation was compromised. Still, relative to earlier clinical research, these studies produced much lower postoperative mortality rates and fewer adverse events for VAD-supported patients. The device was not perfect, but it appeared good enough for an increasing number of heart failure patients with limited treatment options. Thoratec submitted the clinical trial data to FDA officials to support its HeartMate II PMA application for commercial distribution of the device in the United States. In April 2008 the FDA's Circulatory System Devices Panel approved the HeartMate II as a temporary, BTT device; and in January 2010 the device was approved as a permanent, destination therapy.[87] Thoratec had successfully shepherded several cardiac devices into the US medical marketplace and now dominated the global LVAD market.

The Jarvik 2000 Flowmaker Pump

Robert Jarvik was knee-deep in artificial heart research and development during the 1970s and 1980s, most notably with the Jarvik-7 total artificial heart and the infamous Barney Clark permanent implant. Not surprisingly, Jarvik and his colleagues at the University of Utah were tinkering with VADs alongside TAHs, these overlapping lines of research supported by considerable NHLBI grant and contract funding.[88] In terms of design, the pneumatically powered Jarvik-7 TAH consisted of two ventricles, elliptical in shape, which connected at the base to form a spherical heart device. An adaptation of the Jarvik-7 heart to a VAD (using only one ventricle of the Jarvik-7 heart) was implanted in sheep to augment, not replace, heart function. But like other first-generation, pulsatile pumps, Jarvik's auxiliary ventricle had device tethering and pump problems, leading to such adverse events as blood clotting, infection, and valve breakage.[89] No doubt aware of the continuous-flow technology being explored by Wampler and others, Jarvik also toyed with axial flow in cardiac assist devices, which Kolff described as "extremely novel," "very revolutionary," and "most promising."[90] Not much came of this line of research at the University of Utah (which was just as well, since it allowed Jarvik to develop this device later without conflict with Symbion device rights during the 1990s). After the Jarvik-7 heart implant in Barney Clark in 1982–83, Jarvik was predominantly occupied with running Symbion Inc. as chairman and chief executive officer and marketing the company's various products. At the time, Symbion manufactured the Acute Ventricular Assist Device, which was a paracorporeal pulsatile pump for single or biventricular assist based on the Jarvik heart technology. Then in 1987 the Symbion board of directors fired Jarvik, who had long been at odds with the board, vehemently opposing their decision to accept a bid for takeover of Symbion by the investment firm of E. M. Warburg Pincus and Company.[91] Jarvik moved to New York and set up his own device company, Jarvik Research Inc., thereafter focusing his attention almost exclusively on the development of his continuous-flow VAD—the Jarvik 2000 Flowmaker pump.[92]

Jarvik's continuous-flow VAD system encompassed a blood pump, an outflow graft, a percutaneous power cable, a controller, and a power supply. Its technology platform was distinctly different from that of his pneumatic, pulsatile pumps developed in Utah, with their many limitations; for Jarvik, continuous-flow technology represented the future research direction of the field. The Jarvik 2000 is a small, implantable, axial-flow impeller pump, about the size of a C-cell battery. It initially weighed 260 grams, or about a half pound (approximately the weight of the competing HeartMate II) but was eventually reduced to only 90 grams (one-fifth of a pound). Like the HeartMate II, the Jarvik 2000 had only one moving part, a single titanium, vaned impeller that spun on two ceramic blood-immersed bearings. Its

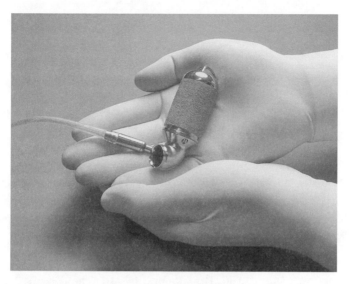

The Jarvik 2000 Ventricular Assist Device, roughly the size of a C-cell battery. Courtesy of Jarvik Heart Inc.

operating speed was the same as that of the HeartMate II device; however, the Jarvik 2000 generated less cardiac output at an approximate flow rate of 7 liters per minute. The Jarvik 2000 was electrically powered, with a direct-current motor contained within the device to generate the electromagnetic force that rotated the impeller. The device received power from an external controller. The Jarvik 2000 was significantly smaller and lighter than any other continuous-flow VAD under development at the time.[93]

The Jarvik 2000 also involved several novel design aspects, such as the surgical placement of the pump. Cardiac surgeons implanted the device directly within the left ventricle, which then pushed blood to an outflow graft attached to the aorta for circulation throughout the body. Jarvik and his co-workers produced various design iterations and improvements, experimenting with different device versions in rigorous bench and animal testing. The percutaneous version of the Jarvik 2000 required the insertion of the power cable through the abdominal wall, while another version explored the use of a transcutaneous (across the skin) energy transfer system coil to avoid having drive lines penetrate the skin.[94] A third Jarvik 2000 prototype incorporated a titanium pedestal, screwed to the skull at the back of the head, as a way of transferring external power and control to the implanted device. Drawing from similar skull-mounted pedestals used with artificial hearing devices, Jarvik and his co-workers hoped to minimize the infection problems typically reported with abdominal percutaneous exit sites.[95]

Next, Jarvik tested different versions of his device at two cardiac centers in the United States and England, first in animals, then in heart failure patients. During the 1990s, Frazier and his Houston surgical research team implanted the abdominal-percutaneous Jarvik 2000 device in 37 calves, while a similar surgical research team at the Oxford Heart Centre, under Dr. Stephen Westaby, implanted the skull-pedestal Jarvik 2000 pump in 30 sheep.[96] In both calves and sheep, the Jarvik 2000 provided good cardiac output with negligible problems of thrombosis, infection, or hemolysis. Animal implantations demonstrated that the device worked well enough; however, the issue of greater system reliability remained, requiring greater bioengineering attention to the durability of the bearings, the flex-fatigue of the electric wires, and the reliability of the electronic system, including the batteries.[97] Still, the data collected from these studies was good, and it strengthened Jarvik's applications to the US FDA and the United Kingdom's Medical Devices Agency for approval to initiate patient trials with the Jarvik 2000 pump.

The first human implants with the experimental device took place in early 2000 in both the United States and England. In April 2000 at THI, Frazier implanted the percutaneous Jarvik 2000 as a BTT device, while two months later at the Oxford Heart Centre, Westaby implanted the skull-pedestal Jarvik 2000 as a permanent implant.[98] Over the next year, Frazier implanted 10 patients with the Jarvik 2000 pump, recording only minor technical problems and no device failures. In 2001 Frazier reported that seven of the patients successfully underwent heart transplantation; three patients died while being supported with the Jarvik 2000.[99] No one left the hospital while supported by the mechanical pump, because of previously established trial restrictions. In contrast, Westaby's first patient, 61-year-old Peter Houghton, did leave the hospital as intended with his permanent Jarvik 2000 implant. In the first year of the trial, Westaby implanted the device in four male patients, three of whom were discharged from the hospital.[100]

Houghton lived an extraordinary seven and a half years with his Jarvik 2000 pump, enjoying improved heart function and a quality of life that allowed him to resume daily activities as well as travel internationally.[101] Sometimes Houghton accompanied Jarvik to medical meetings, showcasing his recovery with the device to audience members.[102] Over the years, Houghton participated in charity walks and hiked for miles in the Swiss Alps and the American West. He even survived a mugging and the abrupt termination of his heart pump while shopping in Birmingham's busy city center. A teenage thief grabbed Houghton's camera bag, which contained the battery powering the implanted pump, ripping its connection from the skull pedestal in the back of Houghton's head. Device alarms sounded loudly, and the frightened perpetrator dropped the bag and fled the scene. Houghton crawled on hands and knees to reach the battery and quickly restored power to his Jarvik 2000 device, reportedly unharmed from the incident.[103] Several years later, in December 2007, Houghton died of kidney failure, with his Jarvik 2000 device still pumping properly; only the external components had been replaced over the years, owing to general wear and tear.[104]

Frazier, who had been implanting various mechanical assist devices since the 1980s at THI, described the Jarvik 2000 pump as a "true assist device."[105] It augmented the

TABLE 6.1
Selected continuous-flow VADs and FDA regulatory status

Device	Description	FDA status
Jarvik 2000 VAD, by Jarvik Heart Inc.	An implantable, axial-flow blood pump	2000 IDE approved
HeartMate II LVAD, by Thoratec Corp.	An implantable, axial-flow blood pump	2003 IDE approved 2008 PMA granted
HeartWare HVAD, by HeartWare International Inc.	An implantable, centrifugal LVAD	2008 IDE approved 2012 PMA granted

Note: FDA = Food and Drug Administration; IDE = investigational device exemption (to use device in US multicenter clinical trials); PMA = premarket approval (to distribute device commercially in the United States); LVAD = left ventricular assist device.

work of a weakened native heart, only partially ejecting blood out of the ventricle, in comparison to the more commonly used (at that time) implantable pulsatile LVADs—the HeartMate and Novacor devices—that more fully replaced the function of the left ventricle. According to Frazier, for some patients, total cardiac output replacement was unnecessary, even undesirable.[106] There was an advantage of augmenting (rather than totally replacing) the work of the weakened left ventricle, thus preserving as much natural function as possible, allowing for continued pulsatility supplied by the native heart, and thus offering the potential for myocardial improvement and recovery. Theoretically, these devices might serve as a bridge to recovery, supporting some patients until their hearts resume sufficient function without need for mechanical support or heart transplantation thereafter. Frazier's comments on the role that the Jarvik 2000 pump might play reiterated the need for a family of mechanical cardiac support devices to serve a diverse patient population.[107] In a positive way, it also differentiated the Jarvik 2000 from the HeartMate II device, which could pump faster and produce greater cardiac output. In the United States, the Jarvik pump remains in clinical trials with FDA Investigational Device Exemption status, while in Europe, the Jarvik 2000 has Conformité Européene Mark certification for commercial use as both a BTT and a permanent cardiac assist device.[108]

Clinical Gains, Ongoing Problems

Continuous-flow VADs forged significant gains in the clinical use of MCSSs, swaying many in the cardiac medical field and society to adopt heart assist pumps as viable life-extending therapy for end-stage heart failure patients. Continuous-flow VADs worked well for many select patients, as clinical trial results demonstrated, and wider market approval and reimbursement expanded their use. Device research teams carefully worked through anticipated challenges of device design, materials, and performance of this newer technology. But as more implant cases took place, clinicians and researchers learned that the technology also imparted its own set of problems.

At first, second-generation device researchers confronted technological challenges that commonly emerged in the building of mechanical pumps. In comparison with first-generation VADs, the continuous-flow pumps were a different technology platform that overcame some, but not all, former device problems. The older, pulsatile VADs were quite large and required considerable surgical intervention; these units required compliance chambers and percutaneous tubes to externally vent displaced air from the pump. Device malfunction or infection was not uncommon, which required subsequent surgery, raised the issue of device durability, and increased the risk of patient morbidity and mortality. In comparison, continuous-flow VADs were smaller, more durable owing to their fewer moving parts, did not need external venting, and were easier to implant in patients, now potentially including children. University-industry research teams identified and resolved many technical or design glitches associated with different VAD models under development through iterative device improvement of bench work, animal testing, and early clinical trials. For example, Michael DeBakey's research team battled power fluctuations and thrombus (blood clot) formation issues with their experimental continuous-flow pump, the MicroMed DeBakey Noon VAD, later renamed the HeartAssist VAD.[109] The team altered this device by using stronger magnets and changing the bearings and the inflow cannula to address these problems.[110] In 2004 MicroMed Inc. executives secured Humanitarian Device Exemption status from FDA administrators for the use of the HeartAssist 5 as an assist device for children, as a step toward marketing the device to a wider BTT patient population.[111]

A newer problem with the second-generation devices related to the low pulsatility of these continuous-flow VADs. Patients implanted with the newer VADs had no palpable pulse, and this had implications in several ways. The first-generation, pulsatile VADs were audible pumps that mimicked the rhythmic contraction of the heart, reinforcing the pulse and the movement of blood through the heart and the body in sound and sensation for the patient. Continuous-flow devices were noticeably quieter, and no difference was felt physically by patients with the nonpulsatile movement of blood. Some individuals may have joked about their nearly pulseless existence, teasing medical staff to try to find their pulse. Using a stethoscope, health care professionals would hear only a hum, or a whirring sound, if the pump was running; a special Doppler blood pressure monitor was needed to detect a continuous-flow VAD patient's pulse. Patients' testimonies of adjusting to, and living with, a VAD emphasize the restorative power of the technology; no longer bedridden, short of breath, or limited in physical activities, they embrace their improved health and return to daily activities, travel, interacting with family, and so forth. No one commented on the lack of pulse sensation; it was inconsequential given the health benefits enjoyed by these end-stage heart failure patients.[112] But in emergency situations, first responders have unintentionally killed unresponsive VAD patients because of their lack of a pulse. According to one EMS worker, "When a patient doesn't have a pulse, their first instinct is to start CPR, but doing chest compressions on an LVAD patient can kill them. In fact, two Floridians have died because first responders did just that."[113] Another EMS professional recalled, "He has no pulse, but his wife won't let us do CPR. What should we do?"[114] With greater use of continuous-flow pumps, more EMS training is being conducted to prepare first responders to interact with, and care for, VAD patients.

The low pulsatility of these devices raises grave new issues and complications for physicians and patients, issues that were absent or unimportant with the use of first-generation VADs.[115] One serious problem was gastrointestinal bleeding as a complication and morbidity for patients implanted with second-generation pumps. The increased risk of gastrointestinal bleeding was a pathophysiological implication of near pulseless flow. In response, clinical researchers revised patient management and prevention strategies, such as setting a lower pump speed in the device.[116] In addition, the recommended anticoagulation regimen based on older, pulsatile VAD cases contributed to gastrointestinal bleeding, and thus it was recommended that the patient be given a lower dose or no warfarin or heparin (anticoagulants).[117] Device management guidelines for optimal pump speed and performance needed ongoing adjustments; how many revolutions per minute (generally 9,000 to 10,000 rpm) were needed to maintain an acceptable pulsatility index (higher than 3.5–4.0) for good cardiac output?[118] Medical practitioners also raised concerns about the long-term use of continuous-flow devices. What were the long-term effects on the body of nonpulsatility; how would it affect other organ function? According to Westaby, its importance was debatable; while the heart needed to contract and relax to function, nonpulsatile circulation of the blood did not seem to impact function of the brain, liver, or kidneys.[119] The field agreed that more clinical research needed to be done to better understand the physiological and psychological implications of these devices in patients. Capturing implant data might contribute to an improved understanding, and thus a national registry of implant cases was organized.

In 2005 the NHLBI sponsored the creation of the Interagency Registry for Mechanically Assisted Circulatory Support (INTERMACS) to track the ongoing use of long-term circulatory assist devices for the purpose of improving clinical practice. All patients receiving FDA-approved VAD implants for long-term support are subjects of INTERMACS, where details are collected regarding survival time, adverse events, device performance, and other issues, for scientific and clinical study of performance characteristics and direct comparisons of devices. This national electronic database unites the efforts of many stakeholders invested in the success of mechanical assist devices, including the NHLBI, the FDA, the CMS, hospitals, patients, physicians, researchers, and industry partners. There are obvious benefits of compiling this data for each group as the field works to develop better, next-generation devices, to determine the best device options for individual patients, to identify predictors of good outcomes and risk factors, to develop "best practice" guidelines to improve patient management, and to ease the burden of reimbursement submissions.[120] There are significant academic, clinical, regulatory, and economic gains to be made from supporting a high-quality national registry of these VAD-supported cases. In many ways overdue, it serves to consolidate and standardize patient data, in stark contrast to earlier less uniform data collection by individual sites, companies, and countries. INTERMACS inspired the formation of an international registry—the International Society for Heart and Lung Transplantation Registry for Mechanically Assisted Circulatory Support (IMACS)—launched in January 2013, that is similarly managed and directly connected to the American database.[121] Researchers can now compare how long and how well patients are living with different VADs in the United States and around the world.

Most recently, VAD researchers are experimenting with a third-generation VAD, a second-generation design of the continuous-flow cardiac assist pumps. These devices are smaller in size and operate with frictionless movement of a rotor or diaphragm.[122] The new design, based on hydrodynamic and magnetic bearings, increases device durability by eliminating heat from friction and the wear of components, but without compromising on blood flow rates and cardiac output. Another design advantage is the further miniaturization of the pump, which means less-invasive surgery and a smaller pocket (if any) in the chest cavity. These new, bearing-free, magnetically suspended pumps promise to be smaller, lighter, and easier to implant than older models.[123]

The HeartWare assist pump was the first device of this newer technology that become commercially available in the United States after FDA officials approved it in 2012.[124] Manufactured by HeartWare International Inc., headquartered in Framingham, Massachusetts, the HeartWare VAD (HVAD) is a small device that is designed to be implanted completely within the pericardial space (the sac surrounding the heart), resulting in an easier and shorter surgery.[125] The thinner and more flexible drive lines of this device suggested lower rates of bleeding and infection. Moreover, its smaller size allows for the device to be used in smaller patients, including some women and children.[126] But does being smaller make it a better device? According to one surgeon, the HVAD is "fussier" than the HeartMate II device and less effective on larger patients.[127] Studies comparing these two devices have published mixed findings. One group studying posttransplant patient outcomes found that both devices worked equally well, while another group reported increased incidences of stroke and gastrointestinal bleeding in HVAD patients.[128] There have also been reports of minor device malfunctions of the HVAD device, but not enough to warrant FDA removal of the pump from the market.[129] The HVAD emerged as a competing alternative to the more clinically entrenched HeartMate II pump in the medical marketplace. (In an attempt to neutralize a potential competitor, Thoratec executives tried to acquire HeartWare International Inc. in a cash and stock deal reported to be worth $282 million in 2009. However the US Federal Trade Commission ruled against the deal, citing antitrust reasons.)[130] Certainly cognizant of the newer VAD technology, Thoratec researchers are developing the HeartMate III, a centrifugal design that uses electromagnetic bearings.[131] A range of other factors, such as institutional preference, device cost and availability, specific patient conditions, and the surgeon's confidence and expertise with one device over others, also contribute to the commercial success of different medical devices.[132]

Securing a Place

Two key turning points leading to increased clinical use of VADs were the favorable results of the REMATCH study and the development of second-generation, continuous-flow assist pumps. The REMATCH trial was a landmark study for several reasons. First, it demonstrated that large RCTs in cardiac device surgery were doable, rigorous, and valuable. The RCT protocol employed in the REMATCH study quelled skepticism that unique surgical variables such as the surgeon's skill and specialized institutional care environments prevented the rigorous testing and comparison of new surgically implanted devices. Favorable LVAD data gathered through the clinical trial provided reassuring assessment for both regulatory and medical evaluation. Second, the REMATCH study marked the technological achievement of cardiac assist pumps. It demonstrated the efficacy and reliability of the HeartMate pump as permanent or destination therapy, extending clinical indications for LVAD technology beyond BTT use to a new patient subset. For this older, sicker patient population, not eligible for cardiac transplantation, LVAD treatment produced better survival outcomes than conventional drug therapy, according to REMATCH results, which secured approval for the device from medical technology regulators and payers. As physician Muriel Gillick commented, it was "virtually a foregone conclusion" that regulatory bodies interested in device safety more than clinical effectiveness would approve LVAD use based on the "high-quality data" gathered in the RCT.[133] In 2002 the FDA Circulatory Systems Devices Panel voted 8 to 2 in favor of approving the HeartMate XVE LVAD as a long-term, destination therapy for transplant-ineligible patients in advanced heart failure.[134] Not long afterward, the CMS approved reimbursement for the use of these devices as destination therapy, effective October 2003.[135] Third, the REMATCH trial provided a benchmark for heart failure devices as destination therapy. The INTrEPID trial, the RELIANT study, and others sought to obtain similarly favorable patient results for their devices or directly tested their devices against the HeartMate XVE LVAD used in the REMATCH study.

The influence of the REMATCH study on the broader adoption or clinical uptake of LVAD technology as destination therapy is more ambiguous. The REMATCH study provided proof of concept for LVADs as destination therapy but faltered in the transition to broad clinical utilization. On the one hand, the REMATCH study reported that patient survival outcomes with LVADs were higher than for patients treated with optimal drug therapy, and this result realized the clinical promise of this technology and fueled further research and development. On the other hand, the quality of the REMATCH results was simply not strong enough to lead to widespread adoption of the technology in its current state. As cardiologist Sharon

Hunt commented, it was "new data [but] old problems." In terms of LVAD patient mortality and device malfunction rates, the REMATCH study reported better results, but "not much" better, according to Hunt.[136] The REMATCH study and the subsequent device trials that it inspired immediately thereafter underscored the inherent limitations of these pulsatile pumps, referred to as first-generation LVAD technology. Survival outcomes of LVAD patients were better than for those treated with optimal medical therapy but still poor.[137] In addition to the device limitations, the LVAD was costly; approved reimbursement did not fully cover hospital expenses. Nonetheless, the REMATCH results suggested that LVAD implantation should be added to the treatment options for this patient population. Cardiologists and cardiac surgeons support multiple treatments in their toolbox to serve individualized patient scenarios. With these REMATCH results in hand, Thoratec executives supported a mass marketing campaign of the HeartMate XVE device to increase awareness of destination therapy for congestive heart failure to both the medical community and the public. But as Gillick states, "Despite the publicity blitz, the LVAD did not catch on" in this immediate post-REMATCH period.[138] The LVAD was an imperfect and expensive technology that, rather than directly displace other treatments, settled on being recognized as a justifiable alternative option for some heart failure patients.[139]

According to INTERMACS, few pulsatile pumps were implanted as destination therapy. Between 2006 and 2009, less than 10 per cent of LVADs were implanted permanently.[140] There was no significant clinical uptake of LVAD technology as destination therapy in the immediate post-REMATCH era. Many heart failure cardiologists did not believe that the risk-benefit ratio for LVADs as destination therapy was favorable enough for most of their patients. The REMATCH results were hardly compelling, with a 23 percent LVAD patient survival outcome at two years and a high incidence of device replacement at 18 months.[141] Formed to assess current LVAD technology challenges and opportunities, a NHLBI Working Group recommended that the next generation of devices aim to deliver a 50 percent survival outcome at two years for LVAD patients, with minimal time in the hospital after implantation. It was their hope that improved technology would become an attractive therapy to treat patients with less advanced, but progressive, heart failure.[142] A less-ill patient population boded well for the device, and it contributed to the blurring of indications for the use of this device. Heart failure patients who improved with LVAD therapy often became the BTT or bridge-to-candidacy group as their transplant eligibility status fluctuated.

The next-generation LVAD that dominated the post-REMATCH era was the nonpulsatile or axial-design device, the continuous-flow rotary pump. This second-generation technology demonstrated improved patient survival and device performance over the older pulsatile systems. The quieter, smaller, and more durable HeartMate II rotary pump represented the new technology. In 2008 the FDA's

Circulatory System Devices Panel approved the continuous-flow Heart Mate II LVAD as a BTT device for sale in the United States.[143] Two years later, the FDA panel approved the HeartMate II pump for permanent or destination therapy after a clinical trial reported a 58 percent survival rate of HeartMate II–implanted patients at two years, compared with a 24 percent survival rate of patients implanted with the older pulsatile LVAD.[144] Clinical uptake of the new HeartMate II device, for both BTT and destination therapy, was significant and almost immediate. According to the INTERMACS database, there was a rise in the number of LVADs implanted as destination therapy—more than 30 percent of total implants—in 2010 and 2011; this increase coincided with FDA approval of the HeartMate II pump for destination therapy in January 2010.[145] In 2011 Thoratec discontinued sale of the older HeartMate XVE LVAD (the device used in the REMATCH trial).[146] In 2012 FDA officials granted PMA to the HeartWare HVAD, which would now compete commercially with the HeartMate II pump for a piece of the American VAD-market pie. By early 2017 the VAD industry had changed significantly when medical device corporate giants Medtronic Inc. and Abbott Laboratories acquired the companies HeartWare International Inc. and Thoratec, respectively, to add these two continuous-flow VADs to their product portfolios.[147]

The use of continuous-flow devices stimulated new basic research questions and clinical applications. Whereas earlier pulsatile technology rigidly imitated the action of the heart, continuous-flow pumps raised the question, Do we need a pulse? Through animal experiments and more clinical cases, Frazier and his research team found that the loss of a clinical pulse did not compromise circulation or other organ function in the body. Still, continuous-flow support seemed to contribute to other patient complications, such as gastrointestinal bleeding, hemorrhagic strokes, and aortic valve insufficiency. Some researchers speculated that diminished arterial pressure pulsatility was the cause. A device that modulates pump speed to create pulses may help resolve some of these complications, but it remains to be worked out what the ideal pulse rate might be.[148] Conflicting findings from studies comparing pulsatile-flow and continuous-flow cardiac assist pumps fuel the debate over what is the better technology, adding to the uncertainty surrounding the use of these devices as long-term and permanent treatment.[149]

The use of continuous-flow pumps prompted new questions and expanded our knowledge of organ functions and the body. The technology generates new "ways of knowing," or the creation of new knowledge as a result of clinical experience with this device. Cardiac surgeon O. H. Frazier calls this type of knowledge gained from device-implanted patients the "soft science" or "applied art" of medicine. One needs to do and observe in humans because the animal model is imperfect and unanticipated reactions or responses to new treatments may occur in patients.[150] For example, one unexpected effect identified in some patients supported by continuous-flow pumps is the return of their diseased heart to its natural size and shape, a case of possible "reverse remodeling." As more clinical evidence bolstered such claims, the arguments of many practitioners to implant support devices in less ill patients became stronger.[151]

The REMATCH research group expanded their study in 2009 to incorporate the newer devices. Not surprisingly, they found that patients implanted with second-generation continuous-flow VADs did significantly better than those who had received first-generation pulsatile VADs, with 46 percent and 11 percent survival results at two years, respectively.[152] The medical field resumed the discussion of mechanical hearts as a valid treatment option in addition to heart transplantation, the gold-standard therapy for chronic heart failure since the 1980s. Could VADs be a "transplant alternative" for heart failure patients who might decline transplantation because of its serious complications of graft failure, rejection, and infection?[153] Members of artificial heart research teams were vocal in this debate, urging the acceptance of their devices, while others cautioned for mindful cost containment and judicious usage.[154] VAD technology was good, but was it really better than a heart transplant? Most cardiac specialists said no, that mechanical devices still have a long way to go to match the long-term outcomes of heart transplant patients. One Swiss research group implied that a "paradigm change" in heart failure therapy was under way as more data continues to be collected on the long-term survival rates of patients with continuous-flow VADs.[155]

Of notable significance, there was an ongoing discussion and a growing perception that mechanical support devices had become a viable and important option for patients in advanced heart failure. Good patient results from these clinical trials contributed to greater clinical uptake as more physicians became aware of the availability, effectiveness, and safety of VADs for a well-selected patient group.[156] According to cardiologists Tara Hrobowski and David Lanfear at Detroit's Henry Ford Heart and Vascular Institute, "LVADs are ready for 'Primetime' as a therapeutic option in and of themselves."[157] Good technology aside, the current "success" of VADs was facilitated by the convergence of interests held by researchers, clinicians, industry, the government, and patients who wanted these devices to work well for various reasons. Like Cheney boasting about his return to a near-normal life, other Heart-Mate II implant patients also told their upbeat stories online at Thoratec's corporate website or personal blogs. Andrea, age 30–39, after her implant, wrote: "I have more energy, mobility and just feel so much better, it is amazing." For Christopher, age 40–49, "The greatest gift that an LVAD has given me is the gift of more time." At two years postimplant, Stephen, age 65–69, commented that "LVAD recipients can travel and do things. (Check out my pictures!)"[158] Such patient testimonies on various Internet sites supported by VAD patients, VAD implant hospital programs, and VAD companies are almost always triumphant in tone. Such sources, while serving as an information portal (with tips and guidelines to "living with an LVAD"), are also constructing a celebratory narrative of a "successful" technology. (The patient testimonials are also interesting for what they do not disclose: motivations for sharing their story, serious risks and complications of LVAD implants, spouse or care-giver experiences, and dying with a LVAD.)[159] Continuous-flow technology worked so well that cardiac surgeon O. H. Frazier confidently stated, "The [total artificial] heart of the future that will replace the failed heart will be a pulseless or continuous-flow pump."[160]

This prediction of a continuous-flow TAH was one of many indicators that the research field had not given up on the quest to build a mechanical heart that can fully replace the natural heart. Aside from the obvious technological challenges, there re-mained much clinical and social resistance to the TAH; the experience of Barney Clark and other Jarvik-7 heart recipients had certainly not been forgotten. The moniker "The Dracula of Medical Technology" still hung in the air, dusted off by the media periodically to remind readers. Differentiating VADs from TAHs was fore-grounded in both the minds of patients and corporate advertisements. Intuitively, it seems preferable to attach a mechanical pump to an intact, partially functioning heart rather than to agree to the irreversible removal of the native heart and totally depend on an implanted mechanical heart. Cheney made it clear to CNN anchor Wolf Blitzer that his pump was *not* an artificial heart, stating, "We don't have those *yet*." Not true. Simultaneously with VAD development, work on TAHs continued; however, by the twenty-first century, the high-cost, labor-intensive endeavor had substantially narrowed the research field so that only one FDA-approved TAH materialized.

CHAPTER SEVEN

Artificial Hearts for the
Twenty-First Century

The real measure of an invention is not just how well it works or how impressively it is engineered, but how it changes our lives. . . . For saving the life of Robert Tools and for changing our perception of what is possible, the AbioCor artificial heart is Time's invention of the year.

"Best Inventions of 2001," *Time*, November 19, 2001

At the turn of the twenty-first century, the battered and long-awaited goal of building an acceptable total artificial heart appeared within reach. In the two decades after the sensational Jarvik-7 heart implant cases, artificial heart research teams worked steadily to improve TAH technology. The realization of ventricular assist devices in the 1990s and the early 2000s offered much encouragement, and the knowledge gained with VADs transferred to TAH research. Equally important, the clinical uptake of VADs contributed to a more hospitable environment for TAHs, reinforcing the view that a spectrum of devices would be worthwhile to treat acute and chronic heart failure patients. One device would not fit all. Cardiologist Marvin Slepian, who was involved in the development of the SynCardia TAH, reminded the profession that the VAD was not a substitute for the TAH and that some patient populations would benefit more from TAHs than from VADs.[1] These were not competitive devices but different therapeutic tools for a heart failure patient population with different cardiac support needs. The more widely used left ventricular assist device compensated for left ventricular dysfunction but required the patient's right ventricle to be functioning appropriately. The use of two VADs to provide biventricular support was sometimes attempted but was problematic for long-term support. While some patients were sustained adequately by VADs, which typically pumped blood at approximately 4 to 6 liters (1 to 1.5 gallons) per minute to assist the native heart, the more powerful TAH provided increased blood flow at 7 to 9 liters per minute for more severely compromised heart failure patients. Ultimately, the end-stage heart disease patient needs a new heart—a donor heart or a TAH—to replace the irreparably damaged native heart and to restore adequate circulatory function. In the case of biventricular heart failure without the immediate option of a cardiac transplant, the TAH was a device possibility to sustain life for some patients.

Less than two decades after the much-publicized and contentious permanent implant cases using the Jarvik-7 heart, the clinical use of TAHs in non-transplant-eligible patients began once again. In the earliest years of the 2000s, the medical literature and the media reported inspiring clinical results with two differently designed mechanical hearts—the AbioCor TAH and the SynCardia TAH. Reporters joked about the resuscitation of this device: "The artificial heart is back and beating," stated a *Technology Review* writer in 1999.[2] At this time the TAH recovered its popular excitement and amazement, partly because of the controlled public relations campaigns of industry and of hospitals that were implanting these newer (and, it was assumed, improved) devices, and partly because of the enduring appeal of life-saving medical technology within American society. *Time* magazine proclaimed the AbioCor TAH one of the best inventions of the year in 2001, celebrating its success in extending the life of Robert Tools, the first AbioCor TAH implant patient.[3] Had a fully implantable TAH finally emerged as a viable clinical option for end-stage heart failure patients? A 2001 *Newsweek* cover portrayed two open hands reverently displaying the plastic and titanium AbioCor TAH under the headline "How Technology Will Heal Your Heart."[4] Such celebratory accounts by the media sustained public optimism and faith in the success—finally—of this technology. Following the clinical and commercial success of mechanical assist pumps, TAH researchers appeared to be on a similar track of overcoming technological and regulatory challenges in the development of these total replacement devices.

This chapter reviews recent events in the development of TAHs to highlight changes and continuities in the development of this seductive technology. As VAD technology gained clinical and commercial ground, TAHs were being developed by other research teams hoping for similar achievements. VAD success did not necessarily preclude TAH success; different patient populations would benefit from these different devices. The AbioCor TAH and the SynCardia–CardioWest TAH were the dominant two TAH devices of this period; both are volume-displacement, pulsatile TAHs; however, they differ in device design, intended use, and commercial viability. The use of these TAH devices in the late twentieth and early twenty-first centuries raised issues that were both old and new. Familiar stakeholders championed the technology, while others voiced concerns, although the concerns were more muted than in the past. In the end, to what extent had the technology improved by the twenty-first century, and was it "good enough" to use clinically? How have TAHs, alongside the success of VADs, affected how medicine and society understand and treat heart failure?

The AbioCor TAH: Persistent Difficulties

The well-publicized Jarvik-7 TAH cases of the 1980s raised the hopes of many that the realization of a clinically acceptable artificial heart was close at hand. Instead, it became clear that many technical and social problems were still unresolved with this controversial technology. There were device criticisms of limited mobility, awkward machine tethering, technology-induced strokes, neurological events, treatment costs, device access, and other concerns. Researchers returned to the laboratory, in large part because artificial heart clinical investigators, National Heart, Lung, and Blood Institute officers, and other stakeholders refused to abandon this line of research. In 1988 the NHLBI offered new TAH-targeted funds, a contentious decision that led NHLBI director Claude Lenfant to cancel and then to reinstate this money in response to political pressure. Bolstered by the recommendations of the NHLBI Review Panel on the artificial heart program and the promising results of the pulsatile VAD systems at this time, the NHLBI awarded sizable five-year funding contracts, approximately $22.6 million in total, to four research groups to develop a long-term, electrically powered, fully implantable TAH.[5] The four university-industry research teams who received this NHLBI funding were the University of Utah; the Hershey

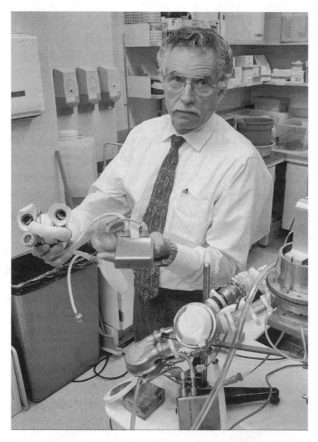

Biomedical engineer Gerson Rosenberg holds the Penn State Electric Total Artificial Heart at Hershey Medical Center of Pennsylvania State University, where he conducted research on mechanical circulatory support systems for roughly four decades. Photo taken June 21, 1999. (AP Photo/John S. Zeedick)

Medical Center of Pennsylvania State University, working with 3M / Sarns Inc.; the Texas Heart Institute and Abiomed Inc. of Danvers, Massachusetts; and the Cleveland Clinic with Nimbus Inc. The NHLBI administrators stipulated that TAH devices under development must be tether-free (to maintain patient mobility), free of percutaneous (through the skin) lines (to eliminate a common source of infection), and durable (to reduce mechanical failure). Each device needed to provide a minimum cardiac output of 8 liters per minute and work continuously for five years without malfunctioning. Also, the units would be placed orthotopically (surgically implanted in the location of the removed diseased heart) and offer battery support for patient mobility. A high bar had been set with these specifications, which in the post-Jarvik-7 heart era seemed absolutely necessary if there was to be any hope of widespread clinical adoption.

In the end, not all research teams were able to meet the NHLBI conditions with their respective devices, owing to the cost and technological difficulties associated with TAH device development. In 1993 the initial NHLBI contracts ended, and afterward, based on the NHLBI-sponsored readiness-testing program of LVADs in the 1980s, the NHLBI provided another round of funding and guidelines for phased-in TAH device testing. Three of the original groups (Penn State–3M, THI–Abiomed Inc., and Cleveland Clinic–Nimbus) received new three-year contracts for Phase I in vitro, or bench, testing of their devices. In 1996 only two of the groups (Penn State–3M and THI–Abiomed Inc.) moved forward into Phase II in vivo, or animal, testing of their respective devices, having met the technical bench-test markers set out by the NHLBI; both teams received four-year follow-up contracts.[6] Then in 2000 Abiomed Inc. acquired the rights to the Penn State TAH and the assets of BeneCor Heart Systems Inc., a company created to commercialize the Penn State TAH when 3M exited as Penn State's industry partner.[7] The last device company standing within the NHLBI-supported group was Abiomed, driven by its CEO and founder David Lederman, an aerospace engineer, and his commitment to the development of the TAH.

Since 1981 Abiomed had provided a commercial suite of cardiac support devices, backed by a skilled and experienced research and development team of aerospace engineers, scientists, and clinicians. In 1982 research scientist Robert Kung joined Abiomed as chief scientist and principal investigator of the AbioCor TAH project. The company's development strategy for cardiac devices was steadfast in its aim to overcome the technological challenges (which sometimes meant acquiring the technology of their competitors) while remaining financially solvent. Contributing to Abiomed's financial stability was the development of its heart-assist product line, notably several commercially successful mechanical circulatory support systems, which included the BVS5000 (Food and Drug Administration–approved in 1992) and the AB5000 (FDA-approved in 2003), both temporary and external circulatory support systems, for which the majority of health care insurers approved coverage. MCSS commercial success and its shared technological platform with total replacement heart devices bolstered Abiomed executives and researchers to continue developing the AbioCor TAH.

The AbioCor TAH was the first self-contained artificial heart system that fit almost entirely within the body. It was the first TAH that did not require component lines to penetrate the patient's skin, which often caused infection; instead it used a transcutaneous (across the skin) energy transfer (TET) system, thus promising improved patient mobility. The AbioCor TAH had four internal components: a plastic and titanium pump weighing about 2 pounds that was implanted orthotopically (in the exact place of the natural heart); an internal controller implanted in the patient's abdomen to regulate the movement of hydraulic fluid in the pump, its speed, and its pump rate; an internal lithium-ion battery, also placed abdominally; and an internal TET coil that received high-frequency power transmitted across the skin from an external TET coil. The AbioCor TAH also had four external components: the external TET coil, connected to either a bedside console or a portable TET module; a TET communication system; portable external batteries; and a bedside computer console that, via the radiofrequency communication system, recorded key information related to the function of the device, such as blood flow.[8]

Between 2001 and 2004, 14 male patients received the AbioCor TAH as a permanent treatment for end-stage heart failure in an FDA-approved, multicenter clinical trial.[9] The goal of the trial was to double the expected survival time of these patients from 30 days to 60 days, with improved quality of life. Patient results ranged from

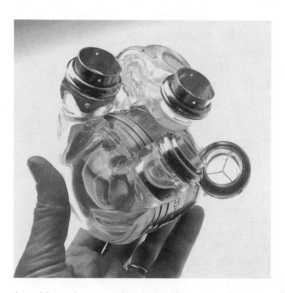

The AbioCor implantable replacement heart, a self-contained total artificial heart developed by Abiomed Inc. and implanted in 14 patients between 2001 and 2004. Shortly thereafter, the company abandoned further development of this device. Courtesy of Jewish Hospital, Louisville, Kentucky.

immediate death to a 17-month survival case. The THI cardiothoracic surgeon O. H. Frazier reported that the pump performed reliably, with only minor technical problems, and that the TET system worked adequately with no interruptions in power.[10] Thromboembolism (blood clots) remained a problem, however, so clinicians adjusted anticoagulation dosages and Abiomed researchers modified the design of the inflow sewing cuff. Not surprisingly, the energy transfer system across the skin reduced infection significantly. But the AbioCor TAH was large, about the size of a cantaloupe, and thus was unusable for women or children. It was also an expensive device, costing approximately $75,000, in comparison to the $50,000 price tag of a VAD.[11] These issues aside, did it really work? Heart surgeons Laman Gray and Robert Dowling at Jewish Hospital–University of Louisville echoed Frazier's assessment of the AbioCor TAH as a reliable, life-saving device that operated well. Dowling called it "user-friendly," stating, "The patients and their families have rapidly adapted to using all components."[12] Gray and Dowling were the surgeons who performed the most AbioCor TAH cases in this clinical study; they implanted seven patients, including the first implant patient, Robert Tools, and the longest-surviving AbioCor TAH recipient, Tom Christerson.

Tools, Christerson, and other AbioCor TAH patients gained media attention, which manifested itself in ways both similar to and different from past newspaper and television coverage. Like earlier experimental TAH cases, these heart implants became human interest stories. Journalists wrote about surgeons and patients thwarting death, the life-sustaining properties of the device, and the inspiring recovery of some AbioCor TAH patients. The articles were not a repeat of the media frenzy surrounding the Jarvik-7 implants of the 1980s. Perhaps the novelty of a mechanical heart had worn off by this time, nearly 20 years later, with the recent clinical achievements of VADs stealing a bit of the thunder. But also, AbioMed executives took unusual steps to control media headlines, while at the same time taking advantage of their public reach. In April 2001 they announced the FDA-approved clinical trial, openly using the media as a way to recruit patients for its new device. In fact, the first implant patient, Robert Tools, had approached the University of Louisville for an AbioCor TAH after reading a news article about the device. Tools fit the strict patient criteria; he was in severe biventricular heart failure, had exhausted all other therapeutic options, and faced imminent death. On July 2, 2001, Tools received his AbioCor TAH at Jewish Hospital. To avoid the University of Utah's clumsiness with the press, Abiomed officers actively managed the flow of information to the public from the hospital. After Tools's surgery, these officers firmly imposed a 30-day "quiet period," restricting medical personnel from discussing the patient's condition. At the initial and only press conference held at Jewish Hospital during this period, surgeons Gray and Dowling identified Tools simply as a diabetic man in his mid-to-late 50s, to shield the family and medical caregivers from unwanted media attention. They also stated that the AbioCor TAH "continue[d] to perform flawlessly" and that their patient was doing better than expected.[13]

Abiomed's containment of hospital reporting on this monumental surgery is remarkable. Medical manufacturers rarely become involved in matters beyond the responsibility of ensuring that their device functions properly. Typically, clinical care issues are the domain of the hospital, with its public relations staff guiding physicians in matters related to the media. Hospitals, not companies, are typically expected to control the release of information, balancing issues of patient privacy and journalists' access to information. Attending physicians are deemed the most qualified to speak about a case, and ethically they represent the best interests of the patient, often consulting with her or him beforehand about media matters. Hospital policies usually guide media interaction, and sometimes patient consent forms outline such policies. Industry's interest lies with the product, with the potential for the foregrounding of economic goals, which may conflict with hospital goals of patient rights and well-being.

In the case of Robert Tools, the hospital and the device company were not always in agreement about when and what patient information should be released to the media. Jewish Hospital had sought publicity for an earlier "first U.S. hand transplant" case, and now, according to *New York Times* reporter Lawrence Altman, hospital officers butted heads with Abiomed executives about not being able to publicize more aggressively the first AbioCor TAH implant in the country.[14] Abiomed CEO David Lederman defended the company's quiet-period media policy as a way to protect patient privacy and to avoid a media circus reminiscent of the Jarvik-7 implants.[15] With permission from Abiomed officers, Jewish Hospital representatives released only terse medical updates on Tools as warranted, such as the doctors' decision to drain fluid accumulating around the battery pack. Otherwise, the information served the patient recovery story: Tools was out of bed, sitting in a chair, and listening to his favorite music.[16] Some journalists and scholars, including Renée Fox and Judith Swazey, suggested that Abiomed's information restrictions had more to do with protecting the company's financial interests than with patient privacy.[17] Bioethicist E. Haavi Morreim, who served as chair of the Independent Patient Advocacy Council, established to assist patients and family participating in the AbioCor TAH trial as well as advise Abiomed executives on pertinent bioethical issues, argued that "moment-by-moment disclosures of enrolled patients' ups and downs should be discouraged," while also acknowledging that a complete media blackout was not desirable either.[18] Commenting on Morreim's argument, clinical ethicist Anne Lederman Flamm suggested that society's interest and curiosity about the TAH played a large part in the criticism of Abiomed's gag order. It was hoped that individuals following the events of the AbioCor TAH trial might reflect upon its benefits and burdens to society; however, "many more probably tuned in to the coverage to see whether the recipient of an artificial heart looks like the Tin Man or still loves his wife," remarked Flamm.[19] Ultimately, the quiet-period policy allowed Abiomed executives to control and to influence the news narrative as predominantly a triumphant story of device success and patient improvement.

Fifty days after the implant operation, the media learned the well-guarded identity of the first AbioCor TAH patient. On August 21, 2001, Robert Tools introduced
himself at a choreographed news conference at Jewish Hospital. Via remote video
hookup, a frail but positive Tools appeared from Gray's office to answer questions
from the media for about 15 minutes. When asked what it was like to beat death with
a mechanical heart, Tools emphatically replied, "It feels great!" Of course death is
inevitable, but Tools stated that "if there is an opportunity to extend (life), you take
it."[20] In the weeks following, the media continued to track Tools's recovery, publishing photos of his more than 20 day trips out of the hospital; Tools even participated
in a *Dateline NBC* interview, which aired in early November 2001.[21] He lived five
months with his artificial heart, battled excessive bleeding from the start, could not
tolerate the usual anticoagulation with heparin or warfarin, and received antiplatelet

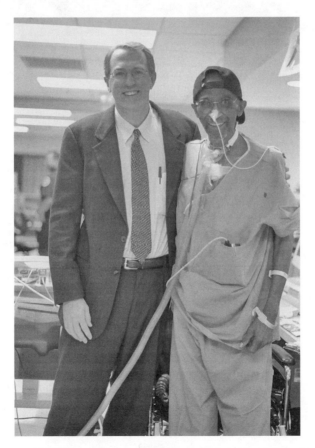

Robert Tools, the first AbioCor artificial heart patient, roughly four weeks after his
surgery, celebrating his birthday in the hospital with University of Louisville cardiac
surgeon Robert Dowling (*left*), July 31, 2001. Tools lived 151 days with an AbioCor
artificial heart. Courtesy of Jewish Hospital, Louisville, Kentucky.

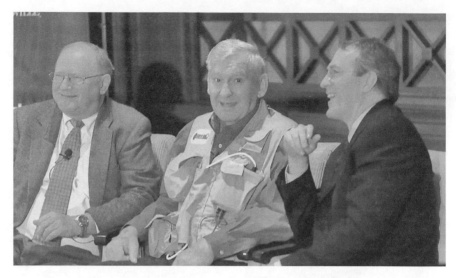

AbioCor heart recipient Tom Christerson (*center*), in a custom vest that holds various external components of his artificial heart, attending a Jewish Hospital press conference on March 12, 2002, roughly six months after his implant surgery, accompanied by University of Louisville cardiac surgeons Laman Gray (*left*) and Robert Dowling. Weeks later, in April 2002, Christerson was discharged from the hospital, returned home, and lived another 10 months with his AbioCor artificial heart. Courtesy of Jewish Hospital, Louisville, Kentucky.

therapy. On postoperative day 61, Tools suffered a transient ischemic attack, and later, on day 130, a much graver cerebrovascular event. He died from multiple organ failure on postoperative day 151; upon autopsy, thrombus was identified on the atrial struts of the AbioCor TAH implanted in the patient.[22] Tools's death did not come as a shock to the American public, since the media had been reporting various stroke-induced "setbacks" in his recovery during the preceding months.[23] Journalists applauded Tools for his role as a "pioneer" and for "making a difference for mankind."[24]

During Tools's convalescence with his mechanical heart, five more patients received AbioCor TAH implants at Jewish Hospital and elsewhere in the United States. On September 13, 2001, Gray and Dowling implanted their second patient, 70-year-old retired businessman Tom Christerson, who made a steady and impressive recovery after some initial problems. The patient had some recurrent aspiration issues, requiring reintubation and a tracheostomy, two episodes of high fever, which were related to a drug (soon discontinued), and rapid onset of renal failure that required hemodialysis. Six months after surgery (postoperative day 182), Christerson was discharged from the hospital to a nearby apartment, and he went home the following month (day 209).[25] Whereas Tools never left Jewish Hospital aside from occasional day trips, Christerson was discharged from the hospital in April 2002. Press releases from

Abiomed and Jewish Hospital emphasized Christerson's improved quality of life with family and friends in his hometown of Central City, Kentucky, with photos of Christerson's outings to his barber, to the local diner, and other places.[26] On the one-year anniversary of his implant operation, the AbioCor TAH team threw a party for Christerson, his family, the hospital staff, and others to celebrate the milestone event. When asked about living with the device for the past year, Christerson responded: "I didn't have any idea it would last this long. I thought it would give me another six months. But I got a year so far. . . . I'm tickled to death with it."[27] Christerson lived a total of 512 days with his artificial heart, more than half of that time spent at home; he was the longest-surviving AbioCor TAH patient in the trial. Christerson died on February 7, 2003, as a result of "device membrane wear."[28] (This device membrane problem was subsequently addressed and was not an issue for the five patients who underwent AbioCor TAH implants after Christerson's death.)

The fifth patient to receive an AbioCor TAH was Philadelphia baker James Quinn, age 51, who, as one of the youngest implant recipients, seemed poised to deliver the resurrecting promise of the artificial heart. Cardiac surgeon Louis Samuels implanted the device on November 5, 2001, at MCP Hahnemann University Hospital, but there were some initial problems. Shortly after the operation, Quinn went into respiratory failure and did not respond to conventional measures, so he received temporary extracorporeal membrane oxygenation support. On the third postoperative day, the medical team discontinued ECMO and Quinn's respiratory issue resolved. However, kidney problems were ongoing from the second to the eighth postoperative days, necessitating hemodialysis.[29] Then the patient settled into a pattern of steady improvement. Roughly a month after his surgery, Quinn told a reporter, "It's just so miraculous. . . . Each day I get stronger. . . . I want to go home. I want to go back to my front porch. That is the future for me, a second chance."[30] At two and one-half months after the operation, Quinn was attending church, playing bingo, going out to the movies, and eating at local restaurants while living at the Hawthorn Suites Hotel, a halfway house for Hahnemann patients before their discharge home. In February 2002, Quinn told the press that after doctors told him that he had less than a week to live, he did not hesitate to undergo the implant operation. "Who was I? An average American guy with no money, retired, very little insurance, not many options. . . . I didn't believe this when it happened. It was like it was sent straight from heaven. No way could I pass it up."[31] Photos of Quinn playing with his grandson at a Hahnemann Hospital press conference now accompanied photos of Christerson eating lobster in a local Louisville restaurant and Tools walking out of Jewish Hospital with his mobile battery pack.[32] Collaborating with the media, Abiomed embraced these AbioCor TAH patient successes, as did the associated site hospitals of the clinical trial. A THI news conference photo of the third implant patient and his doctors—Bobby Harrison, who lived about four months with his AbioCor TAH, seated next to his wife with cardiac surgeons O. H. Frazier and Denton Cooley looking on from behind—also circulated widely during this time.[33]

But then Quinn's recovery turned sour, and with it his decision to accept an artificial heart. Quinn's stay in the nearby adapted hotel suite was short-lived; he was readmitted to the hospital only 20 days after leaving, owing to a severe case of pneumonia. He soon also battled recurrent respiratory problems, a series of strokes, continuing pulmonary hypertension, and other medical problems related to end-stage heart disease.[34] At times he was in great pain, according to his wife. In hindsight, Quinn told one journalist that he should have stuck with his natural heart. "If I had to do it over again . . . I wouldn't do it. No ma'am. I would take my chances on life."[35] The AbioCor TAH had not delivered the quality of life that Quinn had believed it would, and several months before his death, he even talked privately about suing his medical team.[36] His envisioned "miracle" and "second chance" did not happen (despite his earlier optimism); perhaps he was measuring his case against that of Tom Christerson, who was living at home during this time. Quinn lived almost 10 months with his AbioCor TAH. He died in the hospital on August 25, 2002, after suffering a fatal stroke.[37] Less than two months later, his widow, Irene Quinn, filed a lawsuit against Abiomed, Hahnemann Hospital, and others involved in her husband's care, questioning the informed consent process, claiming that she and her husband had been "misinformed and misled" about the risks and benefits of the artificial heart.[38] Months later, Irene Quinn accepted a settlement of $125,000 from all the defendants, and the case never went to court.[39]

In the end, the AbioCor TAH clinical trial perpetuated mixed messages about the viability of implantable mechanical hearts. To the public, the media and Abiomed officers focused their stories on the patient cases with the better outcomes, implying the near-success and the potential of the technology. Aiming to extend life from an estimated 30 days to 60 days in patients who were dying, the AbioCor TAH provided this extension for 10 of the 14 trial patients. The study results validated the mechanical performance of an implantable, electric TAH to sustain life by providing heart function and restoring blood flow to the kidneys, the liver, and other failing organs. It had been anticipated that only three or four lives might have been sustained by the TAH, but device performance had been good enough to support 10 patients beyond their 30 days of expected life. Several patients had commented on a significant improved quality of life after months of suffering, even being bedridden. At the time of surgery, these patients were very ill, in severe heart failure with signs of end–organ dysfunction, for which a device could hardly compensate completely. Not surprisingly, these patients experienced a range of postimplant complications, and individual recoveries varied greatly, raising questions about the expectations of general patient improvement with this treatment course. Not all TAH patients became ambulatory, and four patients died within 24 hours of the implant surgery. There were incidents of excessive bleeding, device failure, blood clotting, cerebrovascular events, and multisystem organ failure. It was enough to influence investigators to stop the clinical trial just shy of its FDA-approved 15 cases. The AbioCor TAH had not surmounted the pump problems that had beleaguered earlier models. Like the Jarvik-7 TAH cases, the AbioCor TAH cases presented an ambiguous depiction of a technology that sort-of worked, for some patients, yet remained experimental. The study did show that the AbioCor TAH, with its electric power source, had advantages over the air-driven Jarvik-7 TAH. One of the most significant trial results for the AbioCor TAH was the performance of the TET system, which virtually eliminated the incidence of infection from penetrating drive lines and delivered a reliable source of power to the implanted device. These were incremental research steps that would test the commitment of Abiomed executives and researchers to continue developing this device.

Lederman was unwavering in his goal of marketing a commercially successful, implantable replacement heart. He referred to the AbioCor TAH as a first-generation device, and its clinical use had yielded much information that would be applied to an improved AbioCor II model. For the rest of the decade, Abiomed researchers worked on improving the firm's TAH device, incorporating the design of the recently acquired Penn State TAH technology, specifically its core energy converter system.[40] The researchers told the media that the AbioCor II device would function better and longer; it would be designed to be 30 percent smaller in size, more than doubling the patient population for its potential use. But no AbioCor II TAH was ever tested in humans. Bench testing of prototypes did not reach the five-year target for its continuous operation. Abiomed researchers were not able to overcome the complications of thromboembolism and atrial "suck-down" events (an encroachment of wall tissue or septum on the inflow cannula, subsequently causing arrhythmias or flow interruption or damage to the left ventricle) that had occurred with the original AbioCor device.[41] By 2009, specialists in cardiac centers had little interest in the device, and Abiomed executives halted the AbioCor TAH project, judging it "commercially unviable" and "prohibitively difficult."[42] Three years later, Lederman died of pancreatic cancer at age 68. With the loss of Lederman, who had long championed the research and development of a TAH, the company shifted its focus away from TAH development to its more popular suite of catheter-based cardiac support devices, notably the Impella system for short-term patient use.[43]

The SynCardia–CardioWest TAH: Not Perfect, but Good Enough

As the AbioCor TAH was being developed, a group of stakeholders in Arizona and Utah formed the startup company CardioWest Technologies, to salvage an older TAH technology for commercial realization. In 1991 the University Medical Center in Tucson and the Medforte Research Foundation of Salt Lake City acquired the Symbion (formerly Jarvik-7) TAH technology after FDA officials withdrew approval for its manufacture because of quality concerns. All Symbion assets were transferred to CardioWest Technologies for continued device development.[44] Instrumental in the formation of CardioWest Technologies were cardiac surgeon Jack Copeland and researcher-veterinarian Don B. Olsen, who had both been involved in clinical cases of the Jarvik-7 (later Symbion) TAH in Tucson and Salt Lake City, respectively, during the 1980s. Based on their experience, they believed in the viability of TAH technology and its bridge role in cardiac replacement for heart failure patients, and they rallied support to prevent the technology from being buried. This older technology survived owing to its continued development by surgeon-researchers familiar with the device, improvements to the device and console unit, better patient care management protocols, the bridge indication for its intended use, and sufficient funding to finance the regulation and clinical trial stages.

CardioWest researchers made slight modifications to the Symbion TAH and renamed it the CardioWest C-70 TAH.[45] It remained an air-driven TAH with three components: the pump unit of two prosthetic ventricles, the connecting drive lines, and an external pneumatic driver. Like earlier iterations, the CardioWest TAH was a volume-displacement, pulsatile, diaphragm pump with two separate ventricles implanted orthotopically in the chest. The group supported research into improved polymeric materials in the fabrication of the pump unit to increase flexibility and durability of the diaphragm. The drive lines attached to the implanted pump and penetrated the patient's skin, exiting through the abdomen to connect to an external drive and monitoring console. Changes were made to the skin button for these drive lines, which were now Dacron covered and attached directly to the air conduits for better fixation, with the hope of limiting friction and infection at the site of skin penetration. The drive line system was in sharp contrast to that connecting power to and monitoring the AbioCor TAH, which had a transcutaneous energy system and a radiofrequency communication system and did not need drive lines. In the case of the CardioWest TAH, its drive lines connected to a large bedside unit consisting of two pneumatic drives (one primary and one backup) and a computer monitoring system. The external console allowed the operator to adjust the patient's heart rate, drive line pressures, systolic percentage, and other features. Again in contrast, the AbioCor TAH was a self-contained and self-regulated system almost entirely implanted in the body. In 1991 CardioWest Technologies decided to manufacture the mechanical heart in one size only—the 70 cc CardioWest TAH—which provided a maximum stroke value of 70 ml to deliver a robust cardiac output of more than 9 liters per minute.[46] The company now sought to implant its device in patients to compile data to submit to the FDA for premarket approval.

In 1992 CardioWest Technologies executives received approval from FDA officials to test the CardioWest TAH in a multicenter PMA clinical trial. From 1993 to 2002, a 10-year nonrandomized study assessed the performance of the CardioWest TAH in 95 advanced heart failure patients with irreversible biventricular failure who were at risk of imminent death (Class IV status). Cardiac surgeons at five different American medical centers, in Chicago, Salt Lake City, Milwaukee, Pittsburgh, and Tucson, participated in the study.[47] In its previous iteration as the Jarvik-7 TAH, this technology had been implanted in transplant-ineligible heart failure patients and presented a myriad of problems. Better clinical outcomes occurred when it was used as a bridge device, which involved less-sick patients requiring shorter-term circulatory support. Copeland was interested in developing the CardioWest TAH to be used in this way, as a temporary biventricular support system to bridge transplant patients.

The study focused only on transplant-eligible patients, whose experience would be measured for rates of survival to transplantation, survival after transplantation, and overall survival to measure success. From the results, Copeland reported encouraging data; more TAH patients survived to and after transplantation than those heart failure patients who had been managed medically (the control group). The study reported a 79 percent survival to transplant in the TAH group in comparison with 46 percent in the control group. This was a higher bridge-to-transplant rate than any other approved bridge device in the world. Similar statistics from single center experiences emerged for patient survival rates after transplantation.[48] The overall improvement in hemodynamic status of these patients after their TAH implants was also encouraging; researchers reported that 75 percent of TAH patients were out of bed one week postimplant, and more than 60 percent of TAH patients were able to walk more than 100 feet another week later. Fewer TAH patients had adverse events than the control group while waiting for their transplant operation. The major problems experienced by the implant patient group were excessive bleeding, infection, and neurological dysfunction. Device malfunction was reported in two patients. Not perfect, but still the results pleased Copeland and his group. The data collected from this clinical study would be good enough to apply for FDA approval of the CardioWest TAH as a BTT device.[49]

At the very moment that the CardioWest TAH seemed poised to move forward, its development came into real jeopardy. In 2001 Tucson's Medical University Center pulled out of CardioWest Technologies, claiming budget cutbacks. So Jack Copeland, Marvin J. Slepian, and biomedical engineer Richard G. Smith formed SynCardia Systems Inc. to complete the clinical trial and market the CardioWest TAH, renamed the SynCardia TAH. The company raised millions of dollars in venture capital and private equity investment to commercialize its device. In 2004 the FDA approved the SynCardia TAH for American sales as a bridge device, based on the safety and efficacy data compiled during the 10-year multicenter clinical trial.[50] In the following decade, another 150 TAH-as-bridge implants took place in 15 medical centers across the United States, with 75 percent of TAH patients surviving to undergo cardiac transplantation.[51] In 2008 Medicare approved reimbursement of the SynCardia TAH, and private insurers did the same shortly thereafter. In 2012 Forbes listed SynCardia Systems as one of "America's most promising companies."[52]

SynCardia researchers and executives continued to improve and expand their TAH product line. The company developed a smaller 50cc TAH that had a lower stroke value of 50 ml to deliver a cardiac output of approximately 6 to 8 liters per minute. It was intended for use in women and adolescents, for whom the 70cc TAH was

TABLE 7.1
Selected total artificial hearts and FDA regulatory status

Device	Description	FDA status
Liotta-Cooley heart, implanted at the Texas Heart Institute	A pneumatic, pulsatile TAH	n/a
Akutsu III heart, implanted at the Texas Heart Institute	A pneumatic, pulsatile TAH	n/a
Phoenix heart, implanted at the University of Arizona Medical Center	A pneumatic, pulsatile TAH	n/a
Jarvik-7 heart, by Kolff Medical-Symbion Inc.	A pneumatic, pulsatile TAH	1981 IDE approved 1990 IDE approval withdrawn
Penn State heart, implanted at the Penn State Hershey Medical Center	A pneumatic, pulsatile TAH	1985 IDE approved
SynCardia–CardioWest heart, by SynCardia Systems Inc.	A pneumatic, pulsatile TAH (an evolution of the Jarvik-7 heart technology)	1992 IDE approved 2004 PMA granted
AbioCor heart, by AbioMed Inc.	An electrohydraulic, pulsatile TAH	2001 IDE approved

Note: FDA = Food and Drug Administration; TAH = total artificial heart; IDE = investigational device exemption (to use device in US multicenter clinical trials); PMA = premarket approval (to distribute device commercially in the United States).

too large. SynCardia researchers significantly improved the driver technology, which became smaller, quieter, and more user friendly over time. Two driver systems became available to power the TAH. The Companion driver system was a new 55-pound hospital-based driver system with a touch screen interface, redundant compressors, and a continuous monitoring system. It was durable, user friendly, and more portable for patient and staff handling in the hospital. Initially supplemental to traditional technology, the Companion driver system eventually replaced the older, 418-pound console upon FDA-approval in 2012. SynCardia also introduced a portable Freedom driver system for use outside the hospital. After receiving FDA approval in 2014, this driver was advertised as the first wearable power supply for a TAH. The Freedom driver weighs 13.5 pounds and fits in a backpack or shoulder bag, with batteries that can be charged through a standard electrical outlet or the cigarette lighter adaptor in a car. A small digital screen displays the patient's heart rate, cardiac output, and fill volume.[53] Not surprisingly, the "heart in a bag" is a costly system at about $125,000 for the unit and $18,000 for annual maintenance expenses. "Still, you can't put a price on freedom," wrote one journalist unable to resist using the cliché.[54] For

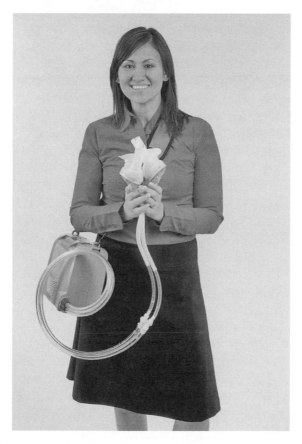

The SynCardia temporary Total Artificial Heart with the Freedom portable driver, a wearable power supply that can be fitted into a backpack or a shoulder bag, offering significant patient mobility in comparison to much larger hospital-based power units for this technology. Courtesy of syncardia.com.

those who can afford it, this driver makes home discharge possible, which would have been unimaginable for patients tethered to large bedside consoles only a decade earlier.

With more than 1,635 SynCardia TAH implants worldwide, SynCardia Systems has developed the most successful total heart replacement device to date. However, while this number of TAH implants is considerably more than the approximate 200 Jarvik-7 TAH implants of the 1980s, it is still only a fraction of the total number of VAD implants (approximately 18,000).[55] SynCardia Systems regularly issues press releases on recovery stories of TAH patients, incorporating the age-old trend of patient testimony to solidify a triumphant narrative. The rising number of TAH patients offers insight into the experience, both positive and negative, of living with this device. In March 2012 39-year-old TAH patient Michelle Johnson left

Cedars-Sinai Medical Center in Los Angeles with her Freedom portable driver to wait for her heart transplant. A single mother of three children, she told reporters, "The SynCardia Total Artificial Heart has given me one more day at life, and that day has turned into weeks and months, allowing me to become healthier for my heart transplant." When asked about being "tethered" to a drive unit, Johnson replied, "The Freedom driver allowed me to leave the hospital and enjoy a better quality of life at home, where I'm able to see my kids and enjoy the closeness of my family. The light weight of the driver allows me to move around with little hassle or strain."[56] Apparently the Freedom driver was portable enough for 40-year-old Randy Shepherd to hike Arizona's Tonto National Forest and to participate in long-distance run-walk courses. In April 2014 Shepherd was the first person with an artificial heart to enter and complete the annual Pat's Run in Tempe, Arizona. He told reporters, "I am hoping by next year at Pat's Run I'll be running it instead of walking it . . . [because] I am hoping to have a donor heart. But if not, I'll be back there with my backpack again and I'm going to do it again next year."[57] That same month, 16-year-old Nalexia Henderson left University of Florida Health Shands Children's Hospital with her SynCardia TAH and portable driver. She was the first Florida resident to receive a TAH and the youngest person to be discharged home with the device. Reporters snapped smiling photos of the teenager leaving the hospital. When asked by reporters what the artificial heart felt like, Henderson replied, "I feel like my normal self. . . . There's nothing bad about the SynCardia [Heart]. You got life."[58] The expressed optimism, happiness to be leaving hospital, and hope for the future was evident among those SynCardia TAH patients using the Freedom driver.

Beyond the media sound bite, more qualitative studies were being conducted by allied health professionals and social scientists to capture the lived experience of patients with implanted mechanical hearts. These studies document the physical and psychosocial needs of the TAH and VAD patient during the wait for a donor heart.[59] Most patients commented that prior to receiving the device implant, their heart failure symptoms had severely limited their life to the point of little enjoyment. Thus the technology represented hope for an improved quality of life in addition to serving as a life-sustaining device. But living with a mechanical heart was certainly different. When asked if the TAH feels any different from having a real heart, Randy Shepherd answered, "Yes. It runs at 135 beats per minute and each beat feels like a small child kicking me in the chest. . . . I let people put their hand on my chest to feel it and the reaction is always astonishment at the force of it. But after 10 months I have gotten quite used to it."[60] While most patients adjusted to the noise of the drive unit or the beeping of batteries and monitors, the tethering of the implanted device to external components was never forgotten. One TAH patient commented, "I know that I am married to this machine now."[61] Another TAH patient said, "I feel completely normal and that's the hardest part because I feel like I could just go home, you know, but I have this 400 pound *thing* hooked up to me."[62]

Health care providers state that one of the greatest obstacles to overcome with TAH technology is the dependence (not necessarily independence) that it requires of patients. Patients living with a SynCardia TAH still must have around-the-clock caregiver attention, and that limitation is one of the predominant psychosocial issues surrounding the use of the device. For example, the switching of drive units requires two people to disconnect and reconnect the drive lines, to ensure quick connection without drive line entanglements.[63] Shepherd commented, "During a driver switch out, from one machine to another, the heart does stop and it is a very unsettling feeling."[64] The benefits of TAHs as life-sustaining devices are certainly articulated by implant patients. But more importantly, their perspectives capture the authentic experience of living with artificial hearts and can benefit health care providers and future patients.

Jack Copeland referred to the Jarvik-7 artificial heart as the "Model T" of its era, which would "inevitably be replaced by better devices."[65] The SynCardia TAH is one such better device, an improved modification of the older heart pump. It has also returned to its original use as a permanent device. In 2012 the FDA granted Humanitarian Use Device status to the SynCardia TAH as destination therapy, allowing the use of this device as a permanent implant for heart failure patients, under the guidance of appropriate institutional review boards.[66] European medical centers had already implanted the TAH as a permanent device, with encouraging results. In 2014 surgeons at the Heart and Vascular Center EKN Duisburg in Germany published the case of a 74-year-old patient who returned to near-normal life at home with his portable Freedom driver, one year after receiving his SynCardia TAH as a permanent implant.[67]

In 2017 the SynCardia TAH is the only TAH approved by the FDA, Health Canada, and the CE (Europe). Whereas the AbioCor TAH showcased a different, arguably more ideal technology platform as a fully implantable unit, it was the older, pneumatic technology that penetrated the market first for use as a BTT device and later for destination therapy. The excitement over the AbioCor TAH was its self-containment, with minimal tethering and greater "forgettability" than the SynCardia TAH. It was the AbioCor TAH, not the SynCardia TAH, that embodied the expectations for the "ideal" TAH. Yet the clunkier SynCardia TAH was the one that realized greater clinical use. Although not the envisioned self-contained, self-regulated mechanical heart, the SynCardia TAH worked well enough to meet a need not met by other devices. When industry support for the AbioCor heart collapsed, the SynCardia heart secured a corner of the market without any real competition. Its realization can be linked to two things: Copeland and Olsen's commitment to the Symbion device and their efforts to continue its development; and SynCardia's improvement of the driver system to provide greater patient mobility and home discharge. In many ways, the older, less ideal TAH had won a war of attrition, outlasting its competitors in a protracted development course influenced by politics, economics, and device championing as much as by the technology itself. Even so, SynCardia executives still battle serious financial problems, struggling to pay the firm's debts and raise needed capital to further develop its technology. In July 2016 SynCardia Systems filed for Chapter 11 bankruptcy protection, and two months later Versa Capital Management LCC, a private equity investment firm based in Philadelphia, acquired the troubled company with reorganization plans to continue operational support.[68]

By the twenty-first century, it seemed that the TAH had moved through its depiction as the Dracula of Medical Technology and the haunting images of Barney Clark tethered to a machine at the bedside to emerge as a viable treatment option for end-stage heart failure patients. Better patient outcomes, better device performance, and improved quality-of-life issues led to more favorable clinical reception for TAHs. The SynCardia TAH was not problem-free, perhaps because it had derived from older pulsatile technology. It was this older technology that may have scared potential buyers away when SynCardia ran into financial problems in 2016.[69] Elsewhere researchers were exploring new technology platforms to build a better TAH within the maturing field of mechanical circulatory support systems.

Future Expectations

For the foreseeable future, a technology-based approach to the treatment of end-stage heart failure will continue, thus assuring a place for mechanical pumps. Both TAHs and VADs will improve in efficiency, become smaller and more durable, and hopefully cause fewer adverse events in patients. VADs as small as pencils might someday be catheter-implanted, eliminating the need for open heart surgery. New TAHs will most likely take advantage of electronics, miniaturization, and the transcutaneous energy transmission system to build a completely implantable self-contained, self-regulated system. Implantable mechanical hearts for people are a clinical reality, with current research striving to build better devices, refine surgical procedures, improve patient selection criteria, and better manage postimplant care. The hope is that mechanical circulatory support devices will improve for biventricular heart failure to parallel heart transplantation as a standard treatment.

Cardiac surgeon O. H. Frazier suggests that future TAHs will adopt continuous-flow technology, based on the success of second-generation, nonpulsatile VADs. In 2011 Frazier implanted a continuous-flow total heart replacement—composed of two modified HeartMate II ventricular assist pumps—into a heart failure patient who lived another five weeks before dying of liver failure caused by severe amyloidosis (abnormal protein build-up).[70] Frazier's research team is developing a separate continuous-flow TAH device—the Bivacor—for total heart placement, which is demonstrating encouraging results in calf experiments.[71] Similarly, bioengineer and clinician Len Golding and his research team at Cleveland Heart Inc., a Cleveland Clinic Innovations spin-off company, are building a continuous-flow TAH and centrifugal blood pump, called the SmartHeart Total Artificial Heart and the Smart-

Heart Left Ventricular Assist Device, respectively. Both share the basic design concepts of a continuous-flow pump and an automatic control system. The SmartHeart TAH is small enough to allow implantation in women and adolescents.[72] Golding began experimenting with rotary pumps back in the mid-1970s when he arrived at the Cleveland Clinic. His intent has always been to simplify device design, miniaturizing the pump unit and reducing the number of moving parts.[73] Both Golding's and Frazier's devices have only one moving part, with no bearings or valves, and initial durability tests have produced promising results. In contrast to the pulsatile, volume displacement, pneumatic hearts, continuous-flow technology is smaller with greater long-term durability.

While the limitations of the pulsatile pump were the size and mechanics of the pump itself, Frazier points out that the challenges of utilizing continuous-flow technology for a TAH are the secondary physiological problems.[74] A continuous-flow device reduces pulsatility, raising questions about the importance of a strong pulse. Frazier and his research team found that the loss of a clinical pulse did not compromise circulation or other organ function in the body. However, there are increasing reports of gastrointestinal bleeding and aortic valve problems in animals and patients that appear to be related to denaturation of the von Willebrand factor (a key component of the clotting system). These devices are in the early stages of development, and the debate over the need for a pulse continues, overlapping with similar discussions and observations about the clinical use of second-generation LVADs. The longer-term (permanent) implant of a total replacement continuous-flow device, in comparison to the implant of shorter-term (bridge) assistive devices, amplifies the pulseless state of the body and any physiological ramifications thereof.[75]

In many cardiac centers, LVADs are a treatment option for patients battling severe heart failure, yet the LVAD remains a late-stage measure, to be used after all other therapies are exhausted. A 2013 advertisement for cardiovascular care at the University of Texas Medical Branch health center, promoting the adage "It's about getting your life back," implied the "last resort" connotation associated with these devices: for John, "the only option appeared to be getting on a heart pump and waiting for a transplant," but instead, he agreed to the recommended bypass graft procedure, which was performed successfully by UTMB surgeons.[76] A hierarchy of therapies exists, and the use of mechanical pumps remains reserved for the sickest of the sick, when other approaches no longer work. Typically, indications for VAD and TAH use are directed to New York Heart Association (NYHA) Class IV or advanced Class III patients. Patients are often asked to make decisions about a TAH or VAD implant when death is imminent and no other treatment options remain. Some patients may embrace these devices as a technological fix to their case. For others, a discussion of mechanical hearts may bring on grief, perhaps owing to their loss of other options or a new awareness of their end-stage status. Describing the response of former vice president Dick Cheney, his cardiologist Jonathan Reiner wrote, "My wife, Charisse, asked me later if the vice president looked sad when I told him he needed a VAD. 'Not sad,' I said, 'just weary.' "[77] Cheney described the idea of a VAD implant as initially "off-putting," but he was dying; conceptually not all patients welcomed the technological fix, some reacting strongly against the invasive nature of a mechanical implant, while others processed its implication as one of the few alternatives left, perhaps the only one. As Cheney later admitted, "It was an option, and I was out of other options."[78]

Artificial hearts may surpass heart transplantation as the more common treatment for end-stage heart failure because of the simple shortage of donor hearts. The supply will never meet the demand for donor hearts, particularly with the increasing prevalence and incidence of heart failure cases. In 2014 an estimated 26 million people worldwide were living with heart failure.[79] In the United States, there are an estimated 5.8 million heart failure patients, of which 100,000 are in advanced heart failure.[80] Roughly 2,200 heart transplants are performed each year in the United States, and almost one in three of those patients have been supported by a mechanical pump as a bridge to transplantation. With more than 3,000 patients on the cardiac transplant waiting list at any one time, long wait times for donor hearts will continue. The promissory nature of life-extending treatments like heart transplantation and mechanical replacement hacked into society's acceptance of the end of life as occurring when one's natural heart failed. For transplant-ineligible heart failure patients, mechanical pumps presented a possible postponement of death. Whether as bridge or destination therapy, the clinical use of mechanical pumps is increasing as improved survival outcomes with their longer-term use are being recorded. In 2016 the International Society for Heart and Lung Transplantation reported a 12-month survival rate of about 80 percent and an 18-month survival rate of 75 percent for patients implanted with continuous-flow pump devices, based on the society's registry data of more than 5,000 patients from 31 countries. These one-year survival rates are approaching similar outcomes for heart transplantation, which reports a one-year patient survival rate of 88 percent. However, five-year-plus survival rates are significantly higher with heart transplantation than with mechanical circulatory support, and adverse events (such as infection, bleeding, respiratory failure, neurological dysfunction, device malfunction, and arterial thromboembolism not affecting the brain) occurred in 59 percent of pump-implant patients.[81]

Artificial hearts remain expensive devices. Greater clinical use of these devices has not significantly reduced manufacturing costs, as had been hoped. At various times in their history, the cost of developing artificial hearts threatened to end the initiative, but it did not. The financial viability of these devices was assured once reimbursement by Medicare and most commercial payers began in the 1990s for VADs. This coverage has slowly increased to include related pump equipment and replacement supplies for implant patients discharged home. Adopting pump implants as a standard of care is resource intensive for hospitals, since it includes the implant surgery, medical management, intensive care unit requirements, hospital stays, and often patient readmission costs. A 2016 Canadian review of the cost effectiveness of long-term mechanical circulatory support reported that patient costs ranged from $85,000 to more than $200,000 for BTT use and from $87,000 to more than $1,250,000 for destination therapy (in 2012 Canadian dollars, per quality-adjusted life year).[82] Such amounts exceed the traditionally accepted thresholds for cost effectiveness: $50,000 to $100,000 per quality-adjusted life year. Mechanical circulatory support incurs higher costs in comparison to direct heart transplantation or many other end-of-life therapies.[83]

One of the greatest obstacles to improving patient outcomes with long-term mechanical support is patient comorbidities. End-stage heart failure patients often have liver and kidney dysfunction or chronic obstructive lung disease, which may not improve after the implantation of a mechanical pump. Why not implant these devices in less-sick patients, before irrevocable deterioration of organ function occurs? Most clinicians support improved patient selection criteria for the various mechanical circulatory support systems now available. But proposing TAH and VAD implantations as an elective surgery for Class III heart failure patients is controversial. The new patient classification of the Interagency Registry for Mechanically Assisted Circulatory Support (INTERMACS) provides greater subdivision of heart disease categories than the NYHA system, aiming to assist with implant decisions. When weighed against implantation risks and current medical management outcomes, implanting these devices in patients earlier in the progression of their heart disease may be appropriate. Cardiac surgeons familiar with the technology may suggest a TAH for heart failure patients who are poor LVAD candidates, perhaps influenced by a retrospective study published in 2001 that reported a 75 percent success rate for BTT CardioWest (SynCardia) TAH-implanted patients, in comparison with a rate of 57 percent and 38 percent of patients implanted with the Novacor LVAS and Thoratec LVADs, respectively.[84] The size parameters of the TAH limit its possibility for some individuals, however, and the complications with TAH implantation such as strokes, infection, bleeding, and renal failure still give many clinicians and patients pause.[85]

By far the greater clinical achievement lies with "partial artificial hearts," or VADs, not TAHs, as life-sustaining devices for heart failure patients. Within this small subset of severe heart failure patients who chose device pump support, more individuals have been (and will be) implanted with a VAD than with a TAH. Of this group, about two-thirds chose VAD implants as bridge devices to heart transplantation, still the gold-standard treatment for heart failure. Since 2006 more than 90 percent of implants involved LVADs (numbering 14,986), in comparison with TAHs (344 in total) at only 2 percent of all implants, according to a 2016 INTERMACS report.[86] These statistics speak to the increasing incidence of isolated left ventricular failure, for which patients receive LVADs before their condition possibly warrants biventricular or total heart mechanical support. Given that the annual number of cardiac transplant operations has stagnated at around 2,200 in the United States, an increasing number of heart failure patients may attribute their last years of life to an LVAD regardless of their pre-implant device strategy.

Artificial Hearts: Allure and Ambivalence

The powerful allure of the potential, the promise, and the "what if" mentality has offset the ambivalence surrounding the development of artificial hearts over the past six decades in America. The tension between the allure and the ambivalence influenced how success was characterized and by whom, demonstrating an interpretative flexibility of "success" when it came to device assessment. The initial aims and ideal capabilities of artificial hearts were compromised by the imperfect nature of the technology, its safety and effectiveness questioned by many in the medical community as well as by the public. The ongoing development of artificial hearts, with its medical uncertainty, variable intensity, and related constituents, demonstrated a degree of acquiescence that was connected to broader values and expectations, individual views of risk and benefits, and professional convictions regarding the technology's development and clinical use. A technological momentum supported device-based treatments, which for twentieth-century American heart patients included artificial valves, pacemakers, implantable cardioverter-defibrillators, stents, and other devices. Mechanical hearts added to this therapeutic armamentarium, offering a mechanical replacement for the failed human heart; many different artificial hearts were built and tested, but the majority of them never moved beyond the laboratory.

The development of artificial hearts is a story of technological challenges and desperate implant cases, therapeutic limitations and experiment-therapy dilemmas, ego wars and gruesome patient complications. Early clinical cases suggest that research goals might have been prioritized over any real therapeutic hopes. A heroic ethos of the period that supported aggressive procedures, surgeon self-confidence, and even lay pressure to do whatever was possible to sustain life influenced these actions. Surgical giant Michael DeBakey, artificial kidney inventor Willem Kolff, and leading heart surgeons Adrian Kantrowitz, Denton Cooley, William S. Pierce, Jack Copeland, O. H. Frazier, George Noon, and others tackled problems of device design, biocompatible materials, and power sources, at the same time managing implant patient complications of infection, bleeding, and thromboembolism. Collaborative relationships, clinical acumen, and social contexts affected research teams and their respective device development routes. Mechanical engineer Victor Poirier commented, "I really had to do a lot of work in the physiology and the interactions of the body," while practicing surgeons like John C. Norman and O. H. Frazier "weren't afraid to take a next step into the darkness and to learn and to understand what the technology was about."[87] It is not coincidental that leading surgeon-researchers such as Michael DeBakey, O. H. Frazier, and Robert Bartlett had extensive practices, which facilitated the movement of ideas from bedside to laboratory and back again. Their research work represented pragmatic action to address the clinical need for mechanical circulatory support devices. But when experimental air-driven and electrically powered artificial hearts were implanted in dying patients, with ambiguous results, debate was fueled in both medical and public venues about the development of this technology.

Media coverage of these early cases contributed to public misgivings surrounding the development and use of artificial hearts. Celebratory reporting bolstered public expectations, but often with mixed messages; journalists reported how mechanical hearts extended the lives of some patients, but not without postoperative complications such as device malfunctions and blood clotting that caused strokes. Media coverage included both adoration and critique of artificial hearts and served to reinforce the allure of this technology while at the same time exposing real patient and societal problems surrounding its use. The clinical experiences were unsettling and in some cases downright disturbing. In the 1980s, a rising momentum to end the development of artificial hearts appeared poised to succeed. In 1982–83, Seattle dentist Barney Clark lived 112 days with his Jarvik-7 TAH, but he was tethered to a massive bedside unit, battled numerous complications, and never left the hospital. Politicians, medical professionals, bioethicists, academics, and industry people weighed in on this experimental technology. The *New York Times* declared the artificial heart "The Dracula of Medical Technology" for long sucking public funds to build an impossible device and called for a stake to be driven through the government-sponsored artificial heart program. Media coverage shaped and reflected the American public's concern about the problem of heart failure and the risks surrounding new devices. Alongside the hope that artificial hearts would offer a technological fix, there emerged a legitimate fear that artificial hearts might make patients worse off. The journalists who reported on this medical technology ranged widely in their scientific expertise and particular story angles, but none were immune to the uncertainty that persisted regarding the clinical use of artificial hearts. In the end, the mixed reporting sustained the ambivalence surrounding the technology.

Many medical practitioners and health policymakers asked, Where should we best direct our attention and resources—preventive measures or therapeutic options? All of this questioning raised the possibility that a limit—whether a technological, economical, or ethical limit—might indeed exist in what therapeutic devices could or should do in medicine. Some critics from within and outside the medical community framed the work on artificial hearts as "misguided" and spoke of "overzealous stakeholders" involved in a "hubris-ridden" endeavor."[88] Yet vocal opposition to artificial hearts did not halt its development. Many artificial heart teams refused to abandon their development, recognizing the clinical need for such devices. Bartlett stated, "As surgeons, we see patients with hopeless conditions every day. It naturally occurs to us that the problem should be solvable."[89] The major clinical problem was severe cardiac failure, and its rising incidence and prevalence was worrisome for medical and political reasons. Private and public funding continued. In the end, those involved in the development of artificial hearts enjoyed some clinical and commercial rewards. Better technology and better outcomes emerged as improved mechanical pumps found use as temporary, BTT devices by the 1990s. In the following decade, medicine and society acknowledged artificial hearts as life-sustaining bridge devices for many heart failure patients, including former vice president Dick Cheney. Motivated by this accepting attitude and the extended "temporary" use of VADs, device researchers and industry pursued the use of mechanical pumps as "permanent," destination therapy.

Although the technological momentum behind the development of artificial hearts drove the project forward, it was not a smooth, linear path. Solving technological challenges and promoting the devices' use came about through a multiple-pronged approach with a wide variety of scientific goals. Research and development edged forward, shifted sideways, and in some cases even abandoned several problematic lines of investigation before finally producing clinically viable devices. Many countries supported artificial heart research programs, including Russia, Germany, Japan, Australia, and Canada. The circulatory support research program at the NHLBI was the largest, best funded, and ultimately the first to develop a successful artificial heart. Since the inception of the program, the NHLBI has awarded hundreds of millions of dollars to academic-industry teams to develop artificial hearts. The field of mechanical circulatory support would never have developed without this government funding. Victor Poirier, inventor of the HeartMate II VAD, commented, "I can truthfully say that if we did not receive government support for the development of this technology it wouldn't exist. . . . Had a private investor been required to do that they would have never done it because the return was just too far away. So it's absolutely critical that the government be involved in this type of research."[90] The American resources, research infrastructure, and culture that embraced technological fixes contributed significantly to the development of artificial hearts.

Do limits exist for what mechanical devices can provide as medical treatment? In the case of artificial hearts, desirability rather than the feasibility or practicality of these devices drove their development. Fighting heart failure with medical devices appealed to an American society battling heart disease, but ambiguous results from clinical cases showed that the technology needed improvement. Debates on issues of cost, access, human experimentation, and quality of life ensued for decades. Uncertainty and dispute constantly beleaguered the development of artificial hearts. Continued technological problems with the devices produced variable government and industry support, provoked public opposition, and sustained divergent views within the medical profession. The contentious history of artificial hearts highlights the ambivalence in American medicine and society about technological fixes when it comes to disease and the body. Artificial hearts were (and are) an aggressive approach to treating heart failure. Various technical, economic, and social obstacles in their history challenged the twentieth-century momentum of technological fixes, testing clinical boundaries and the point at which imperfect devices would be acceptable. In the case of artificial hearts, the uncertainty surrounding this technology did not halt its development but influenced its greater clinical use as an assistive rather than a total replacement device, for technological and conceptual reasons.

Social and cultural circumstances frame response to and understanding of medical innovation; in the case of the artificial heart, it was a new technology wrapped in near-success narratives with problematic clinical outcomes that generated uncertainty and lack of consensus concerning its use. Device implants were invasive therapy without guaranteed benefits for end-stage heart failure patients. Physicians and patients have always faced difficult medical decision making; how vigorously does one intervene to halt disease or thwart death? The 1950s and 1960s ethos of pushing boundaries and engaging in aggressive surgical fixes to battle heart disease supported the development of artificial hearts. The desire and potential to replace worn-out body parts galvanized medical researchers, government agencies, device companies, and patient groups to continue mechanical heart research despite recurrent device challenges and opposition.

There also existed another ethos that was more or less dwarfed by the more dominant, aggressive approach concerning end-stage disease treatment choices in Western medicine. During the 1980s and 1990s, the choice to not do everything gained a moral legitimation; this viewpoint moderated but did not dislodge the curative emphasis in medicine. It reflected the value of comfort and care of patients who are dying or chronically ill, as represented by the hospice care movement, and it highlighted quality of life and the patient's wishes, denoting shared responsibilities for end-of-life medical decision making. Physicians have always been tasked with the judgment call of how vigorously to intervene in treating their patients. The dilemma that a particular intervention may be too much or too little haunts many clinicians, most poignantly as they recognize the futility of sustaining life yet perhaps feel family or patient pressure to take action.[91] In comparison to prevailing views in the 1960s, the twenty-first-century ethos surrounding death and dying within the context of end-stage disease treatment decision making has validated, more persuasively than in previous decades, the choice not to pursue riskier, invasive treatments.[92] But this "do-less" ethos failed to divert major investments in VADs and TAHs during the 1990s and early 2000s, despite the ongoing challenges of the technology, thus highlighting the desirability of life-extending treatments in American medicine and society.

During the course of their development, artificial hearts weathered the various storms of criticism from bioethicists and the press because of the role played by more powerful stakeholders. That is, the influence of key political and industrial entities, the confluence of a significant and effective cohort of researchers, and society's desire for technology to cure trumped the naysayers when it came to the feasibility and desirability of these medical devices. For artificial hearts and other medical technologies, it is clear that stakeholders play unequal roles in shaping the development of new devices, which when bolstered by momentum gain further resiliency. In the end, artificial heart researchers, industry partners, and their political allies were some of the stakeholders who won out over bioethicists, consumer advocate groups, opposing medical colleagues, and others who favored less expensive and less high-technology solutions to the heart failure problem in America.

The launching of artificial heart development took place during a period of significant public investment in science and technology and the ascendancy of technological medicine in Western health care. Situated against the rising prevalence of heart failure in American society, the appeal for new cardiac therapies cheered on its development. Yet the development path of artificial hearts faced innumerable barriers, and the device's clinical and commercial realization was never certain. The status of mechanical circulatory support systems in the early twenty-first century represents decades of incremental medical and bioengineering gains, contested program directions, wavering political support, and capricious industry partnerships. Despite ongoing use of VADs and TAHs, the artificial heart remains an imperfect technology, falling short of its goal of becoming the standard heart failure replacement treatment. What comes out of this historical account of artificial heart development is not a "near-success" device narrative but a case study that speaks to questions of "success," values, expectations, limitations, and uncertainty in a high-technology medical world. Throughout their history, artificial hearts have retained an allure and ambivalence that will continue to shape medical and public debates about the feasibility and sustainability of end-stage disease therapies, particularly given the aging demographic trend.

Institutions and Associations

AEC	Atomic Energy Commission
AHA	American Heart Association
CCF	Cleveland Clinic Foundation
DHEW	Department of Health, Education and Welfare
DHHS	Department of Health and Human Services
DOE	Department of Energy
FDA	Food and Drug Administration
GPO	Government Printing Office
HMD	History of Medicine Division, National Library of Medicine
IITRI	Illinois Institute of Technology Research Institute
NARA	National Archives and Records Administration
NHLBI	National Heart, Lung, and Blood Institute
NHLI	National Heart and Lung Institute
NIH	National Institutes of Health
NLM	National Library of Medicine
NMAH	National Museum of American History
PSU	Pennsylvania State University
SU	Stanford University
UU	University of Utah
VU	Vanderbilt University

Journals and Newspapers

AJC	American Journal of Cardiology
AJPH	American Journal of Public Health
AJS	American Journal of Surgery
Am Heart J	American Heart Journal
Am Herit Inv Tech	American Heritage of Invention and Technology
Am J Cardiol	American Journal of Cardiology
Ann Intern Med	Annals of Internal Medicine
Ann Surg	Annals of Surgery
Ann Thorac Surg	Annals of Thoracic Surgery
Arch Surg	Archives of Surgery
Art Org	Artificial Organs
ASAIO J	American Society for Artificial Internal Organs Journal
BMJ	British Medical Journal
Cardiov Dis	Cardiovascular Diseases
CMAJ	Canadian Medical Association Journal
Heart Transpl	Heart Transplantation
JAMA	Journal of the American Medical Association
J Am Coll Cardio	Journal of the American College of Cardiology
J Am Coll Surg	Journal of the American College of Surgeons
J Cardiov Med	Journal of Cardiovascular Medicine
JHLT	Journal of Heart and Lung Transplantation
JHT	Journal of Heart Transplantation

JTCS	*Journal of Thoracic and Cardiovascular Surgery*
MWN	*Medical World News*
Nat Geogr	*National Geographic*
NEJM	*New England Journal of Medicine*
NYT	*New York Times*
SAMJ	*South African Medical Journal*
Sci Am	*Scientific American*
Soc Sci & Med	*Social Science & Medicine*
T&C	*Technology and Culture*
THI Journal	*Texas Heart Institute Journal*
Trans ASAIO	*Transactions of the American Society for Artificial Internal Organs*
US Cardiol	*U.S. Cardiology*
Wash Post	*Washington Post*

Introduction

Epigraph: Stephanie Lecci, "'The Sound of Life': Woman Lives with Artificial Heart," WUWM Radio, aired 6 Sep 2013.

1. Stephanie Lecci, "Surgeon Cuts Out Heart, So Patient Can Live," WUWM Radio, aired 5 Sep 2013; Lecci, "'Sound of Life.'"

2. Sonya Colberg, "With Device, Geary Man," *Oklahoma City Oklahoman,* 18 Oct 2010; see also "Oklahoma Man 1st in Region to Receive Total Artificial Heart," SynCardia Press Release, 5 Oct 2010.

3. Mark Johnson, "Change of Heart: One Woman's Journal from Near-Death to Life," *Milwaukee Journal Sentinel,* 15 Feb 2014; "Change of Heart: Lifesaving Race against Clock," *Milwaukee Journal Sentinel,* 16 Feb 2014.

4. "First Oklahoman to Receive Total Artificial Heart Dies," *Oklahoma City Oklahoman,* 30 Dec 2011; "In Memory of Total Artificial Heart Patient Troy Golden," SynCardia Press Release, 28 Dec 2011.

5. Jack Copeland, "Mechanical Circulatory Support in Heart Failure," *US Cardiol* 8, no. 1 (2011): 48–49.

6. "Control of Life, Part 3—Manmade and Transplanted Organs Usher in an Era of Rebuilt People," *Life,* 24 Sep 1965.

7. "Rebuilding the Body from Nose to Toes," *Nat Geogr,* Dec 1989.

8. "The Incredible Bionic Man," Smithsonian Channel, aired 20 Oct 2013.

9. Dick Cheney and Jonathan Reiner, *Heart: An American Medical Odyssey* (New York: Scribner, 2013), 280.

10. Andrew Wolfson, "'It Feels Great!' Tools Tells Reporters," *Louisville (KY) Courier-Journal,* 22 Aug 2001; Darla Carter, "Heart Patient Takes Field Trips, Tries Fast Food," *Louisville (KY) Courier-Journal,* 26 Sep 2001; Dick Kaukas, "Artificial Heart Patient Doing Better Than Expected," *Louisville (KY) Courier-Journal,* 17 Jul 2001; *Dateline NBC,* 2 Nov 2001.

11. "Barney Clark Dies on 112th Day with Permanent Artificial Heart," *NYT,* 14 Mar 1983; "The Brave Man with the Plastic Heart," *Life,* Feb 1983, 24–30; "Dr Clark's Death Laid to Failure of All Organs but Artificial Heart," *NYT,* 25 Mar 1983; "Death of a Gallant Pioneer," *Time,* 4 Apr 1983.

12. O. H. Frazier, T. Akutsu, and D. A. Cooley, "Total Artificial Heart (TAH) Utilization in Man," *Trans ASAIO* 28 (1982): 534–35; Denton A. Cooley et al., "Total Artificial Heart in Two-Staged Cardiac Transplantation," *Cardiov Dis* 8, no. 3 (Sep 1981): 317; Denton A. Cooley, "Staged Cardiac Transplantation: Report of Three Cases," *Heart Transpl* 1, no. 2 (Feb 1982): 149–52.

13. Sheryl Gay Stolberg, "Artificial Heart, Artificial Life," *NYT,* 10 Oct 2002; untitled News Service story bulletin, *Wash Post,* 17 Oct 2002.

14. Thomas Schlich, "The Technological Fix and the Modern Body," in *A Cultural History of the Human Body,* ed. Linda Kalof and William Bynum (Oxford, UK: Berg, 2010), 84; Susan E. Lederer, *Flesh and Blood: Organ Transplantation and Blood Transplantation in Twentieth-Century America* (New York: Oxford University Press, 2008); David Hamilton, *A History of Organ Transplantation* (Pittsburgh: University of Pittsburgh Press, 2012); Thomas Schlich, *The Origins of Organ Transplantation* (Rochester, NY: University of Rochester Press, 2010); Nicholas L. Tilney, *Transplant: From Myth to Reality* (New Haven, CT: Yale University Press, 2003).

15. See Shelley McKellar, "Limitations Exposed: Willem J. Kolff and His Contentious Pursuit of a Mechanical Heart," in *Essays in Honour of Michael Bliss: Figuring the Social,* ed. E. A. Heaman, Alison Li, and Shelley McKellar (Toronto: University of Toronto Press, 2008), 400–434.

16. Lederer, *Flesh and Blood,* ix–x, 208–12.

17. "The Dracula of Medical Technology," *NYT,* 16 May 1988.

18. Renée C. Fox and Judith P. Swazey, *Spare Parts: Organ Replacement in American Society* (New York: Oxford University Press, 1992), xv ("spare parts pragmatism," "limitless medical progress," "escalating ardor"), 199 ("courage to fail"), 210 ("the human suffering," "social, cultural, and spiritual harm"). See also Renée C. Fox and Judith P. Swazey, *The Courage to Fail: A Social View of Organ Transplants and Dialysis* (Chicago: University of Chicago Press, 1978).

19. George J. Annas, "Consent to the Artificial Heart: The Lion and the Crocodiles," *Hastings Center Report* 13, no. 2 (Apr 1983): 20–22.

20. W. Bruce Fye, *Caring for the Heart: Mayo Clinic and the Rise of Specialization* (Oxford: Oxford University Press, 2015), 461.

21. "Artificial Heart Research and Development," no date, John Watson Papers, NLM, HMD, Accession 2003-054, box 3, folder: USA-CCCP Collaboration; Valeriy I. Shumakov, "Soviet-American Collaboration on the Development of an Artificial Heart and Mechanical Circulatory Assistance," *Art Org* 7, no. 1 (1983): 110–11.

22. V. I. Shumakov, "Some Achievements from the Soviet-American Cooperation in Circulatory Assistance and the Artificial Heart: 1981–1984," *Art Org* 11, no. 1 (1987): 7.

23. "Leading Causes of Death, 1900–98," U.S. National Office of Vital Statistics, www.cdc.gov.

24. Laura B. Shrestha, "Life Expectancy in the United States," CRS Report for Congress, August 16, 2006, www.aging.senate.gov.

25. Howard A. Rusk, "U.S. Fight on Heart Disease Backed Widely by Citizens: Appropriation by Congress for Research Equals Fund for Potato Bug War," *NYT,* 11 Jul 1948, 27, cited in Eugene Braunwald, "Shattuck Lecture—Cardiovascular Medicine at the Turn of the Millennium: Triumphs, Concerns, and Opportunities," *NEJM* 337, no. 19 (6 Nov 1997): 1360.

26. T. R. Dawber et al., "Epidemiologic Approaches to Heart Disease: The Framingham Study," *AJPH* 41 (1951): 279–86; W. B. Kannel et al., "Factors of Risk in the Development of Coronary Heart Disease—Six-Year Follow-Up Experience: The Framingham Study," *Ann Intern Med* 55 (1961): 33–50; Patrick A. McKee et al., "The Natural History of Congestive Heart Failure: The Framingham Study," *NEJM* 285, no. 26 (23 Dec 1971): 14441–46; Braunwald, "Shattuck Lecture," 1361; Daniel Levy and Susan Brink, *A Change of Heart: How the People of Framingham, Massachusetts, Helped Unravel the Mysteries of Cardiovascular Disease* (New York: Knopf, 2005).

27. Paul Dudley White, *Heart Disease,* 3rd ed. (New York: Macmillan, 1944), 249.

28. David S. Jones, *Broken Hearts: The Tangled History of Cardiac Care* (Baltimore: Johns Hopkins University Press, 2013); Stephen Klaidman, *Saving the Heart: The Battle to Conquer Coronary Disease* (Oxford: Oxford University Press, 2000).

29. Robert O. Bonow et al., *Braunwald's Heart Disease: A Textbook of Cardiovascular Medicine,* 9th ed. (Philadelphia: Elsevier Saunders, 2012).

30. AHA, "About Heart Failure," www.heart.org, accessed 3 Nov 2013.

31. AHA, "Classes of Heart Failure," www.heart.org, accessed 3 Nov 2013.

32. V. L. Roger et al., "Heart Disease and Stroke Statistics—2012 Update: A Report from the American Heart Association." *Circulation* 125, no. 1 (2012): e2–e220; William

T. Abraham and Henry Krum, *Heart Failure: A Practical Approach to Treatment* (New York: McGraw-Hill Medical, 2007), 15–17; White, *Heart Disease,* 763.

33. AHA, "Heart Failure Patients Living Longer, but Long-Term Survival Still Low," 15 May 2013, http://newsroom.heart.org.

34. Piotr Ponikowski et al., "Heart Failure: Preventing Disease and Death Worldwide," *ESC Heart Failure* 1, no. 1 (Sep 2014): 4–25.

35. Salynn Boyles, "AHA: Heart Failure Costs Likely to Soar," *MedPage Today,* 25 Apr 2013; Paul A. Heidenreich et al., "Forecasting the Impact of Heart Failure in the United States: A Policy Statement from the American Heart Association," *Circulation: Heart Failure* 6 (2013): 606–19; CDC, Heart Failure Fact Sheet, www.cdc.gov; Abraham and Krum, *Heart Failure,* 13–15.

36. David S. Jones and Jeremy A. Greene, "The Decline and Rise of Coronary Heart Disease," *AJPH* 103, no. 7 (Jul 2013): 1207–18; Jones, *Broken Hearts.*

37. NHLBI, "Who Is at Risk of Heart Failure?," www.nhlbi.nih.gov, accessed 3 Nov 2013.

38. Anne L. Taylor, "Heart Failure in Women," *Current Heart Failure Reports* 12 (2015): 187–88.

39. NHLBI, "What Causes Heart Failure?," www.nhlbi.nih.gov, accessed 5 Nov 2013.

40. White, *Heart Disease,* 764–96.

41. Fye, *Caring for the Heart;* Jones, *Broken Hearts;* Harris B. Shumacker, *The Evolution of Cardiac Surgery* (Bloomington: Indiana University Press, 1992).

42. Jones, *Broken Hearts,* 28.

43. Christopher Hallowell, "Charles Lindbergh's Artificial Heart," *Am Herit Inv Tech* 1, no. 2 (Fall 1985): 58–62; Lindbergh-Carrel Perfusion Pump, Smithsonian Institution, NMAH, Accession no. 279576.

44. A. Carrel and C. A. Lindbergh, "The Culture of Whole Organs," *Science* 81, no. 211 (21 Jun 1935): 621–23; "'Artificial Heart' Interests Science," *NYT,* 22 Jun 1935, 17; "Lindbergh Details Artificial 'Heart,'" *NYT,* 1 Sep 1935, N1, 3.

45. William L. Laurence, "Carrel, Lindbergh Develop Device to Keep Organs Alive Outside the Body," *NYT,* 21 Jun 1935, 1, 13.

46. "Medicine: Men in Black," *Time,* 13 Jun 1938.

47. Henry E. Sigerist, *American Medicine* (New York: W. W. Norton, 1934), 270, quoted in Schlich, "Technological Fix," 73.

48. These statements by Billroth and Paget are often quoted, as by Lael Wertenbaker, *To Mend the Heart* (New York: Viking Press, 1980), 50; and Robert G. Richardson, *The Scalpel and the Heart* (New York: Charles Scribner's, 1970), 27–28. For more on the history of cardiac surgery, see Shumacker, *Evolution of Cardiac Surgery;* Stephen L. Johnson, *The History of Cardiac Surgery, 1896–1955* (Baltimore: Johns Hopkins Press, 1970). For a broader view on the history of surgery, see Thomas Schlich, "The Emergence of Modern Surgery," in *Medicine Transformed: Health, Disease and Society in Europe, 1800–1930,* ed. Deborah Brunton (Manchester, UK: Manchester University Press, 2004): 61–91; Christopher Lawrence, "Democratic, Divine and Heroic: The History and Historiography of Surgery," in *Medical Theory, Surgical Practice: Studies in the History of Surgery,* ed. Christopher Lawrence (London: Routledge, 1992).

49. See Vivien T. Thomas, *Pioneering Research in Surgical Shock and Cardiovascular Surgery: Vivien Thomas and His Work with Alfred Blalock: An Autobiography* (Philadelphia: University of Pennsylvania Press, 1985).

50. See G. Wayne Miller, *King of Hearts* (New York: Random House, 2000); Harris B. Shumacker Jr., *A Dream of the Heart* (Santa Barbara, CA: Fithian Press, 1999); Thomas

Thompson, *Hearts: Of Surgeons and Transplants, Miracles and Disasters along the Cardiac Frontier* (New York: McCall, 1971); Wertenbaker, *To Mend the Heart;* Shelley McKellar, *Surgical Limits* (Toronto: University of Toronto Press, 2003).

51. Kirk Jeffrey, *Machines in Our Hearts* (Baltimore: Johns Hopkins University Press, 2001), 4–6; see also Lynn Payer, *Medicine and Culture* (New York: Holt, 1988).

52. Fye, *Caring for the Heart,* 204.

53. W. G. Bigelow, *Cold Hearts: The Story of Hypothermia and the Pacemaker in Heart Surgery* (Toronto: McClelland and Stewart, 1984), 40.

54. F. T. Lewis and M. Taufic, "Closure of Atrial Septal Defect with the Aid of Hypothermia: Experimental Accomplishments," *Surgery* 33 (1953): 52.

55. Fye, *Caring for the Heart,* 209.

56. Richardson, *Scalpel and the Heart,* 221–24.

57. Robert Carola, John Harley, and Charles R. Noback, *Human Anatomy and Physiology,* 2nd ed. (Toronto: McGraw-Hill, 1992), 608–9.

58. "Medicine: Historic Operation," *Time,* 18 May 1953; J. H. Gibbon Jr, "Application of a Mechanical Heart and Lung Apparatus to Cardiac Surgery," *Minnesota Medicine* 37, no. 3 (Mar 1954): 171–85; J. D. Hill, "John H. Gibbon, Jr. Part I. The Development of the First Successful Heart-Lung Machine," *Ann Thorac Surg* 34, no. 3 (1982): 337–41; Shumacker, *Evolution of Cardiac Surgery,* 242–43; Shumacker, *Dream of the Heart.*

59. See Johnson, *History of Cardiac Surgery,* 145–58; Dr. R. O. Heimbecker, "Open Heart Surgery Performed by Extra-Corporeal Circulation through Pump Oxygenators," March 1957, University of Toronto Archives, A89-0030, Department of Surgery, box 002, Department Chair Files, file 1.

60. See Wertenbaker, *To Mend the Heart,* 196.

61. M. Kurusz, "May 6, 1953: The Untold Story," *ASAIO J* 58, no. 1 (Jan–Feb 2012): 2–5.

62. By the 1980s, ECMO had gained some clinical use as a mechanical circulatory support system for acute heart failure, and it was the only cardiac support system for children until the recent availability of the Berlin Heart system. See the landmark article R. H. Bartlett et al., "Extracorporeal Membrane Oxygenation (ECMO) Cardiopulmonary Support in Infancy," *Trans ASAIO* 22 (1976): 80–93; Robert H. Bartlett, "Extracorporeal Life Support: Gibbon Fulfilled," *J Am Coll Surg* 218, no. 3 (Mar 2014): 317–27; Robert Bartlett, Project Bionics Pioneer Interview, 20 Apr 2005, NLM, HMD.

63. NHLBI, "What Is Heart Valve Disease?," www.nhlbi.nih.gov, accessed 9 Nov 2013.

64. Shumacker, *Evolution of Cardiac Surgery,* 304–10; Richard A. DeWall et al., "The Evolution of Mechanical Heart Valves," *Ann Thorac Surg* 69 (2000): 1612–21; Vincent L. Gott et al., "Mechanical Heart Valves: 50 Years of Evolution," *Ann Thorac Surg* 76 (2003): S2230–S2239.

65. NHLBI, "What Is Heart Block?," www.nhlbi.nih.gov, accessed 9 Nov 2013.

66. This case reported in M. Zoll, "Resuscitation of the Heart in Ventricular Standstill by External Electrical Stimulation," *NEJM* 247 (1952): 768.

67. Jeffrey, *Machines in Our Hearts,* 56.

68. Denton Cooley, "In Memoriam: Tribute to Åke Senning, Pioneering Cardiovascular Surgeon," *THI Journal* 27, no. 3 (2000): 234–35; Jeffrey, *Machines in Our Hearts,* 90–92.

69. For more on atomic pacemakers, see Victor Parsonnet et al., "Thirty-One Years of Clinical Experience with 'Nuclear-Powered' Pacemakers," *PACE* 29 (Feb 2006): 195; Jeffrey, *Machines in Our Hearts,* 115–17.

70. Jeffrey, *Machines in Our Hearts,* 174–77.

71. Ibid., 235–62; Wilson Greatbatch and Curtis F. Holmes, "History of Implantable Devices," *IEEE Engineering in Medicine and Biology* (Sep 1991): 38–41, 49.

72. Rachel Haase, Marsha Michie, and Debra Skinner, "Flexible Positions, Managed Hopes: The Promissory Bioeconomy of a Whole Genome Sequencing Cancer Study," *Soc Sci & Med* 130 (Apr 2015): 146–53; Tiago Moreria and Paolo Palladino, "Between Truth and Hope: On Parkinson's Disease, Neurotransplantation and the Production of the 'Self,'" *History of the Human Sciences* 18, no. 3 (2005): 55–82.

73. Mads Borup et al., "The Sociology of Expectations in Science and Technology," *Technology Analysis and Strategic Management* 18, 3–4 (Jul–Sep 2006): 285–86; Nik Brown and Andrew Webster, *New Medical Technologies and Society: Reordering Life* (Cambridge, UK: Polity Press), 2004.

74. Adrian Kantrowitz, Project Bionics Pioneer Interview, 19 Apr 2005, NLM, HMD.

75. See Copeland, "Mechanical Circulatory Support," 51; Kantrowitz, interview, 19 Apr 2005, NLM.

Chapter 1 · Multiple Approaches to Building Artificial Hearts

Epigraph: John Buchanan, "The Man Who Invented the 'Kidney,'" *Empire Magazine, Denver Post,* 13 Feb 1966, 10–15, news clipping, UU, MS 654 Willem J. Kolff Collection, box 1, folder 14.

1. Michael E. DeBakey, "The Odyssey of the Artificial Heart," *Art Org* 24, no. 6 (Jun 2000): 406.

2. F. A. Gotch, "The Evolution of the Society," *Trans ASAIO* 25 (1979): 534–38.

3. Jean Kantrowitz, Project Bionics Pioneer Interview, 25 Aug 2015, NLM, HMD.

4. S. McKellar and M. Kurusz, "Reflections and Visions: 50 Years of Presidential Addresses," *ASAIO Journal* 50, no. 6 (Nov–Dec 2004): 629–34.

5. Peter F. Salisbury, "Implantation of Physiological Machines into the Mammalian Organism: Identification of Problems Connected with the Implantation of Artificial Hearts and of Artificial Kidneys: Experimental Results to Date," *Trans ASAIO* 3, no. 1 (Apr 1957): 37–42; S. McCabe, "Pump for Replacement of the Heart," *Trans ASAIO* 5, no. 1 (Apr 1959): 289–92.

6. See Mary-Jo Delvecchio Good, "The Medical Imaginary and the Biotechnical Embrace," in *Subjectivity: Ethnographic Investigations,* ed. Joao Biehl, Byron Good, and Arthur Kleinman (Berkeley: University of California Press, 2007), 362–80; Anneke Smelik, ed., *The Scientific Imaginary in Visual Culture* (Göttingen, Germany: V & R Unipress, 2010).

7. Lesley A. Sharp, *The Transplant Imaginary: Mechanical Hearts, Animal Parts, and Moral Thinking in Highly Experimental Science* (Berkeley: University of California Press, 2014), 9.

8. Salisbury, "Implantation of Physiological Machines," 37–42; McCabe, "Pump for Replacement," 289–92.

9. For more on Kolff and the artificial kidney, see Paul Heiney, *The Nuts and Bolts of Life: Willem Kolff and the Invention of the Kidney Machine* (London: History Press, 2003); J. S. Cameron, *History of the Treatment of Renal Failure by Dialysis* (Oxford: Oxford University Press, 2002); Steven J. Peitzman, *Dropsy, Dialysis and Transplant: A Short History of Failing Kidneys* (Baltimore: Johns Hopkins University Press, 2007); A. B. Weisse, *Conversations in Medicine* (New York: New York University Press, 1984).

10. Declaration of Intention by the Board of Governors, 22 Jul 1965, CCF Archives, folder 3-PR20 Artificial Organs; W. J. Kolff, "Program of Artificial Organs," 1 Aug 1965, ibid.

11. Memorandum by the Board of Governors, 21 Feb 1967, CCF Archives, folder 3-PR20 Artificial Organs; W. J. Kolff to CCF Board of Governors, 17 Feb 1967, UU, MS 654 Willem

J. Kolff Collection, box 381, folder 12; Leonard L. Loveshin to W. J. Kolff, 13 Apr 1967, ibid.; Allen B. Weisse, *Heart to Heart: The Twentieth Century Battle against Cardiac Disease* (New Brunswick, NJ: Rutgers University Press, 2002), 254.

12. Weisse, *Heart to Heart,* 252.

13. Minutes, Meeting of Board of Governors, 14 Dec 1957, CCF Archives, folder 3-PR20 Artificial Organs; W. J. Kolff, Progress Reports, Program of Artificial Organs, ca. 1958–66, ibid.

14. Willem J. Kolff, "An Artificial Kidney inside the Body," *Sci Am* 213, no. 5 (Nov 1965): 41.

15. O. H. Frazier, "In Memoriam: Tetsuzo Akutsu 1922–2007," *THI Journal* 35, no. 1 (2008): 4; S. Takatani, "In Remembrance of Dr. Tetsuzo Akutsu: A Man Who Started Artificial Heart Research," *Journal of Artificial Organs* 11, no. 1 (Apr 2008): 1–3.

16. T. Akutsu and W. J. Kolff, "Permanent Substitutes for Valves and Hearts," *Trans ASAIO* 4 (1958): 230; Josephine Robertson, "Substitute Heart of Plastic Pushed by Clinic Team," *Cleveland Plain Dealer,* 15 Apr 1958; "The Artificial Heart: Progress toward Its Implantation in Man," *JAMA* 185, no. 13 (28 Sep 1963): 24.

17. Years later, Kolff and Akutsu learned that a Soviet scientist, Vladimir Demikhov, had performed a similar experiment in 1937. See George M. Pantalos, "A Selective History of Mechanical Circulatory Support," in *Mechanical Circulatory Support,* edited by T. Lewis and T. R. Graham (London: Edward Arnold, 1995), 6; H. B. Shumacker Jr, "A Surgeon to Remember: Notes about Vladimir Demikhov," *Ann Thorac Surg* 58 (1994): 1196.

18. P. M. Portner, "Permanent Mechanical Circulatory Assistance," in *Heart and Lung Transplantation,* ed. W. A. Baumgartner et al., 2nd ed. (Philadelphia: W. B. Saunders, 2002), 533.

19. W. J. Kolff et al., "Artificial Heart in the Chest and Use of Polyurethane of Making Hearts, Valves and Aortas," *Trans ASAIO* (1959): 298. For an image of the Solenoid heart, see "Off-the-Shelf: The Mechanical Heart," *Machine Design,* 16 Feb 1961, 28.

20. C. S. Houston, T. Akutsu, and W. J. Kolff, "Pendulum Type of Artificial Heart within the Chest," *Am Heart J* (1960): 723. For an image of the Pendulum heart, see "Off-the-Shelf," 29.

21. News Release, 15 Apr 1958, CCF Archives, folder 3-PR20 Artificial Organs; "Early Types of Artificial Hearts," n.d., UU, MS 654 Willem J. Kolff Collection; "Artificial Heart: Progress," 25–26; W. J. Kolff, "The Artificial Heart: Research, Development or Invention?," *Diseases of the Chest* 56 (1969): 314–29.

22. Willem J. Kolff, "An Artificial Heart Inside the Body," *Sci Am* 213, no. 5 (Nov 1965): 45.

23. Sharp, *Transplant Imaginary,* 110.

24. Ibid., 112. See also Lesley A. Sharp, "The Art of Medicine: Bioengineered Bodies and the Moral Imagination," *Lancet* 374 (19 Sep 2009): 970–71.

25. K. W. Hiller et al., "A Servomechanism to Drive an Artificial Heart inside the Chest," *Trans ASAIO* 8 (1962): 125–30; W. J. Kolff et al., "Results Obtained with Artificial Hearts Driven by the N.A.S.A. Servomechanism and the Pathologic Physiology of Artificial Hearts," *Trans ASAIO* 8 (1962): 135–39.

26. T. Akutsu et al., "Silastic Sac-Type of Artificial Heart and Its Use in Calves," *Trans ASAIO* 9 (1963): 281; "New Hearts Are 'In the Bag,'" *MWN,* 11 May 1962, 90–1.

27. "Artificial Heart: Progress," 25–26.

28. W. Seidel et al., "Air-Driven Artificial Hearts inside the Chest," *Trans ASAIO* 7 (1961): 378; K. W. Hiller, W. Seidel, and W. J. Kolff, "Electro-Mechanical Control for an Intrathoracic Artificial Heart," *Academic Journal of Manufacturing Engineering* 2 (1963): 212; S. H. Norton, T. Akutsu, and W. J. Kolff, "Artificial Heart with Antivacuum Bellows," *Trans ASAIO* 8 (1962): 131; E. K. Panayotopoulous et al., "A Special Reciprocating Pump to Drive

an Artificial Heart inside the Chest," *JTCS* 48 (1964): 844; Y. Nosé and W. J. Kolff, "The Intracorporeal Mechanical Heart," *Vascular Disorders* 3 (1966): 25.

29. B. K. Kusserow, "Artificial Heart Research—Survey and Prospectus," *Transactions of the New York Academy of Sciences* 27 (Jan 1965): 309–23.

30. B. K. Kusserow, "A Permanently Indwelling Intracorporeal Blood Pump to Substitute for Cardiac Function," *Trans ASAIO* 4, no. 1 (Apr 1958): 227–29.

31. B. K. Kusserow, "The Use of a Magnetic Field to Remotely Power an Implantable Blood Pump: Preliminary Report," *Trans ASAIO* 6 (Apr 1960): 292–98.

32. F. W. Hastings, W. H. Potter, and J. W. Holter, "A Progress Report on the Development of a Synthetic Intracorporeal Blood Pump," *Trans ASAIO* 8 (1962): 116–17; Adrian Kantrowitz, "The Technological Response to Heart Failure," *SOMA* (October 1986): 7–8.

33. William S. Pierce et al., "Problems Encountered in Experiments during the Development of Our Artificial Intrathoracic Heart," *Trans ASAIO* 8 (1962): 118–24.

34. D. Liotta et al., "Artificial Heart in the Chest: Preliminary Report," *Trans ASAIO* 7 (1961): 318–22.

35. "Artificial Heart: Progress," 27.

36. *Hearings on DHEW Appropriations for 1965, Before the House Subcommittee of Appropriations,* part 2, p. 1926, 1 Jul 1964, 88th Cong. (1964) (statement of Dr. Michael DeBakey).

37. Michael E. DeBakey: An oral history, 23 Nov 1986 and 6 Apr 1992, NLM, HMD, OH 127; Michael E. DeBakey interview, 14 Dec 1998, William S. Stoney Collection, Vanderbilt University Medical Center, Eskind Biomedical Library Special Collections, Collection no. 241, box 01A, folder 6.

38. Renée Fox and Judith P. Swazey, *The Courage to Fail: A Social View of Organ Transplants and Dialysis,* 2nd ed. (New Brunswick, NJ: Transaction, 2002, 141.

39. Liotta et al., "Artificial Heart in the Chest," 318–22.

40. Fox and Swazey, *Courage to Fail,* 173; Domingo Liotta et al., "Prolonged Partial Left Ventricular Bypass by Means of an Intrathoracic Pump Implanted in the Left Chest," *Trans ASAIO* 8, no. 1 (Apr 1962): 90–109; Domingo Liotta et al., "Prolonged Assisted Circulation during and after Heart or Aortic Surgery," *Trans ASAIO* 9 (Apr 1963): 182–85.

41. Fox and Swazey, *Courage to Fail,* 173.

42. Domingo Liotta et al., "Prolonged Assisted Circulation during and after Cardiac or Aortic Surgery," *AJC* 12 (Sep 1963): 339–405; Liotta, "Prolonged Partial Left Ventricular Bypass," 90; Liotta et al., "Artificial Heart in the Chest," 318.

43. In 1964, C. William Hall donated the intracorporeal tube-type pump used in this clinical case to the Smithsonian Institution. Liotta-Hall Intracorporeal Heart Pump, Smithsonian Institution, NMAH, Accession no. 256189.

44. Liotta et al., "Prolonged Assisted Circulation," *AJC,* 339–405; M. E. DeBakey, "Current Directions in the Artificial Heart Program," *Gazzetta Sanitaria* 18, no. 1 (1969): 7; "The Artificial Heart," in *The History of Surgery in Houston,* ed. Kenneth L. Mattox (Austin, TX: Eakin Press, 1998), 348.

45. "Medicine: Half-Heart Replacement," *Time* 82, no. 19 (8 Nov 1963): 50; "Toward an Artificial Heart," *Time* 85, no. 22 (28 May 1965): 55. *New York Times* journalist Robert Plumb did not use the word *success* in his reporting. See Robert K. Plumb, "Blood Pump Used In Heart Victim," *NYT,* 28 Oct 1963, 29.

46. M. E. DeBakey et al., "The Fate of Dacron Vascular Grafts," *Arch Surg* 89 (Nov 1964): 757–82; R. M. O'Neal et al., "Cells Grown on Isolated Intravascular Dacron Hub: An Electron Microscopic Study," *Experimental Molecular Pathology* 90 (Oct 1964): 403–12;

M. M. Stump et al., "Endothelium Grown from Circulating Blood on Isolated Intravascular Dacron Hub," *American Journal of Pathology* 43 (Sep 1963): 361–67.

47. M. E. DeBakey, "Left Ventricular Bypass Pump for Cardiac Assistance," *AJC* 27 (Jan 1971): 11.

48. *Hearings on DHEW Appropriations for 1967, Before the House Subcommittee of Appropriations,* part 5, 21–25, 28–30 Mar 1966, 89th Cong. (1966), p. 490.

49. C. William Hall, Domingo Liotta, and Michael E. DeBakey, "Bioengineering Efforts in Developing Artificial Hearts and Assistors," *AJS* 114 (Jul 1967): 24–25.

50. M. E. DeBakey and C. W. Hall, "Towards the Artificial Heart," *New Scientist* 393 (28 May 1964): 540–41.

51. Ibid., 539.

52. Ibid., 540–41.

53. *Hearings on DHEW Appropriations for 1965,* pp. 1924–25.

54. See Susan E. Lederer, "Transplant Nation: The NIH and the Politics of Heart Transplantation in the 1960s," in *Biomedicine in the Twentieth Century: Practices, Policies, and Politics,* ed. C. Hannaway (Washington, DC: IOS Press, 2008), 151; Domingo Liotta, *Amazing Adventures of a Heart Surgeon: The Artificial Heart: The Frontiers of Human Life* (New York: iUniverse, 2007), 174.

55. Irvine H. Page, "Some Observations on Medical Research," *CA: A Cancer Journal for Clinicians* 16, no. 2 (May–Jun 1966): 123. A pioneer in hypertension research, Page himself navigated lay publicity while adhering to traditional conventions in reporting research results. Page was featured on the cover of *Time* magazine in 1955 for his work on high blood pressure and its possible treatment in the battle against heart disease. See "Medicine: The Chances for Recovery" (cover story), *Time* 66, no 18 (31 Oct 1955); Lawrence K. Altman, "Dr Irvine H. Page Is Dead at 90; Pioneered Hypertension Research," *NYT,* 12 June 1991.

56. Thomas Thompson, *Hearts: Of Surgeons and Transplants, Miracles and Disasters along the Cardiac Frontier* (New York: McCall, 1971), 143–44.

57. Denton A. Cooley, *100,000 Hearts: A Surgeon's Memoirs* (Austin: University of Texas at Austin, 2012), 89.

58. "Medicine: Half-Heart Replacement," 50; "Public Health: A $3 Billion Plan," *Time* 84, no. 26 (18 Dec 1964): 64; "Surgery: Repairing the Royal Aorta," *Time* 84, no. 27 (25 Dec 1964): 52.

59. "Toward an Artificial Heart," 46–55.

60. NIH funding for the research and development of mechanical circulatory support systems primarily began in the 1960s, and it continues today. During the 1970s, the program name changed because of the reorganization of the National Heart and Lung Institute and the expansion of NHLI administrator roles involved in supporting and advancing the development of these devices. The Artificial Heart Program, established in 1964, was renamed the Medical Devices Applications Program in 1970. Two years later, this program became the Division of Technological Applications. In 1973 it was renamed the Cardiovascular Devices Branch in the Division of Heart and Vascular Diseases. In 1974 it was renamed again as the Devices and Technology Branch (DTB) in this division. In 1976 John Watson was appointed chief of DTB, and he delivered program stability and efficiency until his retirement in 2004. Annual Report (A.H.P.) 1 July 1972 to 30 June 1973, NLM, HMD, John Watson Papers, Accession 2003-054, box 2, folder Division of Technological Applications of the NHLI, 1973.

61. Established in 1948, the National Heart Institute was renamed in 1969 the National Heart and Lung Institute and in 1976 the National Heart, Lung, and Blood Institute, re-

flecting its expanded research, treatment, and prevention activities related to diseases of the heart, blood vessels, lung, and blood. "NIH Institutes, Centers, and Offices: A Summary History," National Institutes of Health Office of History, www.history.nih.gov.

62. "Federal Support for the Development of Artificial Heart Devices, Prior to FY 1964," NLM, HMD, John Watson Papers, Accession 2003-054, box 2, folder The Artificial Heart Program at the National Heart Institute, 1964–68.

63. M. J. Strauss, "The Political History of the Artificial Heart," *NEJM* 310 (2 Feb 1984): 334; Barton J. Bernstein, "The Artificial Heart Program," *Center Magazine* 14, no. 3 (1981): 25.

64. *Hearings on DHEW Appropriations for 1964, Before the House Subcommittee of Appropriations,* part 2, 7–8, 13–17 May, 4–5 Jun 1963, p. 1389, 88th Cong. (1963).

65. Thomas A. Preston, "The Artificial Heart," in *Worse than the Disease: Pitfalls of Medical Progress,* ed. Diana B. Dutton (Cambridge: Cambridge University Press, 1988), 94. In a 1998 interview, DeBakey stated that initially the NIH had not wanted an artificial heart program, that Shannon had characterized the research as "soft science," and that Senator Hill's support had been key toward realizing the program. See DeBakey interview, 14 Dec 1998, VU.

66. *Hearings on DHEW Appropriations for 1966, Before the House Subcommittee of Appropriations,* part 3, 4, 8–11, 15, 16, 18, 19, 22 May 1965, p. 501, 89th Cong. (1965), cited in Preston, "Artificial Heart," 94.

67. *Hearings on DHEW Appropriations for 1966,* p. 502.

68. Ibid., p. 505.

69. President's Commission on Heart Disease, Cancer and Stroke, 1963–1965, Michael E. DeBakey Papers, NLM, HMD, MS C 582, box 10, folder 1; Lyndon B. Johnson to Michael E. DeBakey, 9 Mar 1964, LBJ Presidential Library and Museum, White House Central Files, box D91, Name File: "DeBakey, Michael E. (DR)."

70. W. Bruce Fye, *Caring for the Heart: Mayo Clinic and the Rise of Specialization* (Oxford: Oxford University Press, 2015), 261.

71. Johnson to DeBakey, 9 Mar 1964, LBJ Presidential Library and Museum.

72. Strauss, "Political History of Artificial Heart," 334.

73. *Artificial Heart Program Conference Proceedings, 9–13 June 1969,* DHEW, Washington, DC (Washington: GPO, 1970), 2.

74. Annual Report (A.H.P.) 1 July 1972 to 30 June 1973, NLM.

75. Frank Hastings to Senators, 24 Mar 1969, NLM, HMD, John Watson Papers, Accession 2003-054, box 16, folder Congressional Inquiries.

76. Hastings was extremely well-liked and respected by the MCSS community for his earlier research work and for his role as the Artificial Heart Program director. It came as a great shock to the MCSS community when Hastings, at age 52, died unexpectedly in 1971 from a stroke. Quote in chapter taken from Lowell T. Harmison, "Dedication" (to Frank W. Hastings), *Bulletin of the New York Academy of Medicine* 48, no. 2 (Feb 1972): 213.

77. "The National Heart Institute: A Brief History," ca. 1968, NLM, HMD, John Watson Papers, Accession 2003-054, box 2, folder The Artificial Heart Program of the National Heart Institute, 1964–68.

78. *Hearings on DHEW Appropriations for 1967,* p. 490.

79. *Hearings on DHEW Appropriations for 1966,* p. 504.

80. Hastings to Senators, 24 Mar 1969, NLM.

81. "The National Heart Institute: A Brief History," ca. 1968, NLM.

82. Ibid.; Kantrowitz interview, 25 Aug 2015, NLM.

83. *Hearings on DHEW Appropriations for 1967,* p. 480.

278 Notes to Pages 45–49

84. See J. H. Gibbon, "The Artificial Intracorporeal Heart," *Surgery* 9 (1966): 1–5.

85. *Artificial Heart Program Conference Proceedings,* 7; "The National Heart Institute: A Brief History," ca. 1968, NLM.

86. "Summary Operational History of the Artificial Heart Program," 4 Dec 1973, NLM, HMD, John Watson Papers, Accession 2003-054, box 16, folder 5.

87. Bernstein, "Artificial Heart Program," 22.

88. *Hearings on DHEW Appropriations for 1966,* pp. 505–6.

89. Bernstein, "Artificial Heart Program," 24.

90. "Summary Operational History of the Artificial Heart Program," NLM; Institute of Medicine, *The Artificial Heart: Prototypes, Policies and Patients* (Washington, DC: National Academy of Sciences, 1991), 206.

91. See Preston, "Artificial Heart," 100; Strauss, "Political History of Artificial Heart," 334; Bernstein, "Artificial Heart Program," 25.

92. DeBakey, "Odyssey of the Artificial Heart," 407; Bernstein, "Artificial Heart Program," 25.

93. See Robert F Rushmer, *National Priorities for Health: Past, Present, and Projected* (New York: Wiley, 1980).

94. James A. Shannon to Mary Lasker, 26 Jun 1964, Columbia University Libraries Rare Book & Manuscript Library, Mary Lasker Papers, accessed online at The Mary Lasker Papers, Profiles in Science, NLM, at profiles.nlm.nih.gov.

95. Bernstein, "Artificial Heart Program," 25.

96. "The National Heart Institute: A Brief History," ca. 1968, NLM; "Summary Operational History of the Artificial Heart Program," 4 Dec 1973, NLM; Mechanically Assisted Circulation—The Status of the NBLI Program and Recommendations for the Future: Report of the Cardiology Advisory Committee, May 1977, NLM, HMD, John Watson Papers, Accession 2003-054, box 6, folder Research Areas Artificial Heart 1975–79.

97. Thank you to NLM historian Susan Speaker for her insights on NIH director James Shannon and the tensions between basic and applied research programs during this period. Personal communication, 29 Jun 2015. See also James Shannon, "The American Experience with Biomedical Science," in *Health in America: 1776–1976* (Rockville, MD: DHEW, US Public Health Service, Health Resources Administration, 1976), 106; James A. Shannon, MD, interview by Dr. Thomas Kennedy, in *Leaders in American Medicine* (Bethesda, MD: NLM, 1984).

98. Mads Borup et al., "The Sociology of Expectations in Science and Technology," *Technology Analysis and Strategic Management* 18, nos. 3–4 (Jul–Sep 2006): 290.

99. DeBakey, "Current Directions in Artificial Heart Program," 7.

100. DeBakey, "Left Ventricular Bypass Pump," 4–5.

101. Moselle Boland, "Artificial Heart Patient Treated for Possible Swelling of Brain," *Houston Chronicle,* 22 Apr 1966, 1; Martin Waldron, "Booster Pump Used after Heart Surgery," *NYT,* 22 Apr 1966, 1, 22.

102. Martin Waldron, "Lung Rupture Kills Heart Pump Patient," *NYT,* 27 Apr 1966, 1.

103. "A Patient's Gift to the Future of Heart Repair," *Life,* 6 May 1966, 84–92, cited in Thompson, *Hearts,* 144.

104. "3d Texas Patient Gets Heart Pump," *NYT,* 18 May 1966, 29; "Heart Pump Patient Is Dead of Lung Bleeding in Houston," *NYT,* 21 May 1966, 12.

105. Bricker wrote, "It is hard to understand why you will participate in the promotion of a public spectacle that, in my opinion, is an exhibition of extreme poor taste, is not in the

best interest of surgery, and does not serve the best interest of your patient or his family."
Eugene M. Bricker to Michael E. DeBakey, 26 Apr 1966, Michael E. DeBakey Papers, NLM,
HMD, MS C 582, box 8, folder 7, Mechanical Left-Ventricular Bypass Implant—Aftermath,
1966 Apr–Sept. Based at Barnes-Jewish Hospital and Washington University School of
Medicine in St. Louis, Bricker developed numerous surgical procedures for patients with
bladder and cervical tumors, among other urological procedures. Obituary, 2000, VF00889
(Bricker, Eugene M.), Vertical File Collection, Bernard Becker Medical Library Archives,
Washington University School of Medicine.

106. Irvine H. Page, "I Wonder!" (editorial), *Modern Medicine* (20 June 1966): 79–84.
During the 1960s, Page wrote several editorials that initiated greater public discussion within
the medical community on social and moral issues, including the problem of science and
publicity. See also Irvine H. Page, "Medical Ethics," *Science* 153, no. 3734 (22 Jul 1966): 371;
J. Russell Elkington, "Moral Problems in the Use of Borrowed Organs, Artificial and Transplanted," *Ann Intern Med* 60, no. 2 (Feb 1964), 309–13; Irvine H. Page, "Moral Problems of
Artificial and Transplanted Organs," *Ann Intern Med* 61, no. 2 (Aug 1964), 355–63.

107. Michael E. DeBakey to M. M. Geffen, 28 May 1966, Michael E. DeBakey Papers,
NLM, HMD, MS C 582, box 8, folder 7.

108. A censure is a written judgment, condemning the fellow member's action as wrong,
constituting a firm professional reprimand but without any punitive actions, such as proba-
tion, suspension, or expulsion from the medical association. In a letter to the secretary of the
Harris County Medical Society, DeBakey disagreed with the censure, stating, "I am writing
to state again that I deny these charges and that I do not consider this action as evidence that
I have violated the By-laws of the Society." Michael E. DeBakey to Vincent C. Bash, 24 Sept
1966, Michael E. DeBakey Papers, NLM, HMD, MS C 582, box 8, folder 7.

109. Avco artificial heart contract, 1965–1966, Adrian Kantrowitz Papers, NLM, HMD,
MS C 572, box 4, folder 10; and Task Completion Report—Contract PH43-66-7, Feb 1966,
Adrian Kantrowitz Papers, NLM, HMD, MS C 572, box 4, folder 27.

110. Adrian Kantrowitz et al., "Clinical Experience with Permanent Mechanical Circulatory Assistance," *Progress in Cardiovascular Diseases* 10, no. 2 (Sep 1967): 134; Toru Okura
et al., "U-Shaped Mechanical Auxiliary Ventricle," *Arch Surg* 95 (Nov 1967): 821–25; Adrian
Kantrowitz, "Cardiac Assist Devices," *Journal of Extra-Corporeal Technology* (Summer 1972):
16. Many of Kantrowitz's devices, including the mechanical auxiliary ventricle, are deposited
at the Smithsonian Institution, NMAH, Accession no. 290303.

111. Experiment Records, 1964–1966, Adrian Kantrowitz Papers, NLM, HMD, MS C
572, box 7, folders 11–48 and box 8, folders 1–81.

112. Harold M. Schmeck Jr., "Heart Patient Aided by Pump Implanted in Chest 5 Days
Ago," *NYT,* 23 May 1966; Harold M. Schmeck Jr., "Surgeons Report on Heart Pumps,"
NYT, 29 Jul 1966, 14.

113. Kantrowitz, "Cardiac Assist Devices," 16.

114. Adrian Kantrowitz and OR team at Louise Ceraso operation (photo), 18 May 1966,
Profiles in Science: The Adrian Kantrowitz Papers, NLM, HMD, folder Kantrowitz-Avco
auxiliary ventricle (press packet).

115. Kantrowitz, "Cardiac Assist Devices," 16.

116. Adrian Kantrowitz et al., "A Clinical Experience with an Implanted Mechanical
Auxiliary Ventricle," *JAMA* 197, no. 7 (15 Aug 1966): 525–29; Kantrowitz et al., "Clinical
Experience with Permanent," 142. See also "Woman, 63, Dies in Heart Implant," *NYT,* 31
May 1966, 34.

117. Weisse, *Heart to Heart,* 232.

118. DeBakey, "Left Ventricular Bypass Pump," 9–10; "Heart Pump Placed in Mexican Woman," *NYT,* 9 Aug 1966, 15; "Heart Pump Removed from Houston Patient," *NYT,* 19 Aug 1966, 35; "Heart Pump Patient Leaves Hospital in Houston," *NYT,* 7 Sep 1966, 36; "Mexican Heart Patient Operation by DeBakey and Baylor, 1966," Texas Archive of the Moving Image, KHOU-TV Collection.

119. DeBakey, "Left Ventricular Bypass Pump," 6–9.

120. "Statham Instruments Wins Artificial Heart Contract," Press Release (1966), Smithsonian Institution Archives; "Statham to Produce DeBakey Artificial Heart," 27 Jun 1966, Statham Newsletter no. 8, ibid.

121. DeBakey, "Left Ventricular Bypass Pump," 11.

122. Pump cases, 1964–67, Adrian Kantrowitz Papers, NLM, HMD, MS C 572, box R7, folders 3–5; Adrian Kantrowitz, "Origins of Intraaortic Balloon Pumping," *Ann Thorac Surg* 50 (1990): 672–74; S. Scheidt et al., "Intra-Aortic Balloon Counterpulsation in Cardiogenic Shock: Report of a Co-operative Clinical Trial," *NEJM* 288, no. 19 (10 May 1973): 979–84; Adrian Kantrowitz et al., "Intraaortic Balloon Pumping," *JAMA* 203, no. 11 (11 March 1968): 988; Adrian Kantrowitz et al., "Clinical Experience with Cardiac Assistance by Means of Intra-Aortic Phase-Shift Balloon Pumping," *Trans ASAIO* 14 (1968): 344–48.

123. Adrian Kantrowitz, "Initial Clinical Experience with Intraaortic Balloon Pumping in Cardiogenic Shock," *JAMA* 203, no. 2 (8 Jan 1968): 136.

124. Adrian Kantrowitz, "Early Mechanical Left Ventricular Assistance," *ASAIO Journal* (1993): 835.

125. S. D. Moulopoulos, S. Topaz, and W. J. Kolff, "Diastolic Balloon Pumping (with Carbon Dioxide) in the Aorta—A Mechanical Assistance to the Failing Circulation, *Am Heart J* 63 (May 1962): 660–75.

126. Kantrowitz, "Initial Experience with Intraaortic Balloon," 140.

127. See Kantrowitz, "Cardiac Assist Devices," 18; Donald McRae, *Every Second Counts: The Race to Transplant the First Human Heart* (New York: Berkley Books, 2006); Jean Kantrowitz, "The Intra-Aortic Balloon Pump: An Early Chapter in Translational Medicine," *Art Org* 39, no. 6 (2015): 457–72.

128. Eduard Sujansky et al., "A Dynamic Aortic Patch as a Permanent Mechanical Auxiliary Ventricle: Experimental Studies," *Surgery* 66, no. 5 (Nov 1969): 875–82.

129. Haskell Shanks waving as he is discharged from Sinai Hospital of Detroit (photo), 18 Sept 1971, Profiles in Science: The Adrian Kantrowitz Papers, NLM, folder Further Innovations in Diastolic Augmentation, 1968–2008; Clinical Films: Haskell Shanks, 1971, Adrian Kantrowitz Papers, NLM, HMD, MS C 572, boxes 2004-017-048, 2004-017-131, 2004-017-066, and 2004-017-067.

130. In 1972 and 1976, Kantrowitz implanted this device in two more chronic heart failure patients, both of whom died within days with similar infection problems. Kantrowitz suspended further implants of the device and pursued research on infection-resistant percutaneous access devices. Adrian Kantrowitz et al., "Permanent Cardiac Assistance in Chronic Congestive Failure by Means of a Mechanical Auxiliary Ventricle," paper delivered at the Fifth International Symposium on Hemoperfusion and Artificial Organs, Tianjin, China, 20–22 Nov 1983, Smithsonian's NMAH, Division of Medical Sciences, Adrian Kantrowitz file #290303. See also Kantrowitz, "Early Mechanical Left Ventricular Assistance," 836–37; Earl Ubell, "A 'Patch Booster' for a Failing Heart," *NYT,* 19 Sep 1971, E9; "Heart Pump Patient Ailing," *NYT,* 7 Oct 1971, 62.

131. Kantrowitz, "Cardiac Assist Devices," 20.

132. Michael E. DeBakey et al., "Orthotopic Cardiac Prosthesis: Preliminary Experiments in Animals with Biventricular Artificial Heart," *Cardiovascular Research Center Bulletin* 7, no. 4 (Apr–Jun 1969): 127–42.

133. Preston, "Artificial Heart," 101. Similarly argued by Bernstein, "Artificial Heart Program," 25.

134. Strauss, "Political History of Artificial Heart," 336.

135. Adrian Kantrowitz, "The Development of Mechanical Assistance to the Failing Human Heart," *Medical Instrumentation* 10, no. 5 (Sept–Oct 1976): 224–27.

Chapter 2 · Dispute and Disappointment

Epigraph: Mark Bloom (science editor), "Docs: Mechanical Hearts Are Next," *New York News,* 14 Jan 1968, NLM, HMD, John H. Gibbon Papers, MS C313, box 6, folder Heart Transplantation—Printed Material, news clipping.

1. See Thomas Thompson, *Hearts: Of Surgeons and Transplants, Miracles and Disasters along the Cardiac Frontier* (New York: McCall, 1971); Denton A. Cooley, *100,000 Hearts: A Surgeon's Memoir* (Austin: University of Texas at Austin, 2012); Harris B. Shumacker Jr., *The Evolution of Cardiac Surgery* (Bloomington: Indiana University Press, 1992).

2. Jordan D. Haller and Marcial M. Cerruti, "Heart Transplantation in Man: Compilation of Cases—II," *AJC* 24 (Oct 1969): 554–60; Michael E. DeBakey et al., "Human Cardiac Transplantation: Clinical Experience," *JTCS* 58, no. 3 (Sep 1969): 303–17; Denton A. Cooley et al., "Human Heart Transplantation: Experience with Twelve Cases," *AJC* 22 (Dec 1968): 804–10.

3. Michael E. DeBakey, "Human Cardiac Transplantation," *JTCS* 55, no. 3 (March 1968): 449.

4. See "A Patient's Gift to the Future of Heart Repair," *Life,* May 6, 1966, 84–92; and Thompson, *Hearts,* 143–44.

5. See "Artificial Devices," *NYT,* 10 Dec 1967; Harold M. Schmeck Jr., "Lessons of the Heart Transplants," *NYT,* 14 Jan 1968.

6. M. E. DeBakey and Denton A. Cooley, "Successful Resection of Aneurysm of Thoracic Aorta and Replacement by Graft," *JAMA* 152 (20 Jun 1953): 673–76; M. E. DeBakey et al., "Clinical Application of a New Flexible Knitted Dacron Arterial Substitute," *American Surgeon* 24, no. 12 (Dec 1958): 862–69; M. E. DeBakey, "Basic Concepts of Therapy in Arterial Disease (Lasker Award)," *JAMA* 186 (2 Nov 1963): 484–98; Allen B Weisse, *Heart to Heart: The Twentieth-Century Battle against Heart Disease: An Oral History* (New Brunswick, NJ: Rutgers University Press, 2002), 177–202.

7. Gerald Astor, "Medicine's Frontier: Rebuilding the Human Body," *Look,* 30 Jun 1964, 26.

8. Thompson, *Hearts,* 61.

9. M. E. DeBakey and C. W. Hall, "Towards the Artificial Heart," *New Scientist* 393 (28 May 1964): 540–41.

10. M. E. DeBakey, "Left Ventricular Bypass Pump for Cardiac Assistance," *AJC* 27 (Jan 1971): 9–10; "Heart Pump Placed in Mexican Woman," *NYT,* 9 Aug 1966, 15; "Heart Pump Removed from Houston Patient," *NYT,* 19 Aug 1966, 35; "Heart Pump Patient Leaves Hospital in Houston," *NYT,* 7 Sep 1966, 36.

11. Michael E. DeBakey et al., "Orthotopic Cardiac Prosthesis: Preliminary Experiments in Animals with Biventricular Artificial Heart," *Cardiovascular Research Center Bulletin* 7, no. 4 (Apr–Jun 1969): 127–42.

12. Cong. Rec. H26172–75, vol. 153, pt. 19 (2 Oct 2007); Antonio M. Gotto Jr, "Profiles in Cardiology: Michael E. DeBakey," *Clinical Cardiology* 14 (1991): 1007–10.

13. Cooley, *100,000 Hearts,* 87–88.

14. Thompson, *Hearts;* Cooley, *100,000 Hearts;* Shumacker, *Evolution of Cardiac Surgery;* D. G. McNamara, "Denton Cooley's Part in the Evolution of Heart Surgery in the Years 1944–1994," *THI Journal* 21, no. 4 (1994): 252–56.

15. *Twenty-Five Years of Excellence: A History of the Texas Heart Institute* (Houston: Texas Heart Institute Foundation, 1989), 9.

16. Cooley, *100,000 Hearts;* Shumacker, *Evolution of Cardiac Surgery.*

17. Michael E. DeBakey and Denton Cooley, "Surgical Treatment of Mitral and Aortic Stenosis: Results of One Hundred Fifteen Valvotomies," *JAMA* 155, no. 3 (15 May 1953): 235–39; Michael E. DeBakey, Denton A. Cooley, and Oscar Creech Jr., "Surgical Treatment of Aneurysms and Occlusive Disease of the Aorta," *Postgraduate Medicine* 15, no. 2 (Feb 1954): 120–27; Denton A. Cooley et al., "Surgical Repair of Ruptured Interventricular Septum Following Acute Myocardial Infarction," *Surgery* 41 (1957): 930; Denton A. Cooley et al., "Ventricular Aneurysm Following Myocardial Infarction: Results of Surgical Treatment," *Ann Surg* 150 (1959): 595. See also Shumacker, *Evolution of Cardiac Surgery.*

18. "Surgeon to the Duke: Michael Ellis DeBakey," *NYT,* 15 Dec 1964, 38.

19. For one analysis of the "contrasting surgical styles, professional profiles, and political and social outlooks" of Cooley and DeBakey, see Renée C. Fox and Judith P. Swazey, *The Courage to Fail: A Social View of Organ Transplants and Dialysis,* 2nd ed. (New Brunswick, NJ: Transaction, 2002), 177–79.

20. Cooley, *100,000 Hearts,* 115; see also Denton A. Cooley, "Surgical Mentors: Blalock, Brock, and DeBakey," *THI Journal* 36, no. 5 (2009): 433–34.

21. *Twenty-Five Years of Excellence,* 10–19.

22. Thompson, *Hearts,* 61.

23. Ibid., 144–45.

24. See Todd K. Rosengart, "The 1,000th VAD, the Great Rivalry, and the Grand Experiment of the Texas Medical Center," *THI Journal* 41, no. 2 (2014): 114; Denton A. Cooley, "Feuds: Social and Medical," *THI Journal* 37, 6 (2010): 649; Cooley, *100,000 Hearts,* 115.

25. Thompson, *Hearts,* 128–29.

26. Donald McRae, *Every Second Counts: The Race to Transplant the First Human Heart* (New York: Simon and Schuster, 2006), Tony Stark, *Knife to the Heart: The Story of Transplant Surgery* (Toronto: Macmillan, 1996); and Nicholas L. Tilney, *Transplant: From Myth to Reality* (New Haven, CT: Yale University Press, 2003).

27. Susan E. Lederer, *Flesh and Blood: Organ Transplantation and Blood Transfusion in Twentieth-Century America* (Oxford: Oxford University Press, 2008), ix, 208–12.

28. R. R. Lower and N. E. Shumway, "Studies on Orthotopic Homotransplantation of the Canine Heart," *Surgical Forum* 11 (1960): 18–19.

29. Norman Shumway and Richard Lower, "Successful Homotransplantation of the Canine Heart after Anoxic Preservation for Seven Hours," *AJS* 104 (1962): 302–6; Norman Shumway and Richard Lower, "Special Problems in the Transplantation of the Heart," *Annals of New York Academy of Science* 120 (30 Nov 1964): 773–77; Norman E. Shumway, William W. Angell, and Robert D. Wuerflein, "Progress in Transplantation of the Heart," *Transplantation* 5, no. 4 (Jul 1967): S900–S903. See also Shumacker, *Evolution of Cardiac Surgery.*

30. J. D. Hardy et al., "Heart Transplantation in Man: Developmental Studies and Report of a Case," *JAMA* 188 (29 Jun 1964): 1132–40; J. D. Hardy, "The Transplantation of

Organs," *Surgery* 56 (Oct 1964): 685–705; Haller and Cerruti, "Heart Transplantation in Man," 558.

31. "First Year of Cardiac Transplantation," *BMJ* (11 Jan 1969): 65; Shumacker, *Evolution of Cardiac Surgery,* 327; Lederer, *Flesh and Blood,* 201.

32. David K. C. Cooper and Robert P. Lanza, *Xeno: The Promise of Transplanting Animal Organs into Humans* (Oxford: Oxford University Press, 2000), 34–40.

33. David K. C. Cooper, *Open Heart: The Radical Surgeons Who Revolutionized Medicine* (New York: Kaplan, 2010), 336; Michael E. DeBakey interview, 23 Nov 1986, 6 Apr 1992, NLM, HMD, OH 127.

34. Stanford University Medical Center Press Release, 20 Nov 1967, SU, Special Collections and University Archives, Norman Shumway Project (V0222), box 6, vol. 1; see also "Way Is Clear for Heart Transplant," *JAMA* 202, no. 8 (20 Nov 1967): 31.

35. Ibid.

36. "Way Is Clear," 31. See also Carl G. Groth et al., "Historic Landmarks in Clinical Transplantation," *World Journal of Surgery* 24, no. 7 (Jul 2000): 834–43; James I. Fann and William A. Baumgartner, "Norman E. Shumway, Jr (1923–2006)," *JTCS* 142, no. 6 (Dec 2011): 1299–1302.

37. Stanford Medical Center Press Release, 20 Nov 1967; see also "Way Is Clear," 31.

38. Norman Shumway interview, 16 Oct 1997, William S. Stoney Collection, Vanderbilt University Medical Center, Eskind Biomedical Library Special Collections, Collection no. 241, box 01A, folder 31. There is much literature on the debates surrounding how death was to be measured and the influence of heart transplantation on the redefinition of death during the late 1960s, including Helen MacDonald, "Crossing the Rubicon: Death in 'The Year of the Transplant,'" *Medical History* 61, no. 1 (2017): 107–27; Margaret Lock, *Twice Dead: Organ Transplants and the Reinvention of Death* (Berkeley: University of California Press, 2002); Martin S. Pernick, "Brain Death in a Cultural Context: The Reconstruction of Death, 1967–1981," in *The Definition of Death: Contemporary Controversies,* ed. Stuart J. Youngner, Robert M. Arnold, and Renie Schapiro (Baltimore: Johns Hopkins University Press, 1999), 3–33.

39. Maurice Nellen obituary, *Daily Telegraph* (London), 31 Aug 2000, cited in David Hamilton, *A History of Organ Transplantation: Ancient Legends to Modern Practice* (Pittsburgh: University of Pittsburgh Press, 2012), 505n27; W. Bruce Fye, *Caring for the Heart: Mayo Clinic and the Rise of Specialization* (Oxford: Oxford University Press, 2015), 451; Cooper, *Open Heart,* 328–29.

40. Shumway interview, 16 Oct 1997, VU.

41. Donald McRae, "Norman Shumway" (obituary), *Guardian* (London), 15 Feb 2006; McRae, *Every Second Counts,* 301.

42. See C. N. Barnard et al., "Further Experiences with the U.C.T. Mitral, Tricuspid and Aortic Prostheses," *Surgery* 57 (Feb 1965): 211–19; V. Schrire and C. N. Barnard, "The Preoperative Assessment of Mitral-Valve Disease," *SAMJ* 38 (12 Sep 1964): 721–28; C. N. Barnard et al., "Total Aortic Replacement," *Lancet* 2, no. 7313 (26 Oct 1963): 856–59.

43. J. R. Ackermann and C. N. Barnard, "Successful Storage of Kidneys," *British Journal of Surgery* 53, no. 6 (1966): 525–32; J. R. Ackermann, A. J. Fisher, and C. N. Barnard, "Live Storage of Kidneys: A Preliminary Communication," *Surgery* 60, no. 3 (Sep 1966): 720–24; J. R. Ackermann, A. J. Fisher, and C. N. Barnard, "In vivo Kidney Storage: A Preliminary Communication," *SAMJ* 39, no. 35 (25 Sep 1965): 794–96.

44. C. N. Barnard to David M. Hume, 23 Jun 1966, Virginia Commonwealth University, Tompkins-McCaw Library Special Collections and Archives, David M. Hume Vertical

File; "Heart Transplant Operation Performed Here by MCV," *Richmond Times-Dispatch,* 26 May 1968, news clipping, ibid. I am indebted to VCU Archivist Jodi Koste for providing me with these sources; her tremendous archival digging allows me to confirm that Barnard's study period with Hume took place in 1966, and not in 1967 as has been erroneously repeated in some secondary literature.

45. Christiaan Barnard and Curtis Bill Pepper, *One Life* (Toronto: Macmillan, 1969), 323–27.

46. Shumway interview, 16 Oct 1997, VU; Cooper, *Open Heart,* 326, 332; McRae, *Every Second Counts,* 174–76.

47. Barnard and Pepper, *One Life,* 330.

48. C. N. Barnard, "The Operation: A Human Cardiac Transplant: An Interim Report of a Successful Operation Performed at Groote Schuur Hospital, Cape Town," *SAMJ* 41, no. 48 (30 Dec 1967): 1271–74; Cooper, *Open Heart,* 336.

49. C. N. Barnard, "Human Cardiac Transplantation: An Evaluation of the First Two Operations Performed at the Groote Schurr Hospital, Cape Town," *AJC* 22, no. 4 (Oct 1968): 584–96.

50. But Barnard's transplant surgery also alarmed others, as Lederer states, "for crossing the cardiac color line." See Lederer, *Flesh and Blood,* 174–75.

51. Ayesha Nathoo, *Hearts Exposed: Transplants and the Media in 1960s Britain* (Bastingstoke, UK: Palgrave Macmillan, 2009), 65.

52. For immediate professional criticism of the publicity surrounding the procedure, see these editorials: Watts R. Webb, "Cardiac Transplantation and Publicity," *Annals of Thoracic Surgery* 5, no. 4 (Apr 1968): 377–78; Bernard Sandler, "Cardiac Transplantation," *Lancet* (18 May 1968): 1086–87; "Cardiac Transplantation," *Lancet* (10 May 1969). For immediate professional criticism of the procedure, see the following editorials: Lyman A. Brewer, "Cardiac Transplantation: An Appraisal," *JAMA* 205, no. 10 (2 Sep 1968): 101–2; John H. Kennedy, "Cardiac Transplantation—A Current Appraisal," *JAMA* 203, no. 10 (4 May 1968): 892–93; M. H. Pappworth, "Scientific, Technical and Ethical Considerations in Cardiac Transplantation," *BMJ* (16 Mar 1968): 705. See also Nathoo, *Hearts Exposed;* McRae, *Every Second Counts.*

53. Shumway interview, 16 Oct 1997, VU.

54. Adrian Kantrowitz, "America's First Human Heart Transplantation: The Concept, the Planning, and the Furor," *ASAIO Journal* 44, no. 4 (Jul–Aug 1998): 245–46; "Way Is Clear," 31–32.

55. Kantrowitz, "America's First Human Heart Transplantation," 247.

56. Susan E. Lederer, "Transplant Nation: The NIH and the Politics of Heart Transplantation in the 1960s," in *Biomedicine in the Twentieth Century: Practices, Policies, and Politics,* ed. C. Hannaway (Washington, DC: IOS Press, 2008): 158–59.

57. Ibid., 159; Tilney, *Transplant,* 173; Cooper, *Open Heart,* 336.

58. Cooper, *Open Heart,* 336.

59. Ibid., 339.

60. A. Kantrowitz to Robertson C. Scott, 23 Jan 1968, Adrian Kantrowitz Papers, NLM, HMD, MS C572, box 16, folder 82; Adrian Kantrowitz, Project Bionics Pioneer Interview, 19 Apr 2005, NLM, HMD. Respected pediatric cardiologist Helen Taussig criticized Kantrowitz for performing the pediatric heart transplantation and for seeking media attention. Kantrowitz responded, "It would seem to many that we were 'racing to get into the act' . . . [but] our readiness was known by science writers who had followed our work." Helen B. Taussig

to Adrian Kantrowitz, 16 Jan 1968; Adrian Kantrowitz to Helen B. Taussig, 5 Feb 1968, both at Profiles in Science: Adrian Kantrowitz, NLM, HMD, www.profiles.nlm.nih.gov.

61. Cardiac Transplant Operation 12/6/67 (notes), Adrian Kantrowitz Papers, NLM, HMD, MS C572, box 16, folder 88; Slides 6 Dec 1967, ibid., box 12, folders 39–41; Adrian Kantrowitz et al., "Transplantation of the Heart in an Infant and an Adult," *AJC* 22, no. 6 (Dec 1968): 782–90.

62. Kantrowitz, "America's First Human Heart Transplantation," 250; McRae, *Every Second Counts;* Kantrowitz interview, 19 Apr 2005, NLM.

63. N. E. Shumway, E. Dong, and E. B. Stinson, "Surgical Aspects of Cardiac Transplantation in Man," *Bulletin of the New York Academy of Medicine* 45, no. 5 (May 1969): 391.

64. Lawrence E. Davies, "U.S. Heart Patient Dies on 15th Day: Transplant Surgeon Notes Kasperak Had Experienced 'Galaxy' of Complications," *NYT,* 22 Jan 1968, 1.

65. Lawrence E. Davies, "Second Heart Transplant Performed on Coast," *NYT,* 3 May 1968.

66. E. B. Stinson et al., "Initial Clinical Experience with Heart Transplantation," *AJC* 22, no. 6 (Dec 1968): 791–96; Randall B. Griepp et al., "A Two-Year Experience with Human Heart Transplantation," *California Medicine* 113 (August 1970): 17–26. See also "Medicine: Michael Kasperak," *Time,* 19 Jan 1968.

67. "Two Heart Patients Begin Recoveries: Third, on Coast, in Crisis," *NYT,* 5 May 1968.

68. Stinson et al., "Initial Clinical Experience," 796–802; Haller and Cerruti, "Heart Transplantation in Man," 555; Davies, "Second Heart Transplant."

69. Haller and Cerruti, "Heart Transplantation in Man," 556.

70. Fye, *Caring for the Heart,* 452.

71. Edward B. Stinson et al., "Experience with Cardiac Transplantation in Fourteen Patients," *Laval Medical* 41 (Feb 1970): 129; Griepp et al., "Two-Year Experience," 17.

72. Press Conference, May 3, 1968, Texas Archive of the Moving Image, KHOU-TV Collection.

73. Cooley et al., "Human Heart Transplantation," 806.

74. Denton A. Cooley, "Transplantation versus Prosthetic Replacement of the Heart," *Biomaterials, Medical Devices and Artificial Organs* 3, no. 4 (1975): 482; Griepp et al., "Two-Year Experience," 17.

75. DeBakey et al., "Human Cardiac Transplantation," 304; "4 in Texas Given a Woman's Organs," *NYT,* 1 Sep 1968; "Progress Reported on 4 Transplants," *NYT,* 2 Sep 1968; "Transplant Patient Dies," *NYT,* 17 May 1972.

76. DeBakey et al., "Human Cardiac Transplantation," 304; "Patient, 22, Who Received New Heart in '68 Is Dead," *NYT,* 8 Nov 1974.

77. Haller and Cerruti, "Heart Transplantation in Man," 558–59.

78. Ibid., 555–58.

79. Adrian Kantrowitz Papers, NLM, HMD, MS C572, box 17, folders 3 through 8, which all contain lay inquiries. Examples include Ralph Agritelley to Adrian Kantrowitz, 10 Feb 1968; Rhona Saltzman to Adrian Kantrowitz, 14 Feb 1968; Ira Weiner to Adrian Kantrowitz, 22 Feb 1968, all in box 17, folder 4.

80. "First Year of Cardiac Transplantation," 66; Thomas Thompson, "A New and Disquieting Look at Transplant: The Year They Changed Hearts," *Life,* 17 Sep 1971, 56–70; S. Jamieson, E. Stinson, and N. Shumway, "Cardiac Transplantation: New Heart, New Hopes," *Nursing Mirror* 148, no. 25 (21 Jun 1979): 24.

81. Fox and Swazey, *Courage to Fail*, 121.

82. Irving Page, "The Ethics of Heart Transplantation," *JAMA* 207 (6 Jan 1969): 109–13, cited in Fox and Swazey, *Courage to Fail*, 121.

83. Griepp et al., "Two-Year Experience," 26.

84. "Heart Transplantation: Alive and Well at Stanford," *MWN,* 23 Aug 1974, 27.

85. Fye, *Caring for the Heart,* 454; Lawrence Altman, "3 Years of Heart Transplants," *NYT,* 3 Dec 1970, 1.

86. Jean Selgimann, "Saving New Hearts," *Newsweek,* 7 Jan 1980, 39.

87. Fye, *Caring for the Heart,* 451–54.

88. Fox and Swazey, *Courage to Fail,* 60.

89. Shumacker, *Evolution of Cardiac Surgery,* 333.

90. Haller and Cerruti, "Heart Transplantation in Man," 555–57; Fox and Swazey, *Courage to Fail,* 109.

91. Newspaper headlines declared, "Heart Transplant Future Looks Bleak"; "Heart Transplants Diminish: Better Conditions Awaited"; "Heart Transplants Halted at World's Medical Center," as cited in Fox and Swazey, *Courage to Fail,* 113–15, 122.

92. McRae, *Every Second Counts,* 302.

93. "Heart Transplantation: Alive and Well," 25–34; see also William A. Baumgartner et al., "Norman E. Shumway, MD, PhD: Visionary, Innovator, Humorist," *JTCS* 137 (2009): 269–77. See also McRae, *Every Second Counts,* 302.

94. Fye, *Caring for the Heart,* 454.

95. D. Liotta et al., "Artificial Heart in the Chest: Preliminary Report," *Trans ASAIO* 7 (1961): 318–22.

96. Statement of Gerald Maley (Baylor Financial Affairs), 11 Apr 1969, Michael E. De-Bakey Papers, NLM, HMD, MS C 582, box 7, folder 46; Statement of C. William Hall, 11 Apr 1969, ibid., folder 45.

97. Summary of Findings in Baylor Investigation of Clinical Implantation of Artificial Heart (Apr) 1969, Michael E. DeBakey Papers, NLM, HMD, MS C 582, box 7, folder 62; C. William Hall, Domingo Liotta, and Michael E. DeBakey, "Bioengineering Efforts in Developing Artificial Hearts and Assistors," *AJS* 114 (Jul 1967): 24–25.

98. C. William Hall to Michael E. DeBakey, 6 May 1969, and Minutes of the (Baylor-Rice) Medical Engineering Laboratory Committee, 4 Jul 1968, Michael E. DeBakey Papers, NLM, HMD, MS C 582, box 7, folder 39; DeBakey and Hall, "Towards the Artificial Heart," 540–41.

99. Statement of Dr. Michael E. DeBakey to the Executive Committee of the Board of Trustees, 10 Apr 1969, Michael E. DeBakey Papers, NLM, HMD, MS C 582, box 7, folder 41; Summary of Findings in Baylor Investigation of Clinical Implantation of Artificial Heart (Apr) 1969, ibid., folder 62.

100. Summary of Animal Experiments (Mar) 1969, Michael E. DeBakey Papers, NLM, HMD, MS C 582, box 7, folder 36; All Facts Documentable with Irrefutable Evidence—Timeline of Events (Apr) 1969, ibid., folder 58.

101. DeBakey et al., "Orthotopic Cardiac Prosthesis," 127–42. By 1977 DeBakey had concluded that there were too many problems associated with the TAH, and his Baylor research team directed their full attention to ventricular assist devices. Michael E. DeBakey interview, 14 Dec 1998, William S. Stoney Collection, Vanderbilt University Medical Center, Eskind Biomedical Library Special Collections, Collection No. 241, box 01A, folder 6.

102. In a letter to Dr. Hebbel Hoff, chair of Baylor's Special Committee investigating the Karp case, Cooley wrote, "About four months ago I, myself, decided upon a plan to develop

a two stage technique replacing the human heart for irreversible, terminal heart failure and imminent death of the patient. To develop the prosthesis I sought the advice of my colleague, Dr Domingo Liotta, who offered to serve in an advisory capacity." In a similar statement to Baylor's Special Committee, Liotta confirmed, "Approximately 4 months ago Dr Denton Cooley invited him to collaborate in the development of an artificial heart for total replacement." Denton A. Cooley to Hebbel E. Hoff, 21 Apr 1969, Michael E. DeBakey Papers, NLM, HMD, MS C 582, box 7, folder 39; Summary of Dr. Liotta's Participation in the Clinical Application of the Artificial Heart at St. Luke's Hospital, 10 Apr 1969, ibid., folder 42.

103. Confidential and Privileged Report of Special Committee to the Board of Trustees of Baylor College of Medicine, 18 Apr 1969, Michael E. DeBakey Papers, NLM, HMD, MS C 582, box 7, folder 56.

104. Cooley to Hoff, 21 Apr 1969, NLM; Thomas Thompson, "The Texas Tornado vs. Dr. Wonderful," *Life,* 10 Apr 1970, 74; "History of the Texas Heart Institute," www.tmc.edu, accessed 11 Sep 2002.

105. Summary of Dr. Liotta's Participation in the Clinical Application of the Artificial Heart at St. Luke's Hospital, 10 Apr 1969, NLM; "Secret Bypass in the Plastic Heart Row," *MWN,* 9 May 1969, 18; Cooley, *100,000 Hearts,* 139.

106. Advisory Committee of NIH Grant HE-05435 to Michael DeBakey, 8 Apr 1969, Michael E. DeBakey Papers, NLM, HMD, MS C 582, box 7, folder 56; Statement of J. D. Hellums, 12 Apr 1969, ibid., folder 52; Statement of William O'Bannon, 12 Apr 1969, ibid., folder 53.

107. Fox and Swazey, *Courage to Fail,* 123–24.

108. All Facts Documentable with Irrefutable Evidence—Timeline of Events (Apr) 1969, NLM; Cooley, *100,000 Hearts,* 139.

109. Statement of O'Bannon, 12 Apr 1969, NLM.

110. Herbert R. Smith to Michael E. DeBakey, 8 Apr 1969, Michael E. DeBakey Papers, NLM, HMD, MS C 582, box 7, folder 39; All Facts Documentable with Irrefutable Evidence—Timeline of Events (Apr) 1969, NLM.

111. In his autobiography, Cooley stated, "It was amazing that this heart had been keeping Mr Karp alive at all." He goes on to describe the TAH implant as "an arduous task." See Cooley, *100,000 Hearts,* 140–41.

112. Denton A. Cooley, "Staged Cardiac Transplantation: Report of Three Cases," *Heart Transpl* 1, no. 2 (1982): 146.

113. D. A. Cooley et al., "Orthotopic Cardiac Prosthesis for Two-Staged Cardiac Replacement," *Am J Cardiol* 24, no. 5 (Nov 1969): 726.

114. Ibid., 723–24.

115. Ibid., 727; "Doctors Implant Artificial Heart in Surgical First," *Salt Lake Tribune,* 5 Apr 1969; "Artificial Heart Implanted in Man," *NYT,* 5 Apr 1969.

116. Michael DeBakey stated unequivocally that the evidence exposed Cooley's TAH implant as a premeditated act. See Full Transcript of DeBakey's April 10 Report to Executive Committee of the Board of Trustees, 17 Jun 1969, Michael E. DeBakey Papers, NLM, HMD, MS C 582, box 8, folder 1; All Facts Documentable with Irrefutable Evidence—Timeline of Events (Apr) 1969, NLM; Fox and Swazey, *Courage to Fail,* 174–76.

117. "Mechanical Heart Ticks Along as Plea for Donor Continues," *Salt Lake City Tribune,* 6 Apr 1969.

118. "Woman's Heart Transplanted to Replace Man's Plastic One," *NYT,* 8 Apr 1969.

119. Cooley et al., "Orthotopic Cardiac Prosthesis," 727.

120. Ibid., 728; Cooley, "Transplantation versus Prosthetic Replacement," 486; Denton Cooley et al., "Discussion: First Human Implantation of Cardiac Prosthesis for Staged Total Replacement of the Heart," *Trans ASAIO* 15 (1969): 263.

121. "Man Who Got Plastic Heart Dies as Dispute on the Device Looms," *NYT,* 9 Apr 1969. See also Domingo Liotta, *Amazing Adventures of a Heart Surgeon: The Artificial Heart: The Frontiers of Human Life* (New York: iUniverse, 2007).

122. Cooley et al., "Orthotopic Cardiac Prosthesis," 729.

123. Ibid., 728.

124. Michael DeBakey to Dr. Harold Brown, July 1969; and report of a renal specialist submitted to Baylor College of Medicine faculty committee, both cited in Fox and Swazey, *Courage to Fail,* 161 and 157, respectively.

125. "Artificial Heart Implanted in Man," 1; "Doctors Implant Artificial Heart"; "Mechanical Heart Ticks Along"; "Callers Offer to Donate Hearts to Houston Patient," *NYT,* 7 Apr 1969; "Man Who Got Plastic Heart," 1.

126. "Concept of the Artificial Heart Achieves Its First Great Triumph," *NYT,* 8 Apr 1969, 31.

127. Theodore Cooper to Michael E DeBakey, 8 Apr 1969, Michael E. DeBakey Papers, NLM, HMD, MS C 582, box 7, folder 38.

128. Statement of DeBakey, 10 Apr 1969, NLM.

129. "Secret Bypass," 20.

130. Cooley to Hoff, 21 Apr 1969, NLM.

131. Confidential and Privileged Report of Special Committee to the Board of Trustees of Baylor College of Medicine, 18 Apr 1969, NLM.

132. Cooley to Hoff, 21 Apr 1969, NLM.

133. Max B. Shelton, "Artificial Heart Stirs Dispute, Doctor Calm," *Salt Lake Tribune,* Apr 10, 1969.

134. See Cooley, *100,000 Hearts,* 145–46; "Dr Cooley Censured," *Houston Post,* 10 Dec 1969, 3.

135. Statement of DeBakey, 10 Apr 1969, NLM.

136. L. F. McCollum to Theodore Cooper, 9 May 1969, Michael E. DeBakey Papers, NLM, HMD, MS C 582, box 7, folder 38.

137. Denton Cooley to Michael DeBakey (letter of resignation), 2 Sep 1969, Michael E. DeBakey Papers, NLM, HMD, MS C 582, box 7, folder 55; Michael DeBakey to Denton Cooley (letter accepting resignation), 11 Sep 1969, ibid.

138. Statement of Hellums, 12 Apr 1969, NLM; Statement of O'Bannon, 12 Apr 1969, NLM; John Quinn, "The Surgeons Say Artificial Heart Wasn't Ready," *New York Daily News,* 9 Sep 1969, 38, cited in Fox and Swazey, *Courage to Fail,* 149; "Secret Bypass," 19.

139. Confidential and Privileged Report of Special Committee to the Board of Trustees of Baylor College of Medicine, 18 Apr 1969, NLM.

140. See schematic drawings of each device, printed in DeBakey et al., "Orthotopic Cardiac Prosthesis," 128; and Cooley et al., "Discussion: First Human Implantation," 256, cited in Fox and Swazey, *Courage to Fail,* 158–59.

141. O. H. Frazier, Project Bionics Pioneer Interview, 18 Jul 2013, NLM, HMD. See also DeBakey et al., "Orthotopic Cardiac Prosthesis," 127–42; and Cooley et al., "Orthotopic Cardiac Prosthesis," 723–30.

142. Quoted in "Transplants: An Act of Desperation," *Time,* 18 Apr 1969, 56.

143. See transcript of Karp vs. Cooley and Liotta, 493 F 2d 408 (1974), at http://openjurist.org.

144. Statement by Suzanne Anderson, 11 Apr 1969, Michael E. DeBakey Papers, NLM, HMD, MS C 582, box 7, folder 43.

145. Fox and Swazey, *Courage to Fail,* 184.

146. Ibid., 186.

147. Thompson, "Texas Tornado vs. Dr. Wonderful," 72.

148. Michael E. DeBakey, "The Odyssey of the Artificial Heart," *Art Org* 24, no. 6 (2000): 408.

149. McCollum to Cooper, 9 May 1969, NLM.

150. See Liotta's autobiography for his version of events, acknowledging his willing participation and anticipation of DeBakey's reaction. Liotta, *Amazing Adventures,* 181–210.

151. Karp v. Cooley, S.D.Tex., 1972, 349 F.Supp. 827, cited in William J. Curran, "Law-Medicine Notes: The First Mechanical Heart Transplant: Informed Consent and Experimentation," *NEJM* 291, no. 19 (7 Nov 1974): 1015–16; Fox and Swazey, *Courage to Fail,* 190.

152. Curran, "Law-Medicine Notes," 1016.

153. Statement of DeBakey, 10 Apr 1969, NLM.

154. Michael DeBakey to Dr. Harold Brown, July 1969, cited in Fox and Swazey, *Courage to Fail,* 161.

155. Karp v. Cooley, S.D.Tex., 1972, 349 F.Supp. 827, cited in Fox and Swazey, *Courage to Fail,* 194.

156. Ibid., 193.

157. Ibid.

158. Karp vs. Cooley and Liotta, 493 F 2d 408 (1974); "Heart Transplant Pioneer Upheld in Malpractice Suit," *NYT,* 28 Apr 1974, 59.

159. Fox and Swazey, *Courage to Fail,* 194–97.

160. Ibid., 196.

161. Kantrowitz interview, 19 Apr 2005, NLM.

162. In 1978 Denton Cooley donated the artificial heart that had been implanted in Haskell Karp to the Smithsonian Institution, where it is profiled online and loaned out for special events. Deed of Gift, 10 Jan 1978, Smithsonian Institution, NMAH, Division of Medicine and Science, Accession File 1978.1002; Liotta-Cooley Artificial Heart, Smithsonian Institution, NMAH, Accession No. 1978.1002.

163. Thompson, "Texas Tornado vs. Dr. Wonderful," 74.

164. Fox and Swazey, *Courage to Fail,* 197.

165. R. H. Brownstein, "Heart Transplant: Three Views: The Power over Life and Death," *Diseases of the Chest* 54, no. 4 (Oct 1968): 346–48; R. P. Bergen, "Legal Regulation of Heart Transplants," *Diseases of the Chest* 54, no. 4 (Oct 1968): 352–55; L. M. Nyhus, "Human Experimentation and the Surgeon," *Surgery* 64, no. 4 (Oct 1968): 701–5; D. E. Harken, "Heart Transplantation—a Boston Perspective," *AJC* 22, no. 4 (Oct 1968): 449–51; J. Z. Appel, "Ethical and Legal Questions Posed by Recent Advances in Medicine," *JAMA* 205, no. 7 (12 Aug 1968): 513–16; J. K. Perloff, "Transplantation of the Heart—Dissenting Notes of a Cardiologist," *Medical Annals of the District of Columbia* 37, no. 9 (Sep 1968): 484–86; Pappworth, "Scientific, Technical and Ethical Considerations," 705; "When Do We Let the Patient Die?," *Ann Intern Med* 68, no. 3 (Mar 1968): 695–700.

166. DeBakey, "Human Cardiac Transplantation," 449.

167. "Specialists See Need for Artificial Heart," *Chicago Tribune,* 14 Jan 1968, news clipping, NLM, HMD, John H. Gibbon Papers, MS C313, box 6, folder Heart Transplantation—Printed Material. See also T. Akutsu et al., "Artificial Hearts inside the Chest, Using Small Electro-Motors," *Trans ASAIO* 6 (1960): 299; Y. Nosé et al., "Artificial Hearts inside the Pericardial Sac in Calves," *Trans ASAIO* 11 (1965): 255; C. S. Kwan-Gett et al., "Control Systems for Artificial Hearts," *Trans ASAIO* 14 (1968): 284.

168. "Cardiac Transplantation," *Lancet* (May 10, 1969): 973.

169. See Nathoo, *Hearts Exposed.*

170. Jean Kantrowitz, "The Intra-Aortic Balloon Pump: An Early Chapter in Translational Medicine," *Art Org* 39, no. 6 (2015): 457–72.

171. Denton A. Cooley to W. J. Kolff, 22 Jul 1968, UU, MS 654 Willem J. Kolff Collection, box 322, folder 5; Kantrowitz, "America's First Human Heart Transplantation," 250; McRae, *Every Second Counts.*

172. Denton A. Cooley et al., "Cardiac Transplantation as Palliation of Advanced Heart Disease," *Archives of Surgery* 98 (May 1969): 625 (discussion).

173. Cooley, "Transplantation versus Prosthetic Replacement," 487–88.

174. Ibid.

175. Richard R. Lower, "Cardiac Transplantation in Proper Perspective," *Surgery, Gynecology and Obstetrics* 126, 4 (Apr 1968): 838.

176. Norman E. Shumway et al., "Heart Replacement: The Cardiac Chimera vs. Mechanical Man," *Journal-Lancet* 88, no. 7 (Jul 1968): 171.

177. *Hearings before the Subcommittee on Government Research: A Joint Resolution for the Establishment of the National Commission on Health Science and Society,* Mar–Apr 1968 (M.C. 15501) (statement of Dr. Norman Shumway, 22 Mar 1968), US Government Publications (Depository).

178. "Shumway Says Artificial Heart Is 'Dangerous,'" Stanford University Medical Center Press Release, 7 Feb 1986, SU, Special Collections and University Archives, Norman Shumway Project (V0222), box 6, vol. 2.

179. John Langone, "The Artificial Heart Is Really Very Dangerous," *Discover* (Jun 1986): 40.

180. Thomas A. Preston, "Organ Rationing: Jumping the Queue," *MWN,* 12 Jan 1987, 31.

181. "Top Surgeon Sees No Future for Artificial Heart," *NYT,* 14 Feb 1984; "Doctor Says Heart Implant Lethal Publicity Gimmick," *Duluth (MN) News Tribune & Herald,* 29 May 1986, SU, Special Collections and University Archives, Norman Shumway Project (V0222), box 6, vol. 2; Shumway interview, 16 Oct 1997, VU.

182. W. J. Kolff to Mr. and Mrs. Case Kolff, Netherlands, 5 Mar 1984, UU, MS 654 Willem J. Kolff Collection, box 3, folder 5; Una Loy Clark to W. J. Kolff, 12 Mar 1984, ibid., box 353, folder 7.

183. Lecture by Norman E. Shumway to Community Hospital of Monterey Peninsula, 28 Jan 1978, p. 10, SU, Special Collections and University Archives, Norman Shumway Project (V0222), box 6, vol. 3.

184. Shumway interview, 16 Oct 1997, VU.

185. Lecture by Shumway to Community Hospital, 28 Jan 1978, p. 9, SU.

186. Kristen Christopher, "More Versatile Than Artificial Heart: Heart Device Being Developed at Hospital," *Stanford Daily* 182, no. 49 (8 Dec 1982): 3.

187. Stanford Medical Forum, 18 Nov 1992, SU, Special Collections and University Archives, Norman Shumway Project (V0222), box 6, vol. 3.

188. Stanford University Medical Center Press Release, 18 Feb 1987, SU, Special Collections and University Archives, Norman Shumway Project (V0222), box 6, vol. 2.

189. William S. Pierce, "Mechanical Circulatory Assistance—Current State of the Art," *Heart Transplantation* 3, no. 1 (Nov 1983): 7; J. G. Losman, "Human Technology after Cardiac Epigenesis: Artificial Heart versus Cardiac Transplantation," *SAMJ* (24 Sep 1977): 570–72.

190. Shumway et al., "Heart Replacement," 173.

191. "Cardiac Transplantation in Man," statement prepared by the Board on Medicine of the National Academy of Sciences, *JAMA* 204, no. 9 (27 May 1968): 147.

192. Norman E. Shumway, "Transplantation," *THI Journal* 9, no. 4 (Dec 1982): 438; V. A. Gaudiani et al., "Long-Term Survival and Function after Cardiac Transplantation," *Ann Surg* 194, no. 4 (Oct 1981): 381–85; Vaughn A. Starnes and Norman E. Shumway, "General Surgery: Heart and Heart-Lung Transplantation," *Western Journal of Medicine* 146, no. 6 (Jun 1987): 738.

193. Thank you to Bruce Fye for pointing this out; personal communication with author, 23 Nov 2016. See Fye, *Caring for the Heart*, 456–59, 462–63.

194. Eduardo Solis and Michael P. Kaye, "The International Society for Heart Transplantation Registry," *Clinical Transplantation* (1986): 2.

195. David O. Taylor et al., "The Registry of the International Society for Heart and Lung Transplantation: Twenty-First Official Adult Heart Transplant Report—2004," *JHLT* 23, no. 7 (2004): 797.

196. "New Drugs Offer Promise in Battle against Transplant Rejection," Stanford University Medical Center Press Release, 25 Aug 1989, SU, Special Collections and University Archives, Norman Shumway Project (V0222), box 6, vol. 2; "A Promising 'One-Two' Punch in Transplant Rejection Treatment," Stanford University Medical Center Press Release, 30 May 1991, ibid.; "Laboratory Identifies Three Promising Drugs to Help Transplant and Artery Disease Patients," Stanford University Medical Center Press Release, 18 May 1994, ibid.; Spyros Andreopoulos, "Defusing the Immune System," *Stanford Medicine* (Winter 1991): 4–7; "New Antirejection Drugs Anticipated," *JAMA* 264, no. 10 (12 Sep 1990): 1225; "New Vistas in Immunosuppression," *Physician's Weekly*, 21 Aug 1990.

197. Shumway interview, 16 Oct 1997, VU; Denton Cooley interview, 4 May 1997, William S. Stoney Collection, Vanderbilt University Medical Center, Eskind Biomedical Library Special Collections, Collection no. 241, box 01A, folder 5.

198. "The Transplanted Heart: The Ultimate Operation" (cover story), *Time*, 15 Dec 1967; "Gift of a Human Heart: A Dying Man Lives with a Dead Girl's Heart" (cover story), *Life*, 15 Dec 1967.

199. See Lois DeBakey, "Letters: Time to End DeBakey Myth," *Houston Chronicle*, 26 Dec 2004; Cooley, "Feuds," 650; Cooley, *100,000 Hearts*, 144.

200. "The National Heart Institute: A Brief History," ca. 1968, NLM, HMD, John Watson Papers, Accession 2003-054, box 2, folder The Artificial Heart Program of the National Heart Institute, 1964–68; "Summary Operational History of the Artificial Heart Program," 4 Dec 1973, ibid., box 16, folder 5.

201. J. N. Ross et al., "Problems Encountered during the Development and Implantation of the Baylor-Rice Orthotopic Cardiac Prosthesis," *Trans ASAIO* 18 (1972): 168–75, 179.

202. Michael DeBakey died the following year, just shy of his 100th birthday. Denton Cooley died in 2016 at age 96. See Todd Ackerman, "Top Heart Surgeons Cooley and DeBakey Put Their Decades-Old Feud to Rest," *Houston Chronicle*, 28 Nov 2007; Lawrence K. Altman, "The Feud: The Doctors World," *NYT*, 27 Nov 2007, F1–F2; Lawrence K. Altman,

"Dr Michael E DeBakey, Rebuilder of Hearts, Dies at 99," *NYT,* 13 Jul 2008; Lawrence K. Altman, "Dr Denton Cooley, Whose Pioneering Heart Surgery Set Off a 40-Year Medical Feud, Dies at 96," *NYT,* 18 Nov 2016; Cooley, *100,000 Hearts,* 193–98.

Chapter 3 · Technology and Risk

Epigraph: Eugene Dong and Spyros Andreopoulos, *Heart Beat* (New York: Zebra Books, Kensington, 1982), 319. *Heart Beat* was originally published by Coward, McCann, and Geoghegan in 1978.

1. Dong and Andreopoulos, *Heart Beat.* See also Nancy Faber, "What Heart Surgeon Eugene Dong Wants to Transplant Next Is the Medical Establishment," *Time* 9, no. 18 (8 May 1978).

2. Dorothy Nelkin, *Selling Science: How the Press Covers Science and Technology* (New York: W. H. Freeman, 1987), 54.

3. Ibid.

4. Daniel S. Greenberg, *Science, Money and Politics: Political Triumph and Ethical Erosion* (Chicago: University of Chicago Press, 2001).

5. See NHLI Press Release, 2 Mar 1972, UU, Willem J. Kolff Collection, MS 654, box 300, folder 10; Final Report, "Biomedical Engineering Support," 15 Jun 1979, ibid., box 173, folder 11; E. W. Fowler to Seaborg, 4 Dec 1968, DOE, Office of History and Heritage Resources, RG 326, AEC Commissioner G. T. Seaborg Office Files, box 206, file 6.

6. See Barron H. Lerner, *When Illness Goes Public: Celebrity Patients and How We Look at Medicine* (Baltimore: Johns Hopkins University Press, 2006), 180–200; Renée C. Fox and Judith P. Swazey, *Spare Parts: Organ Replacement in American Society* (Oxford: Oxford University Press, 1992); Barton J. Bernstein, "The Misguided Quest for the Artificial Heart," *Technology Review,* Nov–Dec 1984, 13–19, 62–63; "The Pursuit of the Artificial Heart," *Medical Heritage* 2 (1986): 80–100; Albert R. Jonsen, "The Artificial Heart's Threat to Others," *Hastings Center Report* (Feb 1986): 11; George J. Annas, "No Cheers for Temporary Artificial Hearts," *Hastings Center Report* 15, no. 5 (Oct 1985): 27–28; Arthur L. Caplan, "'To Mend the Heart': Ethics and High Technology: 3, The Artificial Heart," *Hastings Center Report* 12, no. 1 (Feb 1982): 22–24.

7. Bernstein, "Misguided Quest," 13–19, 62–63; "Pursuit of the Artificial Heart," 80–100; Fox and Swazey, *Spare Parts,* 153, 193.

8. Howard P. Segal, *Technological Utopianism in American Culture* (Chicago: University of Chicago Press, 1985). See also Patrick Kupper, "From Prophecies of the Future to Incarnations of the Past: Cultures of Nuclear Technology," in *Cultures of Technology and the Quest for Innovation,* ed. Helga Nowotny (New York: Berghahn Books, 2006), 155–66.

9. Angela Creager, *Life Atomic: A History of Radioisotopes in Science and Medicine* (Chicago: University of Chicago Press, 2013). See also Katherine Jane Zwicker, "Radiation, Researchers and the United States Atomic Energy Commission: Biomedical Research from the Early Twentieth Century to the Early Cold War," PhD diss., University of Edmonton, 2012.

10. On the expanding role of the government in scientific research and development programs, see Alfred K. Mann, *For Better or for Worse; The Marriage of Science and Government in the U.S.* (New York: Columbia University Press, 2000). See also Robert Pool, *Beyond Engineering: How Society Shapes Technology* (Oxford: Oxford University Press, 1999).

11. For general peacetime use of the atom, including health initiatives, see Richard G. Hewlett, *Atoms for Peace and War, 1953–61: Eisenhower and the Atomic Energy Commission* (Berkeley: University of California Press, 1989); John Krige, "Atoms for Peace: Scientific Internationalism and Scientific Intelligence," *Osiris* 21 (2006): 161–81; Martin Mann, *Peacetime*

Uses of Atomic Energy, 3rd rev. ed. (New York: Crowel, 1975), especially chapter 9, "Atoms for Health," which includes discussion of the nuclear pacemaker and the heart pump. For more detailed accounts of the use of radioisotopes, see Creager, *Life Atomic;* Angela Creager, "Nuclear Energy in the Service of Biomedicine: The U.S. Atomic Energy Commission's Radioisotope Program, 1946–1950," *Journal of the History of Biology* 39 (2006): 649–84; Soraya Boudia, "Radioisotopes 'Economies of Promises': On the Limits of Biomedicine in Public Legitimization of Nuclear Activities," *Dynamis* 29 (2009): 241–59; Nestor Herran, "Isotope Networks: Training, Sales and Publications, 1946–1965," *Dynamis* 29 (2009): 285–309; Angela N. H. Creager, "Radioisotopes as Political Instruments, 1946–1953," *Dynamis* 29 (2009): 219–39; Alison Kraft, "Between Medicine and Industry: Medical Physics and the Rise of the Radioisotope, 1945–65," *Contemporary British History* 20, no. 1 (March 2006): 1–35.

12. The contribution of technological uncertainty among scientists and engineers to controversy and breakdown is also explored by Thomas R. Wellock, "Engineering Uncertainty and Bureaucratic Crisis at the Atomic Energy Commission, 1964–1973," *T&C* 53 (Oct 2012): 846–84.

13. Boudia, "Radioisotopes 'Economies of Promises,'" 255. See also Paul Boyer, *By the Bomb's Early Light: American Thought and Culture in the Dawn of the Atomic Age* (Chapel Hill: University of North Carolina Press, 1985); Carolyn Kopp, "The Origins of the American Scientific Debate over Fallout Hazards," *Social Studies of Science* 9, no. 4 (1979): 403–22; Joop van der Plight, *Nuclear Energy and the Public* (Cambridge: Blackwell, 1992); Catherine Caufield, *Multiple Exposures: Chronicles of the Radiation Age* (London: Secker & Warburg, 1989); J. S. Walker, *Permissible Dose: A History of Radiation Protection in the 20th Century* (Berkeley: University of California Press, 2000).

14. F. W. Hastings, W. H. Potter, and J. W. Holter, "A Progress Report on the Development of a Synthetic Intracorporeal Blood Pump," *Trans ASAIO* 8 (1962): 116–17.

15. William E. Mott, "Nuclear Power for the Artificial Heart" (lecture), 17 Oct 1973, UU, MS 654 Willem J. Kolff Collection, box 168, folder 3.

16. "Isotopic Engine for Circulatory Support Systems," report prepared by the Division of Isotopes Development, 7 Dec 1966, DOE, Office of History and Heritage Resources, RG 326, Secretariat Files, 1972–74, box 7740, file 5.

17. *Hearings on DHEW Appropriations for 1966, Before the House Subcommittee of Appropriations,* part 3, 4, 8–11, 15, 16, 18, 19, 22 May 1965, p. 505, 89th Cong. (1965); Alice L. Buck, "A History of the Atomic Energy Commission," DOE, Jul 1983, 6; Richard G. Hewlett and Oscar Anderson, *The New World: A History of the Atomic Energy Commission,* vol. 1, *1939–1946* (1962; repr., Berkeley: University of California Press, 1990); Richard G. Hewlett and Francis Duncan, *Atomic Shield: A History of the Atomic Energy Commission,* vol. 2, *1947–1952* (1962; repr., Berkeley: University of California Press, 1990); Richard G. Hewlett and Jack M. Holl, *Atoms for Peace and War: Eisenhower and the Atomic Energy Commission,* vol. 3, *1953–1961* (Berkeley: University of California Press, 1989).

18. "AEC Picks Four Firms for Design Studies of Radioisotope-Powered Heart Pump Engine," AEC Press Release, 12 May 1967, NARA, RG 128 Joint Committee on Atomic Energy, Isotope Powered Heart Prosthetic.

19. Edward G. English to file, 13 Mar 1968, DOE, Office of History and Heritage Resources, RG 326, Secretariat Files, 1966–72, box 7740, file 5.

20. Artificial Heart Assessment Panel, *The Totally Implantable Artificial Heart: Economic, Ethical, Legal, Medical, Psychiatric, Social Implications: A Report* (Bethesda, MD: National Institutes of Health, 1973), 38–39.

21. "Isotopic Engine for Circulatory Support," DOE.

22. R. Hollingsworth to John T. Conway, 29 Jan 1968, NARA, RG 128, Joint Committee on Atomic Energy, Isotope Powered Heart Prosthetic.

23. Eugene Fowler to G. T. Seaborg, 11 Sep 1970, NARA, RG 128, Joint Committee on Atomic Energy, Isotope Powered Heart Prosthetic.

24. "Totally Implantable Nuclear Heart Assist and Artificial Heart," Feb 1972, John Watson Papers, NLM, HMD, Accession 2003-054, box 1.

25. Circulatory Support System Program Report, 12 Sep 1967, DOE, Office of History and Heritage Resources, RG 326, AEC Commissioner G. T. Seaborg Office Files, box 206, file 6.

26. E. E. Fowler to Chairman Seaborg, 21 Nov 1968, DOE, Office of History and Heritage Resources, RG 326, AEC Commissioner G. T. Seaborg Office Files, box 206, file 6.

27. See "Various Atom Uses Explored by A.E.C.," *NYT,* 28 Aug 1969; AEC Annual Reports for 1966 to 1971, DOE, Office of History and Heritage Resources.

28. Society of Nuclear Medicine, "What Is Nuclear Medicine?," http://interactive.snm .org, accessed Nov 14, 2011; Henry N. Wagner Jr., ed. *Principles of Nuclear Medicine,* 2nd ed. (Philadelphia: Saunders, 1995), chap. 1 "Nuclear Medicine: What It Is, What It Does," 1–8.

29. Seymour Shwiller to file, 10 Jul 1970, NARA, RG 128 Joint Committee on Atomic Energy, Isotope Powered Heart Prosthetic.

30. I thank Matthew Eisler for this information. See also Greenberg, *Science, Money and Politics,* 172–76.

31. Charles J. Zwick to Clinton P. Anderson, 22 Mar 1968, DOE, Office of History and Heritage Resources, RG 326, Secretariat Files, 1972–74, box 7740, file 5.

32. Jim Ramey to Ed Bauser, 17 Sep 1970; Elliot L. Richardson to John O. Pastore, 27 Mar 1972, both in NARA, RG 128, Joint Committee on Atomic Energy, Isotope Powered Heart Prosthetic.

33. Circulatory Support System Program Report, 12 Sep 1967, DOE.

34. Clinton P. Anderson to Charles J. Zwick, 23 Feb 1968, DOE, Office of History and Heritage Resources, RG 326, Secretariat Files, 1972–74, box 7740, file 5.

35. Seymour Shwiller to file, 10 Jul 1970, NARA.

36. W. E. Mott to Edward J. Bauser, 6 Mar 1972, DOE, Office of History and Heritage Resources, RG 326, Secretariat Files, 1972–74, box 7844, file 7.

37. Shwiller to file, 10 Jul 1970, NARA.

38. E. E. Fowler to Chairman Seaborg, 22 May 1970, DOE, Office of History and Heritage Resources, RG 326, AEC Commissioner G.T. Seaborg Office Files, box 206, file 8.

39. E. E. Fowler to Chairman Seaborg, 2 Jul 1970, DOE, Office of History and Heritage Resources, RG 326, AEC Commissioner G.T. Seaborg Office Files, box 206, file 8.

40. Fowler to Seaborg, 11 Sep 1970, NARA.

41. Fowler to Seaborg, 2 Jul 1970, DOE.

42. Seymour Shwiller to file, 13 Jan 1971, NARA, RG 128 Joint Committee on Atomic Energy, Isotope Powered Heart Prosthetic.

43. The Westinghouse engine required 26 watts of nuclear energy, in comparison to the TRW engine that required 40 watts to power its particular blood pump model. Clarence Dennis to file, 8 Aug 1973, John Watson Papers, NLM, HMD, Accession 2003-054, box 17, C. Dennis Files.

44. AEC Annual Report for 1971, p. 153, DOE; Seymour Shwiller to Edward J. Bauser, 6 Dec 1971, NARA, RG 128, Joint Committee on Atomic Energy, Isotope Powered Heart

Prosthetic; Clarence Dennis to file, 13 Sep 1973, John Watson Papers, NLM, HMD, Accession 2003-054, box 17, folder AEC-C. Dennis Files, 1968–76.

45. Mott, "Nuclear Power for the Artificial Heart," 17 Oct 1973, UU; L. Smith et al., "Development of the Implantation of a Total Nuclear-Powered Artificial Heart System," *Trans ASAIO* 20 (1974): 732.

46. Pu-238 is primarily an emitter of alpha particles, which have high energy but very low penetrating power and can be stopped by a thin piece of paper or even skin. Pu-238 also emits penetrating gamma and neutron radiation, but engineers argued that this radiation could be readily shielded from recipients by good capsule and engine design. The heat from the isotope capsule was to be stored and released as required (although no specifications indicated how, in relation to the human duty cycle) to power the thermal engine.

47. See Shelley McKellar, "Limitations Exposed: Willem J. Kolff and His Contentious Pursuit of a Mechanical Heart," in *Essays in Honour of Michael Bliss: Figuring the Social,* ed. E. A. Heaman, Alison Li, and Shelley McKellar (Toronto: University of Toronto Press, 2008), 400–434.

48. Mott, "Nuclear Power for the Artificial Heart," 17 Oct 1973, UU.

49. L. Smith et al., "Development of the Implantation," 732; D. K. Backman et al., "The Design and Evaluation of Ventricles for the AEC Artificial Heart Nuclear Power Source," *Trans ASAIO* 19 (1973): 542–52. In 1998 Willem Kolff closed his Utah lab and the Smithsonian Institution accepted 352 objects of historical significance related to Kolff's artificial organs research program, including material related to the AEC Atomic Heart. See Test Rig for the Atomic Energy Artificial Heart, Smithsonian Institution, NMAH, ID no. 1998.0035.042.02.

50. Westinghouse also subcontracted specific tasks outside of Philips and the University of Utah. At the Cleveland Clinic, Dr. Yukihiko Nosé's team studied the surgical fit of the proposed device to provide dimension limits to both Philips and Kolff. The most significant outsourcing of production surrounded the radioisotope Pu-238. This required the cooperation of the Savannah River Laboratory (where the plutonium-238 was produced), the Los Alamos Scientific Laboratory (where the powder from Savannah was purified and formed into a solid cylinder), the Mound Laboratory (where the cylinder was encapsulated), and TRW Inc. (where the encapsulating materials were fabricated). See Mott, "Nuclear Power for the Artificial Heart," 17 Oct 1973, UU.

51. Annual Report (to AEC)—Biomedical Engineering Support, 15 Jul 1972, UU, MS 654 Willem J. Kolff Collection, box 164, folder 2; Mott, "Nuclear Power for the Artificial Heart," 17 Oct 1973, UU.

52. D. A. Hughes et al., "Nuclear-Fueled Circulatory Support Systems XII: Current Status," *Trans ASAIO* 20 (1974): 741; John C. Norman et al., "An Implantable Nuclear-Fueled Circulatory Support System: I. Systems Analysis of Conception, Design, Fabrication and Initial in vivo Testing," *Ann Surg* 176, no. 4 (Oct 1972): 494.

53. NHLI Press Release, 2 Mar 1972, UU; Robert Reinhold, "Nuclear Heart Pump: 'Moon Shot' for Medicine," *NYT,* 21 Mar 1972; Frank Carey, "Atomic Booster: Artificial Heart? It's on Its Way," *Salt Lake Tribune,* 3 Mar 1972; "Atomic Engine Developed for Artificial Heart," *Houston Chronicle,* 3 Mar 1972.

54. John C. Norman et al., "An Implantable Nuclear Fuel Capsule for an Artificial Heart," *Trans ASAIO* 14 (1968): 204–9; Norman et al., "Implantable Nuclear-Fueled Support System," 492–501. See also Medical Devices Applications Report, 1972, John Watson Papers, NLM, HMD, Accession 2003-054, box 13.

55. Norman et al., "Implantable Nuclear-Fueled Support System," 494.

56. William E. Mott, "Comparison of NHLI and AEC Nuclear-Powered Artificial Heart Systems," 29 Mar 1972, UU, MS 654 Willem J. Kolff Collection, box 332, folder 8.

57. Norman et al., "Implantable Nuclear-Fueled Support System," 499; Medical Devices Applications Report, 1972, NLM.

58. Victor Poirier, Project Bionics Pioneer Interview, 2 Feb 2012, NLM, HMD.

59. "Totally Implantable Nuclear Heart Assist," Feb 1972, NLM.

60. T. C. Robinson, S. S. Kitrilakis, and L. T. Harmison, "The Development of an Implanted Left Ventricular Assist Device and Rankine Cycle Power Systems," *Trans ASAIO* 18 (1970): 165–71; Norman et al., "Implantable Nuclear-Fueled Circulatory System," 492–502.

61. "The Program on the Development of an Artificial Heart: An Evaluation," 29 Nov 1974, NLM, HMD, Clarence Dennis Papers, MS C 574, box 6, folder 18.

62. "Totally Implantable Nuclear Heart Assist," Feb 1972, NLM.

63. During the late 1960s and early 1970s, the Illinois Institute of Technology Research Institute (IITRI) in Chicago was one such recipient of NHLI contract funding for its services as an artificial heart test and evaluation facility. There were no IITRI reports of any device "successes." I thank Dr. Mark D. Johnston, whose father, Dr. Clare C. Johnston, supervised this work at the IITRI, for bringing this to my attention. Personal communication with author, 30 Jun 2016; NHLI Annual Reports, 1971, 1972, and 1973, National Institutes of Health, Office of NIH History.

64. Artificial Hearts News Release, 6 Oct 1972, UU, MS 654 Willem J. Kolff Collection, box 300, folder 10.

65. M. T. Johnson to E. E. Fowler, 5 Apr 1972, DOE, Office of History and Heritage Resources, RG 326, Secretariat Files, 1966–72, box 7844, file 7.

66. William E. Mott, Comment on NHLI Announcements of March 2, 1972, 15 Mar 1972, NLM, HMD, Clarence Dennis Papers MS C 574, box 7, folder 23—U.S. AEC, 1972–1975.

67. Artificial Hearts News Release, 6 Oct 1972, UU.

68. Hughes et al., "Nuclear-Fueled Circulatory Support Systems," 742.

69. Peter Barton Hutt, "A History of Government Regulation of Adulteration and Misbranding of Medical Devices," *Food, Drug and Cosmetic Law Journal* 44 (1989): 102; James Harvey Young, *Pure Food: Securing the Federal Food and Drugs Act of 1906* (Princeton, NJ: Princeton University Press, 1989).

70. Margaret Harris, "Legislation to Regulate Medical Devices," *Biomaterials, Medical Devices and Artificial Organs* 3, no. 3 (1975): 263; Hutt, "History of Government Regulation," 99–117; Richard A. Merrill, "Regulation of Drugs and Devices: An Evolution," *Health Affairs* 13, no. 3 (1994): 47–69; Rodney R. Munsey, "Trends and Events in FDA Regulation of Medical Devices over the Last Fifty Years," *Food and Drug Law Journal* 50, Special Issue (1995): 163–77; Daniel Schultz, "Regulating Medical Devices," in *Perspectives on Risk and Regulation: The FDA at 100,* ed. Arthur Daemmrich and Joanna Radin (Philadelphia: Chemical Heritage Foundation, 2007), 52–64.

71. Harris, "Legislation to Regulate Medical Devices," 262.

72. Kirk Jeffrey, *Machines in Our Hearts: The Cardiac Pacemaker, the Implantable Defibrillator, and American Health Care* (Baltimore: Johns Hopkins University Press, 2001), 191.

73. *Hearings on Medical Device Amendments of 1975, Before the House Committee on Interstate and Foreign Commerce, Subcommittee on Health and the Environment,* 94th Cong. 199 (28–31 Jul 1975).

74. Richard D. Lyons, "Faulty Devices Linked to Deaths," *NYT,* 7 Sep 1969; "Parley Backs Medical Devices Law," *NYT,* 8 Sep 1969.

75. Theodore Cooper, "Device Legislation," *Food, Drug and Cosmetic Law Journal* (Apr 1971): 170.

76. *Medical Devices: A Legislative Plan,* 1970, DHEW.

77. Ibid.

78. See the Pure Food and Drug Act of 1906; Hutt, "History of Government Regulation," 99–117; Harris, "Legislation to Regulate Medical Devices," 261–75.

79. Hutt, "History of Government Regulation," 110, 113.

80. Cooper, "Device Legislation," 171–72.

81. David M. Link, "Cooper Committee Report and Its Effect on Current FDA Medical Device Activities," *Food, Drug and Cosmetic Law Journal* (Oct 1972): 626.

82. *Hearings on Medical Device Amendments of 1975,* p. 220; Harold M. Schmeck Jr., "Law on Faulty Health Devices Urged," *NYT,* 15 Sep 1973.

83. *Hearings on Medical Devices, Before the House Committee on Interstate and Foreign Commerce, Subcommittee on Public Health and the Environment,* 93rd Cong. 188 (23–24 Oct 1973); *Hearings on Medical Device Amendments of 1975,* p. 220; Lawrence K. Altman, "Pacemaker Users Affected by Recall Are Notified," *NYT,* 15 Jun 1974; David Burnham, "G.A.O. Assails FDA over Pacemakers," *NYT,* 13 Mar 1975; David Burnham, "Safety Lag Seen on Pacemakers," *NYT,* 20 Mar 1975.

84. See Susan Foote, *Managing the Medical Arms Race: Public Policy and Medical Device Innovation* (Berkeley: University of California Press, 1992): 117–18; Jane E. Brody, "Pressure Grows for U.S. Rules in Intrauterine Devices," *NYT,* 4 Jun 1973; "Birth Curb Group Acts on IUD Risk," *NYT,* 30 May 1974; "FDA Links Rise in Deaths to Birth Device," *NYT,* 22 Aug 1974.

85. For more on the criticism of the Dalkon Shield and its manufacturer, see *Hearings on the Regulation of Medical Devices (Intrauterine Contraceptive Devices), Before the Committee on Government Operations,* 93rd Cong. (30 May–1 June, 12–13 Jun 1973). See also Morton Mintz, *At Any Cost: Corporate Greed, Women and the Dalkon Shield* (New York: Pantheon, 1985); Susan Perry and Jim Dawson, *Nightmare: Women and the Dalkon Shield* (New York: Macmillan, 1985); Nicole J. Grant, *The Selling of Contraception: The Dalkon Shield Case, Sexuality, and Women's Autonomy* (Columbus: Ohio State University Press, 1992).

86. Foote, *Managing the Medical Arms Race,* 120.

87. *Hearings on Medical Devices,* p. 215, cited in Harris, "Legislation to Regulate Medical Devices," 267–68.

88. *Hearings on Medical Devices,* p. 214; Jeffrey, *Machines in Our Hearts,* 194.

89. No overarching trade organization represented the industry as a whole until the creation, in direct response to increased regulation, of the Health Industry Manufacturers Association in 1976. As a national trade association representing manufacturers of medical devices, diagnostics, and health information systems, it represents the industry before Congress and regulatory agencies like the FDA on issues of interest to members. See Jeffrey, *Machines in Our Hearts,* 192–93; Foote, *Managing the Medical Arms Race,* 120.

90. Harold M. Schmeck Jr., "FDA to Control Medical Devices," *NYT,* 29 May 1976; Patricia E. Weil, "From Toothbrush to Pacemaker: The FDA Is Moving In," *NYT,* 31 Dec 1978.

91. Foote, *Managing the Medical Arms Race,* 121; Suzanne Junod, "Commemorating the 40th Anniversary of the 1976 Medical Device Amendments," *Food and Drug Law Journal* 72, no. 1 (2017): 26–31.

92. Richard E. Clark, "Medical Device Regulation: Current and Future Trends," *Ann Thorac Surg* 29, no. 4 (Apr 1980): 298.

93. Clark, "Medical Device Regulation," 299.

94. Ulrich Beck, *Risk Society: Towards a New Modernity* (London: Sage, 1992); Ulrich Beck, *World Risk Society* (Cambridge, UK: Polity Press, 1999); Anthony Giddens, *Runaway World: How Globablization Is Reshaping Our Lives* (London: Profile Books, 1999).

95. Mott, "Nuclear Power for the Artificial Heart," 17 Oct 1973, UU.

96. Ibid.; William E. Mott to Willem J. Kolff, 8 May 1973, UU, MS 654 Willem J. Kolff Collection, box 168, folder 3.

97. Robert J. Duffy, *Nuclear Politics in America: A History and Theory of Government Regulation* (Lawrence: University of Kansas Press, 1997), 49–80; Caufield, *Multiple Exposures.*

98. See David J. Rothman, *Strangers at the Bedside: A History of How Law and Bioethics Transformed Medical Decision Making* (New York: Basic Books, 1991); Albert R. Jonsen, *The New Medicine and the Old Ethics* (Cambridge, MA: Harvard University Press, 1990).

99. Artificial Heart Assessment Panel, *Totally Implantable Artificial Heart,* 1.

100. Ibid., 194–96.

101. Ibid., 104.

102. Ibid., 104–5, 106–7.

103. Ibid., 107–12.

104. National Council on Radiation Protection and Measurements, Report No. 39, 15 Jan 1971, cited in "Program on the Development of an Artificial Heart," 29 Nov 1974, NLM. A rem (an acronym for *roentgen equivalent man*) is the dose of ionizing radiation that will produce a biological effect approximately equal to that caused by one roentgen of x-ray or gamma-ray radiation. Taken from US Nuclear Regulatory Commission, Office of Nuclear Material Safety and Safeguards, Jul 1976.

105. "Program on the Development of an Artificial Heart," 29 Nov 1974, NLM.

106. Helen Caldicott, *Nuclear Power Is Not the Answer* (New York: New Press, 2006), 44.

107. Artificial Heart Assessment Panel, *Totally Implantable Artificial Heart,* 111–17.

108. Victor Parsonnet et al., "Thirty-One Years of Clinical Experience with 'Nuclear-Powered' Pacemakers," *PACE: Pacing and Clinical Electrophysiology* 29 (Feb 2006): 195.

109. Cardiac Pacemaker, Press Release, 2 Feb 1966; George F. Murphy Jr to John T. Conway, 24 May 1966, both in NARA, RG 128, Joint Committee on Atomic Energy.

110. Cardiac Pacemaker, Press Release, 10 Jun 1969, NARA, RG 128 Joint Committee on Atomic Energy. This press release generated moderate press coverage, including Jane E. Brody, "Nuclear-Powered Heart Pacemaker Tested in Dog," *NYT,* 11 Jun 1969; Larry McCarten, "A-Power Offers Hope for Hearts," *Seattle Post-Intelligencer,* 17 Jun 1969.

111. P. Laurens et al., "Stimulateur cardiaque à energie nucleaire," *Annales de Cardiologie et d'Angeiologie* (Paris) 20, no. 4 (Jul–Aug 1971): 395–96; Jeffrey, *Machines in Our Hearts,* 115.

112. Carole M. Wilson to Hon. Clifford P. Case (US Senate), 5 Nov 1971, John Watson Papers, NLM, HMD, Accession 2003-054, box 1, Pacemakers 1971–72.

113. Milton Shaw to Senator Russell B. Long, 12 Jan 1972, NARA, RG 128, Joint Committee on Atomic Energy, Cardiac Pacemaker; AEC Response to Letters to Members of Congress concerning Availability of Nuclear Powered Pacemakers, 24 Nov 1971, DOE, Office of History and Heritage Resources, RG 326, Secretariat Files, 1966–72, box 7844, file 7.

114. Jeffrey, *Machines in Our Hearts,* 115.

115. Ibid., 116.

116. Ibid., 115.

117. Final Report—Generic Environmental Statement on Routine Use of Plutonium-Powered Cardiac Pacemaker, Jul 1976, John Watson Papers, NLM, HMD, Accession 2003-054, box 11.

118. Wilson Greatbatch quoted in Jeffrey, *Machines in Our Hearts,* 116.

119. Final Report on Routine Use of Plutonium-Powered Cardiac Pacemaker, Jul 1976, NLM, appendix.

120. Ibid.

121. Ibid.

122. Jadwiga Pawicki to Senator Schweiker, 7 Feb 1975, NARA, RG 326, Records of the AEC, Division of Biomedical and Environment Research, box 81, General Correspondence Files 1956–1975.

123. Alfred E. Mann to Donald E. Johnson, 8 Feb 1972, DOE, Office of History and Heritage Resources, RG 326, Secretariat Files, 1966–72, box 7844, file 7.

124. Victor Parsonnet, "Editorial: Nuclear-Powered Pacemakers," *Medical Instrumentation* 7, no. 3 (May–Aug 1973): 170.

125. Jeffrey, *Machines in Our Hearts,* 116.

126. The last nuclear pacemaker was implanted in January 1983. Victor Parsonnet et al., "A Decade of Nuclear Pacing," *PACE: Pacing and Clinical Electrophysiology* 7 (Jan–Feb 1984): 90.

127. Parsonnet et al., "Thirty-One Years of Clinical Experience," 200.

128. Donald Cole to file, 1 May 1975, NARA, RG 326, Records of the AEC, Division of Biomedical and Environment Research, box 81, General Correspondence Files 1956–1975.

129. Nuclear Pacemaker Clinical Evaluation and Patient Agreement, no date, John Watson Papers, NLM, HMD, Accession 2003-054, box 14.

130. Artificial Heart Assessment Panel, *Totally Implantable Artificial Heart,* 121–23.

131. Ibid., 123.

132. Mott (AEC) to Kolff, 8 May 1973, UU.

133. See Boyer, *By the Bomb's Early Light;* Spencer R. Weart, *Nuclear Fear: A History of Images* (Cambridge, MA: Harvard University Press, 1988); Caufield, *Multiple Exposures.*

134. Artificial Heart Assessment Panel, *Totally Implantable Artificial Heart,* 132.

135. Lee Clarke, "Explaining Choices among Technological Risks," *Social Problems* 35, no. 1 (Feb 1988): 23.

136. Hughes et al., "Nuclear-Fueled Circulatory Support Systems," 741–42; Clarence Dennis to file, 20 Nov 1974, NLM, HMD, Clarence Dennis Papers, MS C 574, box 2, folder 2—General Correspondence, 1974 Oct–Dec.

137. "Program on the Development of an Artificial Heart," 29 Nov 1974, NLM.

138. Ibid.

139. John A. Hill (OMB) to Hon Frank E. Moss (Senator), 30 Dec 1974, UU, MS 654 Willem J. Kolff Collection, box 171, folder 7.

140. Clarence Dennis to William E. Mott (AEC), 7 Jun 1974, NLM, HMD, Clarence Dennis Papers, MS C 574, box 6, folder 10—(U.S. AEC/Dr. William Mott), 1974.

141. James Liverman, director DBER, to Senator Jake Garn (Sen., Utah), 14 Mar 1975, NARA, RG 326, Records of the AEC, Division of Biomedical and Environment Research, box 81 General Correspondence Files 1956–1975; Clarence Dennis to file, 1 Nov 1974, NLM, HMD, Clarence Dennis Papers, MS C 574, box 2, folder 2—General Correspondence, 1974 Oct–Dec.

142. In 1977 ERDA was reorganized, along with other activities, into the DOE. Many AEC scientists working on the artificial heart were reassigned to other projects. See Duffy,

Nuclear Politics in America, 103–22; Glenn T. Seaborg, *The Atomic Energy Commission under Nixon: Adjusting to Troubled Times* (New York: St. Martin's Press, 1993).

143. Robert W. Wood (ERDA) to W. Kolff, 9 May 1975, UU, MS 654 Willem J. Kolff Collection, box 169, folder 7.

144. W. J. Kolff to Mayor E. J. Garn, Salt Lake City, 22 Nov 1974, NARA, RG 326, Records of the AEC, Division of Biomedical and Environment Research, box 81 General Correspondence Files 1956–1975; W. Kolff to J. V. Tunney (Senate, CA), 24 Jan 1975; Allan T. Howe (Rep., UT) to W. Kolff, 2 May 1975, both in UU, MS 654 Willem J. Kolff Collection, box 169, folder 8; W. Kolff to Robert W. Wood (ERDA), 2 Jun 1975, ibid., folder 7.

145. Final Report—ERDA Artificial Heart Program Review, Aug 1976, John Watson Papers, NLM, HMD, Accession 2003-054, box 1.

146. Kolff to G. McKay (Rep., Utah), E. J. Garn (Sen., Utah), O. Hatch (Sen., Utah), D. Marriott (Rep., Utah), F. Church (Sen., Idaho), 15 Mar 1977, UU, MS 654 Willem J. Kolff Collection, box 170, folder 3.

147. Smithsonian Institution, NMAH, Willem J. Kolff Collection (vertical files), box 1, folder 10; Final Report, 1979, UU, MS 654 Willem J. Kolff Collection, box 173, folder 9.

148. Dennis to Mott (AEC), 7 Jun 1974, NLM.

149. "Mechanically Assisted Circulation—The Status of the NHLBI Program and Recommendations for the Future," Report of the Cardiology Advisory Committee, May 1977, John Watson Papers, NLM, HMD, Accession 2003-054, box 6, folder Research Areas Artificial Heart 1975–79.

150. For device approvals, consult the FDA webpage, www.fda.gov, under "medical devices."

151. See Frank E. Samuel Jr., "Safe Medical Devices Act of 1990," *Health Affairs* 10, no. 1 (Spring 1991): 192–95; Foote, *Managing the Medical Arms Race,* 218–20.

152. Amid statements that the new FDA process was too burdensome and time-consuming, one regulatory pathway exploited by industry has been the 501(k) process, which allows new devices of "substantial equivalence" to previously approved devices to circumvent rigorous evaluation for safety and effectiveness—a loophole, according to many commentators, that allows unsafe devices to be used clinically with terrible results. See Brent M. Ardaugh, Stephen E. Graves, and Rita F. Redberg, "The 501(k) Ancestry of a Metal-on-Metal Hip Implant," *NEJM* 368, no. 2 (10 Jan 2013): 97–100; Institute of Medicine, *Medical Devices and the Public's Health: The FDA 501(k) Clearance Process at 35 Years* (Washington, DC: National Academies Press, 2011).

153. See Vakhtang Tchantchaleishvili et al., "Plutonium-238: An Ideal Power Source for Intracorporeal Ventricular Assist Devices? *ASAIO Journal* 58 (2012): 550–53; Victor Poirier, "Will We See Nuclear-Powered Ventricular Assist Devices?" *ASAIO Journal* 58 (2012): 546–47.

154. Foote, *Managing the Medical Arms Race,* 121.

155. W. A. Morton et al., "Impact of Regulations on Artificial Organs Research," *Trans ASAIO* 29 (1983): 773.

156. M. J. Strauss, "The Political History of the Artificial Heart," *NEJM* 310, no. 5 (2 Feb 1984): 335.

157. In the immediate years following its publication, *Heart Beat* received some attention from local newspapers and the Stanford community, including cardiac surgeon Norman Shumway, who railed about "the fantastic danger inherent in any device driven by radioactive materials" and how his department colleague wrote a book about the perils of the

misguided enthusiasm. Norman E. Shumway, lecture to Community Hospital of Monterey Peninsula, 28 Jan 1978, pp. 9–10, SU, Special Collections and University Archives, Norman Shumway Project (V0222), box 6, vol. 3; Faber, "What Dong Wants to Transplant Next"; Newgate Callendar, "Crime" (book review), *NYT,* 2 Apr 1978, BR10.

158. McKellar, "Limitations Exposed," 400–434.

159. "The Dracula of Medical Technology," *NYT,* 16 May 1988.

Chapter 4 · Media Spotlight

Epigraph: Press Release no. 99-124, Committee on Science and Technology, US House of Representatives, 22 Jan 1986, NLM, HMD, John Watson Papers, Accession 2003-054, box 5, folder Congressional Hearing, 5 Feb 1986 (folder 2 of 2).

1. Bert Hansen, "America's First Medical Breakthrough: How Popular Excitement about a French Rabies Cure in 1885 Raised New Expectations for Medical Progress," *American Historical Review* 103, no. 2 (1998): 375.

2. Barron H. Lerner, *When Illness Goes Public: Celebrity Patients and How We Look at Medicine* (Baltimore: Johns Hopkins University Press, 2006), 179.

3. Fay A. LeFevre to W. J. Kolff, 17 Oct 1961, UU, MS 654 W. J. Kolff Collection, box 380, folder 5; W. J. Kolff to Research Projects Committee, Cleveland Clinic, 12 Jan 1965, ibid., box 380, folder 2; W. J. Kolff, Proposal: Institute of Artificial Organs for the Cleveland Clinic Foundation, 5 May 1965, ibid., box 381, folder 1; W. J. Kolff, Progress Report over the Year 1966, Program of Artificial Organs in the Research Division, CCF Archives, folder 3-PR20 Artificial Organs; Board of Governors Memorandum, 21 Feb 1967, ibid.

4. W. J. Kolff to Board of Governors, Cleveland Clinic Foundation, 17 Feb 1967, UU, MS 654 Willem J. Kolff Collection, box 381, folder 12.

5. Don B. Olsen, *True Valor: Barney Clark and the Utah Artificial Heart* (Salt Lake City: University of Utah Press, 2015), 73–77.

6. Allen Weisse, *Heart to Heart: The Twentieth Century Battle against Cardiac Disease—An Oral History* (New Brunswick, NJ: Rutgers University Press, 2002), 254.

7. J. C. Fletcher to W. J. Kolff, 11 Apr 1967, UU Archives, Faculty Files: Willem Kolff; W. J. Kolff to James C. Fletcher, 26 Apr 1967, ibid.

8. R. L. Stephens et al., "Portable/Wearable Artificial Kidney (WAK)—Initial Evaluation," *Proceedings of the European Dialysis Transplantation Association* 12 (1976): 511–18.

9. Institute for Biomedical Engineering: Some of Its Projects; Some of Its People, University of Utah, 1981, UU Archives, Accession 475 Vice President for Health Sciences Records 1945–1960, box 22, folder 12. See also Trudy McMurrin, "Artificial Organs Research at the University of Utah Medical Center," in *Medicine in the Beehive State, 1940–1990,* ed. Henry P. Plenk (Salt Lake City: University of Utah Press, 1992), 453–59.

10. "Artificial Organ Pioneer Says Star Wars Siphoning Funds," *Review: Federation of American Health Systems* 19, no. 4 (Jul–Aug 1986): 23.

11. In 2015, a 10-pound WAK device, powered by 9 volt batteries and worn around the waist, developed by nephrologist-inventor Victor Gura, was in an FDA-approved exploratory clinical trial; however, it is still years away from becoming a routine dialysis practice. Victor Gura et al., "A Wearable Artificial Kidney for Patients with End-Stage Renal Disease," *JCI Insight* 1, no. 8 (2 Jun 2016), pii: e86397; J. P. Kooman, "Creating a Wearable Artificial Kidney: Where Are We Now?," *Expert Review of Medical Devices* 12, no. 4 (Jul 2015): 373–76; A. Davenport, C. Ronco, and V. Gura, "From Wearable Ultrafiltration Device to Wearable Artificial Kidney," *Contributions in Nephrology* 171 (2011): 237–42.

12. See Shelley McKellar, "Limitations Exposed: Willem J. Kolff and His Contentious Pursuit of a Mechanical Heart," in *Essays in Honour of Michael Bliss: Figuring the Social,* ed. E. A. Heaman, Alison Li, and Shelley McKellar (Toronto: University of Toronto Press, 2008), 400–434.

13. W. J. Kolff, "Artificial Organs—Forty Years and Beyond," *Trans ASAIO* 29 (1983): 7.

14. Clifford Kwan-Gett to Willem J. Kolff, 11 Dec 1982, William C. DeVries Papers, NLM, HMD, MS C 588, box 2, folder 14; Willem J. Kolff to William DeVries, 14 Dec 1982, ibid.

15. Kolff, "Artificial Organs—Forty Years," 11–13; Willem J. Kolff, "Artificial Organs beyond the First 40 Years," *Life Support Systems* 2 (1984): 1–14.

16. William DeVries interview, 10 Aug 2010, NLM, HMD, Accession no 2010-021.

17. Many of the experimental devices developed in Kolff's lab are housed at the Smithsonian Institution, NMAH, donated in 1998 by Willem Kolff, including a Soft Shell Mushroom Artificial Heart, ID no. 1998.0035.039.01; an Electrohydraulic Artificial Heart, ID no. 1998.0035.169; and a Right Side Ventricular Assist Device, ID no. 1998.0035.050.

18. Departmental Report, UU, MS 654 Willem J. Kolff Collection, box 149, folder 2; Robert Jarvik, "The Total Artificial Heart," *Sci Am* (Jan 1981): 79; Allan T. Howe (House of Rep., Utah) to W. Kolff, 2 May 1975, UU, MS 654 Willem J. Kolff Collection, box 169, folder 8.

19. Departmental Report, UU; Artificial Heart Press Release, 22 Dec 1982, UU, MS 654 Willem J. Kolff Collection, box 7, folder 9; Proposal: Program Project Grant NIH HE-13738-01, Appendix: Administrative Arrangements—Dr. Kwan Gett, Nov 1970, UU, MS 654 Willem J. Kolff Collection, box 142, folder 6; Jarvik, "Total Artificial Heart," 79.

20. D. J. Lyman et al., "The Development and Implantation of a Polyurethane Hemispherical Artificial Heart," *Trans ASAIO* 17 (1971): 456–63; C. Kwan-Gett et al., "Artificial Heart with Hemispherical Ventricles II and Disseminated Intravascular Coagulation," *Trans ASAIO* 17 (1971): 474–81; C. S. Kwan-Gett et al., "Results of Total Artificial Heart Implantation in Calves," *JTCS* 62, no. 6 (Dec 1971), 880–89.

21. Departmental Report, UU.

22. Olsen, *True Valor,* 105, 130–31, 248–50.

23. Jarvik, "Total Artificial Heart," 79; R. Jarvik et al., "Venous Return of an Artificial Heart Designed to Prevent Right Heart Syndrome," *Annals of Biomedical Engineering* 2, no. 4 (Dec 1974), 335–42; R. K. Jarvik et al., "Recent Advances with the Total Artificial Heart," *NEJM* 298, no. 7 (Feb 1978), 404–5.

24. James Salter, "Two Great Surgical Teams Race for the Man-Made Heart," *Life,* Sep 1981, 36.

25. Manual for Calf Sitters, UU, MS 654 Willem J. Kolff Collection, box 221, folder 7.

26. H. Oster et al., "Survival for 18 Days with a Jarvik-Type Artificial Heart," *Surgery* 77, no. 1 (Jan 1975), 113–17.

27. Table I: Historical (Animal) Records of Total Artificial Heart Research at the University of Utah, UU, MS 654 Willem J. Kolff Collection, box 174, folder 1.

28. Don B. Olsen interview, 14 Jun 1983, NLM, HMD, Judith Swazey Artificial Heart Interviews, Acc. 766.

29. Table: Longest Surviving Animals with a Total Artificial Heart (over 100 Days) at the University of Utah, UU, MS 654 Willem J. Kolff Collection, box 226, folder 1.

30. Robert Jarvik et al., "Surgical Position of the Jarvik Artificial Heart," *JHT* 5, no. 3 (May–Jun 1986): 185; DeVries interview, 10 Aug 2010, NLM.

31. William C. DeVries to Willem Kolff, 12 Sep 1978, William C. DeVries Papers, NLM, HMD, MS C 588, box 2, folder 27.

32. Table: Longest Surviving Animals, UU.

33. W. L. Hastings et al., "A Retrospective Study of Nine Calves Surviving Five Months on the Pneumatic Total Artificial Heart," *Trans ASAIO* 27 (1981): 71–76.

34. Renée C Fox and Judith P. Swazey, *Spare Parts: Organ Replacement in American Society* (Oxford: Oxford University Press, 1992), 104.

35. Artificial Heart Program in Other Centers—Purchase Equipment through Kolff Associates document, UU, MS 654 Willem J. Kolff Collection, box 294, folder 1; Jacques G. Losman to W. J. Kolff, 28 Dec 1980, ibid.; W. J. Kolff to Robert L. Replogle, 3 Sep 1980, ibid.; W. J. Kolff to Denton Cooley, 19 Jan 1982, ibid.

36. According to DeVries, he was the first person on the team to suggest a patient implant, roughly six months after he rejoined the Utah program. William C. DeVries interview, 3 Jun 1999, William S. Stoney Collection, Vanderbilt University Medical Center, Eskind Biomedical Library Special Collections, Collection no. 241, box 01A, folder 7; For simultaneous development of VAD technology, see P. M. Portner, "Permanent Mechanical Circulatory Assistance," in *Heart and Lung Transplantation,* ed. W. A. Baumgartner et al., 2nd ed. (Philadelphia: W. B. Saunders, 2002), 536–40.

37. "Mechanical Heart Test," *Hanford (CA) Sentinel,* 23 Jul 1980; "Utah Doctors to Try Mechanical Heart," *Dallas Times Herald,* 23 Jul 1980; "Temporary Heart Implant Is Sought," *Denver Rocky Mountain News,* 23 Jul 1980; "Artificial Heart Ready for Test," *Fresno (CA) Bee,* 23 Jul 1980; "Surgeons Are Ready for Mechanical Heart Transplant," *Cheyenne (WY) Tribune,* 23 Jul 1980; "Mechanical Heart Transplant Surgery Due," *Sherman (TX) Democrat,* 23 Jul 1980.

38. W. J. Kolff to John Watson, NHLBI, 23 Jul 1980, UU, MS 654 Willem J. Kolff Collection, box 292, folder 1.

39. John Watson to file, memorandum, 7 Jan 1981, NLM, HMD, John Watson Papers, Accession 2003-054, box 4.

40. DeVries interview, 10 Aug 2010, NLM.

41. Ibid.

42. Jarvik, "Total Artificial Heart," 74, cited in Fox and Swazey, *Spare Parts,* 105.

43. Don B. Olsen to Larry Smith, 11 May 1979, UU, MS 654 Willem J. Kolff Collection, box 354, folder 1.

44. Olsen interview, 14 Jun 1983, NLM.

45. Cited in Fox and Swazey, *Spare Parts,* 180.

46. Ibid.

47. E. J. Eichwald et al., "Case Study: Insertion of the Total Artificial Heart" (ca. Mar 1981), UU, MS 654 Willem J. Kolff Collection, box 350, folder 7.

48. Margery W. Shaw, ed., *After Barney Clark: Reflections on the Utah Artificial Heart Program* (Austin: University of Texas Press, 1984), 195–201.

49. Fox and Swazey, *Spare Parts,* 172–74.

50. Eichwald et al., "Case Study," UU.

51. Data collected from the IDE-approved clinical studies is used to support a premarket approval (PMA) application or a premarket notification (510[k]) submission to FDA, necessary for widespread distribution.

52. Victor Zafra (FDA) to Lee M. Smith (Kolff Associates), 29 Mar 1981, UU, MS 654 Willem J. Kolff Collection, box 350, folder 10.

53. Victor Zafra (FDA) to Lee M. Smith (Kolff Associates), 10 Sep 1981, UU, MS 654 Willem J. Kolff Collection, box 534, folder 5.

54. Denton A. Cooley, "A Brief History of the Texas Heart Institute," *THI Journal* 35, no. 3 (2008): 235–39; Courtney J. Gemmato et al., "Thirty-Five Years of Mechanical Circulatory Support at the Texas Heart Institute," *THI Journal* 23, no. 2 (2005): 168–77.

55. O. H. Frazier, "In Memoriam: Tetsuzo Akutsu 1922–2007," *THI Journal* 35, no. 1 (2008): 4; S. Takatani, "In Remembrance of Dr. Tetsuzo Akutsu: A Man Who Started Artificial Heart Research," *Journal of Artificial Organs* 11, no. 1 (Apr 2008): 1–3.

56. T. Akutsu and W. J. Kolff, "Permanent Substitutes for Valves and Hearts," *Trans ASAIO* 4 (1958): 230; Josephine Robertson, "Substitute Heart of Plastic Pushed by Clinic Team," *Cleveland Plain Dealer,* 15 Apr 1958; "The Artificial Heart: Progress toward Its Implantation in Man," *JAMA* 185, no. 13 (28 Sep 1963): 24.

57. Salter, "Two Great Surgical Teams," 35.

58. Denton A. Cooley et al., "Total Artificial Heart in Two-Staged Cardiac Transplantation," *Cardiov Dis* 8, no. 3 (Sep 1981): 306.

59. K. Cheng et al., "The Design and Fabrication of a New Total Artificial Heart," *Cardiov Dis* 4, no. 1 (1977): 7–17; Salter, "Two Great Surgical Teams," 35.

60. See A. K. Vakamudi et al., "Vascular Compliance Studies in Awake Total Artificial Heart Implanted Calves," *Trans ASAIO* 24 (1978): 606–15; Y. Kito et al., "Vasoactive Drug Testing in Calves Following Total Artificial Heart Implantation," *Cardiov Dis* 2, no. 3 (1975): 285–95; T. Honda, "One 25 Day Survivor with Total Artificial Heart," *JTCS* 69, no. 1 (Jan 1975): 92–101; E. C. Henson, "Alterations in the Lungs of Sheep after Implantation of the Akutsu Total Artificial Heart," *JTCS* 65, no. 4 (1973): 629–34; Cheng et al., "Design and Fabrication," 7–17.

61. Cooley et al., "Total Artificial Heart," 310.

62. Marie-Claude Wrenn, "The Artificial Heart Is Here," *Life*, Sep 1981, 31.

63. O. H. Frazier, T. Akutsu, and D. A. Cooley, "Total Artificial Heart (TAH) Utilization in Man," *Trans ASAIO* 28 (1982): 534–35; Cooley et al., "Total Artificial Heart," 317; Denton A. Cooley, "Staged Cardiac Transplantation: Report of Three Cases," *Heart Transpl* 1, no. 2 (Feb 1982): 149–52.

64. Cooley et al., "Total Artificial Heart," 317, 318; The Akutsu III TAH that was implanted in Willebrordus Meuffels was donated by Denton Cooley to the museum collection of the Royal College of Surgeons, London. Akutsu III TAH, Hunterian Museum, Royal College of Surgeons, Object number RCSIC/R11.

65. "Artificial Heart Is Implanted in Man at Houston Hospital," *NYT,* 24 Jul 1981; John Noble Wilford, "Mechanical Heart Given Man in Texas," *NYT,* 25 Jul 1981; "Experimental Heart Sustains Houston Patient for 2d Day," *NYT,* 26 Jul 1981; "Man Kept Alive by Artificial Heart Gets Real One," *NYT,* 27 Jul 1981; "Improvement Is Noted for Recipient of Heart," *NYT,* 28 Jul 1981; "Heart Recipient Is Dead in Houston," *NYT,* 3 August 1981.

66. "The Artificial Heart Is Here," *Life,* Sep 1981, 29.

67. *Threshold,* Twentieth Century Fox, 1981 (93 min.); Les Ericson, "Film: The Arts" (review of *Threshold*), UU, MS 654 Willem J. Kolff Collection, box 291, folder 1; "Fox Dusts Off Its Shelved Artificial Heart Movie," *Salt Lake City Deseret News,* 16 Jan 1983; "Film: 'Threshold,' a Hospital Drama," *NYT,* 21 Jan 1983; Harold M. Schmeck Jr., "The Heart of 'Threshold' and Beyond," *NYT,* 21 Jan 1983; Terry Orme, "'Threshold'—The Artificial Heart Implant as Fiction," *Salt Lake Tribune,* 17 Mar 1983; Christopher Hicks, "'Threshold' Tells a Story Close to Utah's Heart," *Salt Lake City Deseret News,* 18 Mar 1983.

68. "Artificial Heart Is Here," 36.

69. Salter, "Two Great Surgical Teams," 34.

70. Minutes of Kolff Associates Board of Directors' meeting, 27 Jul 1981, UU, MS 654 Willem J. Kolff Collection, box 534, folder 5.

71. Denton A. Cooley to W. J. Kolff, 10 Aug 1981, UU, MS 654 Willem J. Kolff Collection, box 322, folder 6.

72. John Dwan to Willem J. Kolff, 25 Jun 1982, UU Archives, Accession 92-62, box 20450; Willem J. Kolff to Dale Lott, 21 Jun 1982, ibid.; "Dale Lott Cheering for Man Who Got Heart He Wanted," *Salt Lake Tribune,* 5 Dec 1982.

73. "Dying Man Begs U. For Heart," *Salt Lake Tribune,* 16 Mar 1982.

74. Chase N. Peterson, VP Health Sciences, to IRB Members, 18 Mar 1982, UU Archives, Accession 475, box 2, folder 7; Minutes of the Artificial Heart Subcommittee, 3 Mar 1982, ibid.

75. "Floridian Waits as Lawyer Fights U. on Jarvik Rules," *Salt Lake Tribune,* 21 Mar 1982; "U. Surgeon Visits Doctors of Dying Floridian," *Salt Lake Tribune,* 23 Mar 1982; "CBS' Slurs against Medical Center Lacked Osgood's Rhyme, Reason," *Salt Lake Tribune,* n.d., all three in UU, MS 654 Willem J. Kolff Collection, box 292, folder 8.

76. The decision had not been unanimous. Three of 12 IRB members voted against expanding the patient category for TAH implants, and the pushy, determined Willem Kolff approached these members, asking them to defend their negative vote. Kolff had overstepped badly; IRB member Ernst Eichwald identified Kolff's behavior as "clearly unethical." Ernst Eichwald to David Gardiner, 14 Apr 1982; W. J. Kolff to David Gardner, 23 Apr 1982; and W. J. Kolff to Ernst Eichwald, 24 Apr 1982, all from UU Archives, Accession 475, box 2, folder 7.

77. Artificial Heart Fact Sheet, 3 Sep 1982, UU, MS 654 Willem J. Kolff Collection, box 350, folder 7.

78. Robert G. Wilson to John Bosso, 19 Oct 1982, UU Archives, Accession 475, box 2, folder 7.

79. "Lott Abandons Quest for Artificial Heart," *Salt Lake Tribune,* 28 May 1982. See also "A Volunteer for Utah's First Artificial Heart," *Hastings Center Report* 12, no. 2 (Apr 1982), 2.

80. Peterson to IRB Members, 18 Mar 1982, UU Archives.

81. W. J. Kolff to Chase N. Peterson, VP, 3 Apr 1981, UU, MS 654 Willem J. Kolff Collection, box 292, folder 1; Gerry Casey (Manchester, England) to W. J. Kolff, 1 May 1984, ibid., box 354, folder 1; Mrs. Milan Ganser (North Dakota) to W. J. Kolff, 23 Aug 1982, ibid.; J. M. Flake (Provo, Utah) to W. J. Kolff, 3 Feb 1981, ibid.; Patricia Bullwinkel (Freeport, NY) to W. J. Kolff, 21 Oct 1980, ibid.

82. Mrs. John I. McKillip (Lima, Ohio) to W. J. Kolff, 7 Oct 1975, UU, MS 654 Willem J. Kolff Collection, box 354, folder 1.

83. "Artificial Heart Is Here," cover page.

84. Frank W. Martin, "Utah Surgeon William DeVries Seeks a Patient Who Could Live with a Man-Made Heart," *People* 18 (19 Jul 1982): 30–31.

85. Lawrence K. Altman, "Heart Team Drawing Lessons from Dr Clark's Experience," *NYT,* 17 Apr 1983, 1.

86. Jeffery Anderson to Terrance Block, 6 Apr 1982 and 5 May 1982, William C. DeVries Papers, NLM, HMD, MS C 588, box 2, folder 9.

87. Meetings re: Dr. Clark, 1982–83, William C. DeVries Papers, NLM, HMD, MS C 588, box 2, folder 13.

88. Una Loy Clark to Robert H. Ruby, MD, 12 Mar 1987, UU, MS 670, Barney Clark Collection, box 1, folder 30.

89. Willem J. Kolff, "Mankind and Life with Artificial Organs,' unpublished, p. 5, UU, MS 654 Willem J. Kolff Collection, box 2, folder 4.

90. Shaw, *After Barney Clark,* 195–201.

91. Clark to Ruby, 12 Mar 1987, UU.

92. DeVries interview, 10 Aug 2010, NLM.

93. Minutes of the Evaluation Committee Meeting, 30 Nov 1982, William C. DeVries Papers, NLM, HMD, MS C 588, box 2, folder 13.

94. George J. Annas, "Consent to the Artificial Heart: The Lion and the Crocodiles," *Hastings Center Report* 13, no. 2 (Apr 1983): 20–22.

95. In a 1999 interview, DeVries explained how he implanted the TAH in Barney Clark, including sewing in the device connections, "popping" in the ventricles, and then de-airing the device, which he contended was the most difficult part. See DeVries interview, 3 Jun 1999, VU.

96. Olsen, *True Valor,* 308–20; William C. DeVries et al., "Clinical Use of the Total Artificial Heart," *NEJM* 310, no. 5 (2 Feb 1984), 273–78.

97. Artificial Heart Subcommittee Report, 27 Dec 1983, UU Archives, Accession 475, box 3, folder 5.

98. Pamela A. Dew et al., "Mechanical Failures of the Pneumatic Utah-100 and Jarvik Total Artificial Hearts," *ASAIO Transactions* 35, no. 3 (Jul–Sep 1989): 697–99; Olsen, *True Valor,* 329–30.

99. Progress Report on Dr. Barney Clark, 17 Jan 1983, UU, MS 654 Willem J. Kolff Collection, box 351, folder 3.

100. Una Loy Clark to Birdie and Erie Baurman, 17 Jan 1983, UU, MS 670, Barney Clark Collection, box 2, folder 1.

101. John T. Watson to William DeVries, 8 Feb 1983, William C. DeVries Papers, NLM, HMD, MS C 588, box 2, folder 14.

102. Lawrence K. Altman, "Recipient of Artificial Heart Calls the Ordeal Worthwhile," *NYT,* 3 Mar 1983; George Annas, "The Unknowns of the Mechanical Heart," *NYT,* 23 Aug 2001.

103. Audio file excerpt from the 1 Mar 1983 videotape interview with Barney Clark can be found at www.history.com.

104. Una Loy Clark to Birdie and Erie Baurman, 9 Mar 1983, UU, MS 670, Barney Clark Collection, box 1, folder 30.

105. Artificial Heart Subcommittee Report, 27 Dec 1983, UU Archives.

106. DeVries, "Clinical Use of Total Artificial Heart," 273–78; William C. DeVries, "The Permanent Artificial Heart: Four Case Reports," *JAMA* 259, no. 6 (12 Feb 1988): 849–59; William C. DeVries and Lyle D. Joyce, "The Artificial Heart," *Clinical Symposia—CIBA* 35, no. 6 (1983).

107. Chase Nebeker Peterson, *The Guardian Poplar: A Memoir of Deep Roots, Journey, and Rediscovery* (Salt Lake City: University of Utah Press, 2012), 176–77.

108. Artificial Heart Press Releases, UU, MS 670, Barney Clark Collection, box 7, folder 8.

109. "Utah Doctors Separate Siamese Twins Linked at Brain," *NYT,* 31 May 1979.

110. Kathy Fahy, "Newsmen Hang on Every Report during the Seven-Hour Operation," *Salt Lake City Deseret News,* 2 Dec 1982.

111. Chase N. Peterson, "A Spontaneous Reply to Dr Lawrence Altman," in Shaw, *After Barney Clark,* 129.

112. Lawrence K. Altman, "Reflections on a Reporter," in Shaw, *After Barney Clark,* 116.

113. Lawrence K. Altman, "The Doctor's World: Publicity and Medicine: The Human Factors," *NYT,* 1 Jan 1985.

114. See Peterson, *Guardian Poplar,* 177.

115. *NYT,* 3, 4, 5 Dec 1982; *Salt Lake City Deseret News,* 3, 4, 5 Dec 1982.

116. *NYT,* 6, 12, 15 Dec 1982.

117. *Newsweek,* 13 Dec 1982; *Time,* 13 Dec, 14 Mar 1983.

118. "The Brave Man with the Plastic Heart," *Life,* Feb 1983, 24–30.

119. "Barney Clark Dies on 112th Day with Permanent Artificial Heart," *NYT,* 14 Mar 1983; "Dr Clark's Death Laid to Failure of All Organs but Artificial Heart," *NYT,* 25 Mar 1983; "Death of a Gallant Pioneer," *Time,* 4 Apr 1983.

120. Ronni L. Scheier, "Robert K. Jarvik, M.D.: Inventor, Lecturer, 'Hero,'" *American Medical News* (11 Dec 1987): 9–10; "Interview: Artificial Heart Programs to Grow: Jarvik," *Hospitals* (20 Jun 1986): 70–71; "Jarvik, Robert K(offler)," *Current Biography* (Jul 1985): 22–44.

121. Laurence Gonzales, "The Rock'n'Roll Heart of Robert Jarvik," *Playboy,* Apr 1986, 84–87, 128, 146–54; Kristin McMurran, "There's Nothing Artificial about the Way Robert Jarvik's Heart Beats for His Brainy Bride-to-Be," *People,* 27 Jul 1987, 47–50.

122. Joshua Hyatt, "King of Hearts: Has Jarvik Found a Heart of Gold?," *Inc.,* May 1986, 51.

123. Scheier, "Robert K. Jarvik, M.D.," 9.

124. "I Have Him Back Again," *Newsweek,* 10 Dec 1984, 77.

125. DeVries et al., "Clinical Use of Total Artificial Heart," 278. See also Shaw, *After Barney Clark.*

126. Notes from University of Utah Medical Center IRB news conference, 23 Sept 1983, William C. DeVries Papers, NLM, HMD, MS C 588, box 2, folder 19.

127. Prepared Statement, University of Utah Medical Center IRB news conference, 23 Sept 1983, William C. DeVries Papers, NLM, HMD, MS C 588, box 2, folder 19.

128. Gary M. Chan to William DeVries, 12 Jan 1984; and William DeVries to Gary Chan, 31 Jan 1984, William C. DeVries Papers, NLM, HMD, MS C 588, box 2, folder 19.

129. Artificial Heart Fact Sheet, 3 Sep 1982, UU; W. J. Kolff to David P. Gardner, 9 Feb 1983, UU, MS 654 Willem J. Kolff Collection, box 350, folder 19; David P. Gardner to Una Loy Clark, n.d., ibid.; DeVries interview, 3 Jun 1999, VU.

130. Humana Heart Institute Press Conference Transcript, 31 Jul 1984, William C. DeVries Papers, NLM, HMD, MS C 588, box 5, folder 15.

131. DeVries admitted to "not parting on good terms with Kolff," who ensured that DeVries did not leave Utah with any research materials and equipment. Field Notes: Schroeder Implant, 29 Nov–4 Dec 1985, NLM, HMD, The Artificial Heart Case Study, Documents and Tapes of Judith Swazey, Renée Fox and Judith Watkins, 1966–87, Acc. 767; DeVries interview, 10 Aug 2010, NLM; Lawrence K. Altman, "The Doctor's World: The Artificial Heart Mired in Delay and Uncertainty," *NYT,* 25 Oct 1983; "Utah Surgeon Moving Heart Implant Program to Kentucky," *NYT,* 1 Aug 1984.

132. Humana Heart Institute Press Conference Transcript, 31 Jul 1984, NLM.

133. Ibid. See also Fox and Swazey, *Spare Parts,* 119.

134. Lawrence K. Altman, "The Doctor's World: Publicity and Medicine: The Human Factors," *NYT,* 1 Jan 1985.

135. W. J. Kolff to F. David Rollo, 22 Jul 1982, UU, MS 654 Willem J. Kolff Collection, box 396, folder 2; W. J. Kolff to C. Peterson et al., 3 Dec 1982, ibid.; W. J. Kolff to William Gay, 2 Aug 1984, ibid.

136. John Langone, "The Artificial Heart Is Really Very Dangerous," *Discover,* Jun 1986, 44; Arnold S. Relman, "Privatizing Artificial-Heart Research," *Wall Street Journal,* 26 Dec 1984, 11; Fox and Swazey, *Spare Parts,* 117–21.

137. Lawrence K. Altman, "Health Care as Business: Experts Ask Whether Emphasis on Profits Could Dilute the Ideal of Medical Research," *NYT,* 27 Nov 1984.

138. Fox and Swazey, *Spare Parts,* 120.

139. Lawrence K. Altman, "Implant Patient Claims Success; He Feels 'Super,'" *NYT,* 10 Dec 1984; DeVries interview, 10 Aug 2010, NLM.

140. DeVries, "Permanent Artificial Heart," 851–53. From the family's perspective, see the Schroeder Family, *The Bill Schroeder Story* (New York: William Morrow, 1987).

141. Gideon Gil, "The Artificial Heart Juggernaut," *Hastings Center Report* 19, no. 2 (Mar–Apr 1989): 24.

142. Altman, "Implant Patient Claims Success."

143. DeVries, "Permanent Artificial Heart," 851–53; Schroeder Family, *Bill Schroeder Story.*

144. "High Spirits on a Plastic Pulse," *Times,* 10 Dec 1984, 60–62, 64, 67; Lawrence K. Altman, "Heart Recipient 'Feeling Good,' Requests a Beer," *NYT,* 28 Nov 1984; and Lawrence K. Altman, "Heart Patient Briefly Leaves Bed," *NYT,* 30 Nov 1984.

145. "Bill Schroeder's Artificial Heart," *Life,* May 1985, 33–43.

146. Ibid., 37.

147. Lawrence K. Altman, "Learning from Baby Fae," *NYT,* 18 Nov 1984; and any number of bioethics texts, including Gregory E. Pence, *Classic Cases in Medical Ethics,* 2nd ed. (New York: McGraw-Hill, 1995); Ronald Munson, *Raising the Dead: Organ Transplants, Ethics, and Society* (New York: Oxford University Press, 2002).

148. DeVries, "Permanent Artificial Heart," 851–53.

149. Lawrence K. Altman, "Stroke Is Linked to Clot Formed in Artificial Heart," *NYT,* 16 Dec 1984; "Heart Recipient Suffers a Stroke: Doctor Reports Partial Recovery," *NYT,* 14 Dec 1984; "Heart Recipient Loses Enthusiasm, Doctor Reports," *NYT,* 17 Dec 1984.

150. DeVries, "Permanent Artificial Heart," 852.

151. "Son Gives Heart Patient a Wedding Preview," *Chicago Tribune,* 16 Mar 1985; "Schroeder Takes Heart at Record," *Los Angeles Times,* 17 Mar 1985.

152. "Bill Schroeder's Artificial Heart," 41.

153. Patient Murray Haydon, 1985–86, "Chronological Order of Events" (text slide), William C. DeVries Papers, NLM, HMD, MS C 588, box 10, folder 4; DeVries, "Permanent Artificial Heart," 854; Jarvik-7 Artificial Heart (that had been implanted in Murray Haydon), Smithsonian Institution, NMAH, Accession no. 2010.0200.

154. Fox and Swazey, *Spare Parts,* 127.

155. Haydon Family Statement, n.d., William C. DeVries Papers, NLM, HMD, MS C 588, box 4, folder 20.

156. B. L. Koul et al., "Clinical Application of the Total Artificial Heart," *Life Support Systems* 3, suppl. 1 (1985): 195–99; Barnaby J. Feder, "Swedish Team Uses U.S. Device in Heart Implant: Artificial Heart Used in Sweden," *NYT,* 10 Apr 1985, A11, A13.

157. Barnaby J. Feder, "Sweden's Heart Implant Recipient Linked to Police and Tax Inquiries," *NYT,* 11 Apr 1985, A18.

158. Koul et al., "Clinical Application of Total Artificial Heart," 195–99.

159. Ibid.

160. Cited in Fox and Swazey, *Spare Parts,* 131; "Heart Patient Steps forward Grateful for Extended Life," *NYT,* 20 Jul 1985, 8.

161. "Leif Stenberg, Swedish Heart Recipient, Dies," *NYT*, 22 Nov 1985, B9; Gil, "Artificial Heart Juggernaut," 24–55; Fox and Swazey, *Spare Parts*, 130–31, 175.

162. DeVries, "Permanent Artificial Heart," 855.

163. Fox and Swazey, *Spare Parts*, 132.

164. "Voices from Across the USA—How Do You Feel about Artificial Heart Transplants?," *USA Today*, 27 Nov 1984.

165. Dorothy Gilliam, "What If . . . ," *Washington Post*, 13 Dec 1982, cited in Lerner, *When Illness Goes Public*, 197.

166. Una Loy Clark to W. Kolff, 12 Mar 1984, UU, MS 654 Willem J. Kolff Collection, box 353, folder 7.

167. "Remarks from Dr Jack Copeland," *Tucson Arizona Daily Star*, 10 Jun 2010; see also Angela Gonzales, "Artificial Heart Pioneer Jack Copeland Leaving UA," *Phoenix Business Journal*, 29 Jun 2010.

168. Becky Pallack, "UA Losing Copeland, 'Star' of Heart Surgery: World-Famous Doctor Accepts Professorship with UC–San Diego," *Tucson Arizona Daily Star*, 10 Jun 2010.

169. Jack G. Copeland et al., "The Total Artificial Heart as a Bridge to Transplantation: A Report of Two Cases," *JAMA* 256, no. 21 (5 Dec 1986): 2991–92. See also Cecil C. Vaughn et al., "Interim Cardiac Replacement with a Mechanical Heart: Staged Cardiac Transplantation," *THI Journal* 13, no. 1 (March 1986): 45–52; "When Life Is on the Line," *Newsweek*, 18 March 1985, 85–88.

170. Deborah Glazer, "The Artificial Heart: Technical Marvel, Medical Breakthrough," draft, NLM, HMD, John Watson Papers, Accession 2003-054, box 21, folder Human Artificial Heart Implant at the Arizona Heart Institute.

171. W. J. Kolff to Jack Copeland, 7 Mar 1985, UU, MS 654 Willem J. Kolff Collection, box 322, folder 9.

172. G. J. Annas, "The Phoenix Heart: What We Have to Lose," *Hasting Center Report* 15 (Jun 1985): 15–16; and M. King, "Experts Question Increased Use of Jarvik-7 as Temporary Tool," *Louisville Times*, 12 Feb 1986, A1, both cited in Fox and Swazey, *Spare Parts*, 130.

173. Inventor Kevin Cheng continued to develop his air-driven Phoenix Heart, implanting improved prototypes in calves, until he ran out of funding in 1989. His lack of success in securing federal or private funding related to the lack of appeal of another air-driven heart pump, deemed "old technology." No Phoenix Heart model was ever implanted in a human after Thomas Creighton. See "Artificial Heart's Inventor Unable to Finance Testing," *Los Angeles Times*, 30 Jul 1989.

174. Copeland et al., "Total Artificial Heart as a Bridge," 2992–93. See also Vaughn et al., "Interim Cardiac Replacement," 45–52.

175. "Michael Drummond Is Dead at 30; Temporarily Used Artificial Heart," *NYT*, 9 Jul 1990, news clipping, NLM, HMD, John Watson Papers, Accession 2003-054, box 1, folder The Artificial Heart Program in the USA, 1980–92.

176. Bridge implants were done in 39 centers—20 centers in North America and 19 centers outside of North America—according to Kristen E. Johnson et al., "Use of Total Artificial Hearts: Summary of World Experience, 1969–1991," *ASAIO Journal* 38, no. 3 (Jul–Sep 1992): M488.

177. See Jarvik et al., "Surgical Position of Jarvik-7 Artificial Heart," 185.

178. Johnson et al., "Use of Total Artificial Hearts," M486–M492.

179. Ibid., M488.

180. There is a history of neurological complications associated with cardiac surgery; neurological complications are second only to heart failure as a cause of morbidity and mortality following heart surgery. In the course of using surgical clamps, surgeons might dislodge plaque particles in arteries, and the particles may travel to the brain, causing stroke. The hazards of arterial air embolism, caused by the heart-lung machine, that induces stroke in surgical patients were identified in the 1960s. In managing postoperative care, the physician exercises judicious use of blood thinners to balance the risk of stroke against significant bleeding in patients. A short-term syndrome of cognitive impairment related to the use of the heart-lung machine, dubbed "pumphead," is marked by temporary memory loss, impaired vision, and slurred speech in postoperative patients. See Sid Gilman, "Cerebral Disorders after Open-Heart Operations," *NEJM* 272 (1965): 489–98; "Neurological Complications of Open Heart Surgery," *Annals of Neurology* 28, no. 4 (Oct 1990): 475–76.

181. Johnson et al., "Use of Total Artificial Hearts," M489.

182. Ibid., M491.

183. Olsen, *True Valor,* 254.

184. Donald R. Owen, acting president of Kolff Associates Inc., to Clarence Dennis, 11 Jan 1974, NLM, HMD, Clarence Dennis Papers, MS C 574, box 7, folder 28; Willem Kolff to Dr. William Patridge, vice-president for research, University of Utah, 2 Feb 1977, UU, Willem J. Kolff Collection, MS 654, box 243, folder 5.

185. Olsen, *True Valor,* 254.

186. "Academic Capitalism Helping Create Bionic Valley in Utah," *Review: Federation of American Health Systems* (Jul–Aug 1986): 25.

187. History and Description of Kolff Associates Inc., 31 Jul 1981, UU, MS 654 Willem J. Kolff Collection, box 533, folder 1.

188. Conversation with Peter Frommer, NIH, 1 Feb 1977, memo to file, UU, MS 654 Willem J. Kolff Collection, box 533, folder 3; memo to file, 22 Jun 1984, ibid., box 551, folder 1.

189. Olsen, *True Valor,* 256; DeVries interview, 3 Jun 1999, VU.

190. Minutes of Kolff Associates Board of Directors' meeting, 11 May 1982, UU, MS 654 Willem J. Kolff Collection, box 534, folder 5.

191. Kolff to Gay, 2 Aug 1984, UU; Olsen, *True Valor,* 255–56.

192. Kolff Medical Inc. Annual Report for 1983, William C. DeVries Papers, NLM, HMD, MS C 588, box 7, folder 6. See also M. J. Strauss, "The Political History of the Artificial Heart," *NEJM* 310 (2 Feb 1984): 336.

193. Memo to file, 22 Jun 1984, UU. The controversy over the vacuum forming is also cited in Paul Heiney, *The Nuts and Bolts of Life: Willem Kolff and the Invention of the Kidney Machine* (Stroud, UK: Sutton, 2002), 208.

194. Kolff's Four Companies, Oct 1984, UU, MS 654 Willem J. Kolff Collection, box 309, folder 11; Kolff to Robert Reeves, 18 Jan 1985, ibid., box 551, folder 1; Kolff to Winslow Young, 5 Mar 1986, ibid., folder 2.

195. The name Symbion was derived from *symbiosis* and *bionic,* which Jarvik felt better described company products. Memo to file, 22 Jun 1984, UU.

196. Robert Jarvik interview, 4 Aug 1986, NLM, HMD, The Artificial Heart Case Study, Documents and Tapes of Judith Swazey, Renée Fox, and Judith Watkins, 1966–87, Acc. 767, folder: Jarvik & Symbion.

197. The first Canadian case occurred in May 1986. University of Ottawa Heart Institute surgeon Wilbert Keon implanted a Jarvik 7-70 artificial heart in 41-year-old Noella Leclair as a bridge-to-transplant. Seven days later, Leclair was successfully transplanted with a donor

heart. Keon's team received intensive implant training in Utah months before. A London, Ontario, transplant team from University Hospital at the University of Western Ontario attended training sessions in Salt Lake City on March 18, 1986, after purchasing Symbion's Acute Ventricular Assist Device (AVAD). The device was never used at University Hospital; some device components now reside in the Medical Artifact Collection at Western, donated by Dr. Gordon Campbell, former department head for Biomedical Engineering at University Hospital. I thank Dr. Campbell for contacting me and sharing University Hospital's history with the Symbion AVAD with me. See Jane Defalco, "The Heart of the Matter: Ottawa Surgeons Make History and Create a Controversy," *CMAJ* 135 (1 Sep 1986): 510–13.

198. Hyatt, "King of Hearts," 51.

199. Kolff to Gay, 2 Aug 1984, UU.

200. "Top Surgeon Sees No Future for Artificial Heart," *NYT,* 14 Feb 1984.

201. Howard Witt, "Soul-Searching over Artificial Hearts Intensifies," *Chicago Tribune News,* 10 Aug 1986; "The Artificial Heart Is Really Dangerous," *Discover* 7, no. 6 (Jun 1986): 38.

202. Jarvik interview, 4 Aug 1986, NLM; "Artificial Heart Is Really Dangerous," 38.

203. Philip E. Oyer et al., "Development of a Totally Implantable, Electrically Actuated Left Ventricular Assist System," *AJS* 140 (Jul 1980): 17–25; V. A. Starnes and N. E. Shumway, "Heart Transplantation—Stanford Experience," *Clinical Transplantation* (1987): 7–11.

204. R. K. Jarvik et al., "Development of the INERAID Artificial Ear," *Advances in Otorhinolaryngology* 37 (1987): 174–77; "Symbion Inc Has Sold Technology," *Salt Lake City Deseret News,* 11 Jul 1989; Edward B. Diethrich et al., "A New Ventricular Assist Device for Acute Cardiac Failure: Report of Initial Use for Biventricular Support," *Perfusion* 2 (1987): 145–61; Timothy B. Icenogle et al., "Thromboembolic Complications of the Symbion AVAD System," *Art Org* 13, no. 6 (1989): 532–38; Hyatt, "King of Hearts," 51.

205. Jarvik interview, 4 Aug 1986, NLM.

206. "Withdrawal Asked in Bid for Symbion," *NYT,* 16 Apr 1987.

207. "Symbion Board Ousts Jarvik," *NYT,* 27 Apr 1987; Mike King, "Jarvik Fired as Chairman of Mechanical-Heart Firm," *Louisville (KY) Courier-Journal,* 28 Apr 1987, B6.

208. See Lawrence K. Altman, "Artificial Heart Thrives as Bridge to a Real One," *NYT,* 28 Apr 1987.

209. "Smithsonian to Get Transplant's Artificial Heart," *Sioux Falls (SD) Argus-Leader,* 21 May 1987; "Jarvik-7 Artificial Heart Donated to Smithsonian," *Chicago Sun-Times,* 18 Jun 1987; Jarvik-7 Artificial Heart (that had been implanted in Michael Drummond), Smithsonian Institution, NMAH, Accession no. 87.0474.

210. "The Dracula of Medical Technology," *NYT,* 16 May 1988.

211. John Watson, Project Bionics Pioneer Interview, 25 Aug 2015, NLM, HMD.

212. See Daniel Callahan, "The Artificial Heart: Bleeding Us Dry," *NYT,* 17 Sep 1988.

213. James Colgove, "The McKeown Thesis: A Historical Controversy and Its Enduring Influence," *American Journal of Public Health* 92, no. 5 (May 2002): 725–29; Bill Bynum, "The McKeown Thesis," *Lancet* 371 (23 Feb 2008): 644–45.

214. W. Bruce Fye, *Caring for the Heart: Mayo Clinic and the Rise of Specialization* (Oxford: Oxford University Press, 2015), 476–79.

215. See David J. Rothman, *Strangers at the Bedside: A History of How Law and Bioethics Transformed Medical Decision Making* (New York: Basic Books, 1991); and Albert R. Jonsen, *The New Medicine and the Old Ethics* (Cambridge, MA: Harvard University Press, 1990).

216. Barron Lerner, *The 25th Anniversary of Barney Clark's Artificial Heart,* blog, 1 Dec 2007, http://hnn.us.

217. Rothman, *Strangers at the Bedside*, 3.

218. Lerner, *When Illness Goes Public*, 16.

219. Lerner, *25th Anniversary*. See also Barron Lerner, *The Good Doctor: A Father, a Son, and the Evolution of Medical Ethics* (Boston, MA: Beacon Press, 2014).

220. See Harry Schwartz, "Cut the Red Tape: Implant at Full Speed," *NYT*, Aug 17, 1984, A25; Arthur L. Caplan, "Should Doctors Move at a Gallop?," *NYT*, Aug 17, 1984, A25; Gregory E. Pence, "Artificial Hearts: Barney Clark," in Pence, *Classic Cases in Medical Ethics*, 272–92.

221. DeVries interview, 10 Aug 2010, NLM.

222. Arthur L. Caplan, "'To Mend the Heart': Ethics and High Technology, 3: The Artificial Heart," *Hastings Center Report* 12, no. 1 (Feb 1982): 22–24.

223. Annas, "Consent to the Artificial Heart," 20–22.

224. Eichwald et al., "Case Study," UU.

225. Ibid.; Special Consent for Artificial Heart Device Implantation and Related Procedures, 24 May 1982, UU, MS 654 Willem J. Kolff Collection, box 350, folder 7; Zafra to Smith, 29 Mar 1981, UU; the consent form is reprinted in Shaw, *After Barney Clark*, 195–201.

226. DeVries interview, 10 Aug 2010, NLM.

227. Shaw, *After Barney Clark*, 191.

228. Other bioethical issues raised included patient selection criteria, measurements for evaluating success, and experimental volunteers. See Denise Grady, "Summary of Discussion on Ethical Perspectives," in Shaw, *After Barney Clark*, 42–52.

229. George J. Annas, "No Cheers for Temporary Artificial Hearts," *Hastings Center Report* 15, no. 5 (Oct 1985): 27–28; Annas, "Phoenix Heart," 15–16.

230. Ellen J. Flannery, "Should It Be Easier or Harder to Use Unapproved Drugs and Devices?," *Hastings Center Report* 16, no. 1 (Feb 1986): 17–23; "The Man with the Illegal Heart," *NYT*, 9 March 1985.

231. Lerner, *When Illness Goes Public*, 194.

232. "Barney Clark and Lord Tennyson," *NYT*, 25 Mar 1983.

233. "Prolonging Death Is No Triumph," *NYT*, 16 Dec 1982; "Hearts and Technology," *NYT*, 27 Nov 1984.

234. "The Glamorous Artificial Heart," *NYT*, 15 Jan 1983.

235. Albert R. Jonsen, "The Artificial Heart's Threat to Others," *Hastings Center Report* 16, no. 1 (Feb 1986): 9–11.

236. Gil, "Artificial Heart Juggernaut," 24–31.

237. Thomas A. Preston, "The Case against the Artificial Heart," *Utah Holiday*, Jun 1983, 39–49; Thomas A. Preston, "The Artificial Heart," in *Worse Than the Disease: Pitfalls of Medical Progress*, ed. Diana B. Dutton (New York: Cambridge University Press, 1988), 91–126.

238. Barton J. Bernstein, "The Misguided Quest for the Artificial Heart," *Technology Review* (Nov–Dec 1984): 13–19, 62–63; "The Pursuit of the Artificial Heart," *Medical Heritage* 2 (1986): 80–100.

239. Fox and Swazey, *Spare Parts*, 107.

240. Ibid., 153, 193.

241. Report of the Artificial Heart Working Group, 21 May 1981, NLM, HMD, John Watson Papers, Accession 2003-054, box 4.

242. Ibid., emphasis added.

243. Artificial Heart and Assist Devices: Directions, Needs, Costs, Societal and Ethical Issues, NLM, HMD, John Watson Papers, Accession 2003-054, box 15; DHEW Publication no. (NIH) 85-2723, May 1985.

244. Jonsen, "Artificial Heart's Threat to Others," 11.

245. Artificial Heart and Assist Devices, NLM; DHEW Publication no. (NIH) 85-2723, May 1985, p. 35.

246. Lawrence K. Altman, "Strong Curbs Urged in Wake of Unsanctioned Heart Implant," *NYT,* 10 Mar 1985.

247. Marlene Cimons, "Panel, Urging More Oversight, Backs Jarvik-7," *Los Angeles Times,* 21 Dec 1985.

248. Mike King, "FDA Scrutiny of Artificial Heart Amounts to 'Trip to the Woodshed,'" *Louisville Courier Journal,* 23 Dec 1985; Philip M. Boffey, "More Implants of Artificial Hearts Are Urged by U.S. Health Panel," *NYT,* 22 Dec 1985.

249. *Status of the Artificial Heart Program: Hearings before the House Subcommittee on Investigations and Oversight of the Committee on Science and Technology,* 99th Cong. 37, 210 (5 Feb 1986).

250. Ibid., p. 31.

251. Ibid., p. 17; Copeland attracted attention in the late 1990s for performing an aortic valve replacement on a 98-year-old patient. See Fye, *Caring for the Heart,* 498.

252. *Status of the Artificial Heart Program*; also repeated in DeVries interview, 10 Aug 2010, NLM.

253. *Status of the Artificial Heart Program,* p. 160.

254. Ibid., p. 301.

255. Lawrence K. Altman, "U.S. Panel Gives Heart Implant Firm Backing," *NYT,* 24 May 1985; Cristine Russell, "U.S. Urged to Sponsor Development of Fully Implantable Artificial Heart," *Washington Post,* 24 May 1985, A4.

256. Jonsen, "Artificial Heart's Threat to Others," 11.

257. The four research groups were the University of Utah, the Hershey Medical Center of Pennsylvania State University working with 3M/Sarns Inc., the Texas Heart Institute and Abiomed Inc. of Danvers, MA, and the Cleveland Clinic with Nimbus Inc. See T. Sloane Guy, "Evolution and Current Status of the Total Artificial Heart: The Search Continues," *ASAIO Journal* 44 (1998): 30; Portner, "Permanent Mechanical Circulatory Assistance," 534–35.

258. Claude Lenfant interview transcript, 24 Oct 1988, NLM, HMD, The Artificial Heart Case Study, Documents and Tapes of Judith Swazey, Renée Fox, and Judith Watkins, 1966–87, Acc. 767.

259. Ibid.; Watson interview, 25 Aug 2015, NLM.

260. Philip M. Boffey, "Panel Appeals for Funds in Artificial Heart Work," *NYT,* 20 May 1988; Lawrence K. Altman, "Artificial Heart in Turmoil," *NYT,* 17 May 1988; Malcolm W. Browne, "U.S. Halts Funds to Develop Self-Contained Heart Implant," *NYT,* 13 May 1988.

261. Philip M. Boffey, "Federal Agency, in Shift, to Back Artificial Heart," *NYT,* 3 Jul 1988; "Battling with Congress over Priorities on Heart," *NYT,* 8 Jul 1988; Lenfant interview transcript, 24 Oct 1988, NLM.

262. "Senators Doctors Kennedy and Hatch," *NYT,* 15 Jul 1988.

263. "FDA Recalls Jarvik Heart, Scolds Firm," *Salt Lake Tribune,* 12 Jan 1990; News Release from Symbion, 14 Mar 1990, UU, MS 654 Willem J Kolff Collection, box 551, folder 3.

264. Gary Cole to William DeVries, 2 May 1991, William C. DeVries Papers, NLM, HMD, MS C 588, box 7, folder 10; William DeVries to Gary Cole, 20 May 1991, ibid.

265. In total, DeVries implanted seven Jarvik-7 hearts—four cases as permanent implants and three cases as temporary, bridge-to-transplant implants. William DeVries to Allan Lansing, 15 Jun 1988, William C. DeVries Papers, NLM, HMD, MS C 588, box 6, folder 3; DeVries interview, 10 Aug 2010, NLM.

266. Statement by Jack Copeland, no date, Smithsonian Institution, NMAH, Accession file 87.0474.

267. Marsha F. Goldsmith, "Silver Anniversary Celebrated for Penn State Heart," *JAMA* 273, no. 24 (1995): 1891–92; *The Artificial Heart: Past, Present and Future—Celebrating 25 Years at Penn State,* Symposium Brochure, 2 May 1995.

268. Associated Press, "U.S. Will End Artificial Heart Research Funds," *Los Angeles Times,* 12 May 1988, 1A, cited in Gil, "Artificial Heart Juggernaut," 27.

269. Robert Bartlett, "Commentary," in *50 Years of Artificial Organs from Discovery to Clinical Use: Annotated Reproductions of the 25 Landmark Papers,* ed. Robert H. Bartlett and Shelley McKellar (Boca Raton, FL: ASAIO, 2004), 39; Robert Bartlett, personal communication, 22 Jul 2014.

270. Peer Portner, "Commentary" (unpublished), intended for *50 Years of Artificial Organs,* submitted to S. McKellar on 3 May 2004.

271. L. D. Joyce et al., "Response of the Human Body to the First Permanent Implant of the Jarvik-7 Total Artificial Heart," *Trans ASAIO* 29, no. 1 (Apr 1983): 81–87.

272. Fox and Swazey, *Spare Parts,* 208, 210.

273. Peer Portner, "Commentary."

274. Dorothy Nelkin, *Selling Science: How the Press Covers Science and Technology* (New York: W. H. Freeman, 1987), 52.

275. Gil, "Artificial Heart Juggernaut," 24.

276. Jarvik interview, 4 Aug 1986, NLM.

277. See Gil, "Artificial Heart Juggernaut," 28.

278. In 1985, the FDA awarded IDE approval for the clinical use of the pneumatic Penn State TAH for six patients to be implanted by Pierce's team as a BTT at Penn State's Hershey Medical Center. See J. A. Magovern et al., "Bridge to Heart Transplantation: The Penn State Experience," *JHT* 5, no. 3 (1986): 196–202; "2nd Such Device to Be Licensed: 'Penn State Heart' Implanted 1st Time," *Los Angeles Times,* 18 Oct 1985; "Inventor of New Artificial Heart Is Pleased with Its Performance," *NYT,* 24 Oct 1985; Lawrence K. Altman, "Penn State Medical Team Is Ready to Implant 6 Mechanical Hearts," *NYT,* 23 Mar 1985.

279. Mark Roth, "Doctors Elated by Luck of No Strokes," *Pittsburgh Post-Gazette,* 4 Nov 1985, 16.

280. The Unger heart, also known as the "Ellipsoidheart," was designed by Dr. Felix Unger, who spent two years (1974–75) working in Willem Kolff's lab at the University of Utah and afterward continued his work at the Cardiac Surgery Center in Salzburg, Austria. The Berlin TAH was developed by cardiac surgeon Emil S. Büecherl, who led the German artificial heart program and performed the first TAH implant operation in Germany in 1986. F. Unger et al., "Artificial Heart and Cardiac Transplantation: Report on the First European Combined Procedure," *Art Org* 12, no. 1 (1988): 51–55; Felix Unger, "Current Status and Use of Artificial Hearts and Circulatory Assist Devices," *Perfusion* 1 (1986): 155–63; "New Artificial Heart Is Tried," *NYT,* 16 Dec 1986; E. S. Büecherl, "The Artificial Heart Research Program in Berlin, Germany," *JHT* 4, no. 5 (Sep–Oct 1985): 510–17; R. Hetzer and E. Hennig,

"Mechanical Circulatory Support: The Berlin Heart Goes on and on . . . ," *European Heart Journal* 34, no. 35 (Sep 2013): 2720–21.

281. Gary M. Cole to William DeVries, 5 Aug 1991, William C. DeVries Papers, NLM, HMD, MS C 588, box 7, folder 8; Symbion News Release, 2 Aug 1991, ibid.

282. In 2001 CardioWest Technologies Inc. was acquired by SynCardia Systems Inc., a company formed by Jack Copeland, biomedical engineer Richard G. Smith, and Dr. Marvin J. Slepian to commercialize the SynCardia–CardioWest total artificial heart. In 2004 the FDA granted PMA status to the SynCardia heart for bridge-to-transplantation use. It remains the only commercially available total artificial heart on the market in the United States, Canada, and Europe. DeVries interview, 10 Aug 2010, NLM; Jack Copeland et al., "The CardioWest Total Artificial Heart Bridge to Transplantation: 1993 to 1996 National Trial," *Ann Thorac Surg* 66, no. 5 (Nov 1998): 1662–69.

283. David J. Rothman, *Beginnings Count: The Technological Imperative in American Health Care* (New York: Oxford University Press, 1997), 4.

Chapter 5 · Clinical and Commercial Rewards

Epigraph: Philip E. Oyer et al., "Development of a Totally Implantable, Electrically Actuated Left Ventricular Assist System," *AJS* 140 (Jul 1980): 25.

1. See Robert H. Bartlett, "Extracorporeal Life Support: Gibbon Fulfilled," *J Am Coll Surg* 218, no. 3 (Mar 2014): 317–27.

2. P. L. Allison et al., "Devices and Monitoring during Neonatal ECMO: Survey Results," *Perfusion* 5, no. 3 (1990): 193–201.

3. See C. S. Almond et al., "Berlin Heart EXCOR Pediatric Ventricular Assist Device Investigational Device Exemption Study: Study Design and Rationale," *Am Heart J* 162, no. 3 (Sep 2011): 425–35.

4. For more on the concept of a "niche construction," see David S. Jones, "Surgical Practice and the Reconstruction of the Therapeutic Niche: The Case of Myocardial Revascularization," in *Technological Change in Modern Surgery: Historical Perspectives on Innovation,* ed. Thomas Schlich and Christopher Crenner (Rochester, NY: University of Rochester Press, 2017), 185–225.

5. O. H. Frazier, John M. Fuqua, and David N. Helman, "Clinical Left Heart Assist Devices: A Historical Perspective," in *Cardiac Assist Devices,* ed. Daniel J. Goldstein and Mehmet C. Oz (Armonk, NY: Futura, 2000), 6; Frank D. Altieri and John T. Watson, "Implantable Ventricular Assist Systems," *Art Org* 11, no. 3 (1987): 237–38.

6. Peter Frommer to DHVD Associate Director for Cardiology, 17 May 1976, memorandum, NLM, HMD, John Watson Papers, Accession 2003-054, box 5; Report of the Cardiology Advisory Committee, Mechanically Assisted Circulation—The Status of the NHLBI Program and Recommendations for the Future, May 1977, ibid.

7. P. M. Portner, "Permanent Mechanical Circulatory Assistance," in *Heart and Lung Transplantation,* ed. W. A. Baumgartner et al., 2nd ed. (Philadelphia: W. B. Saunders, 2002), 534.

8. Financial History of NHLBI Circulatory Assist/Artificial Heart Program, 23 Jan 1986, NLM, HMD, John Watson Papers, Accession 2003-054, box 5; Deborah P. Lubeck and John P. Bunker, "The Artificial Heart Cost, Risks, and Benefits," in *Background Paper #2: Case Studies of Medical Technologies: The Implications of Cost-Effectiveness Analysis of Medical Technology* (Washington, DC: US GPO, 1982), 14.

9. Request for Proposal: Left Heart Assist Blood Pumps, 1977, DHHS, NIH-NHLBI; Request for Proposal: Development of Electrical Energy Converters to Power and Control

Left Heart Assist Devices, 1977, ibid.; Request for Proposal: Development of an Implantable Integrated Electrically Powered Left Heart Assist System, 1980, ibid.; Frazier, Fuqua, and Helman, "Clinical Left Heart Assist Devices," 6.

10. Victor Poirier, Project Bionics Pioneer Interview, 2 Feb 2012, NLM, HMD.

11. "New Balloon Pump for Cardiac Therapy," *Health Services and Mental Health Administration Health Reports* 86, no. 4 (Apr 1971): 327–29; Igor Gregoric and Christian A. Bermudez, "Current Types of Devices for Mechanical Circulatory Support," in *Mechanical Circulatory Support: A Companion to Braunwald's Heart Disease,* ed. Robert L. Kormos and Leslie W. Miller (Philadelphia: Saunders, 2012), 106–8.

12. The Penn State Heart, n.d., PSU, Special Collections Library, PSUA 435, Milton S. Hershey Medical Center Records, box 10, folder PS Heart Media Packet.

13. William S. Pierce et al., "Complete Left Ventricular Bypass with a Paracorporeal Pump: Design and Evaluation," *Ann Surg* 180, no. 4 (Oct 1974): 418–26.

14. Wayne E. Richenbacher and William S. Pierce, "Assisted Circulation and the Mechanical Heart," in *Heart Disease: A Textbook of Cardiovascular Medicine,* ed. Eugene Braunwald, 5th ed. (Philadelphia: W. B. Saunders, 1997).

15. Pierce et al., "Complete Left Ventricular Bypass," 426 (discussion).

16. Penn State Ventricular Assist Device and Artificial Heart, PSU.

17. William S. Pierce et al., "Prolonged Mechanical Support of the Left Ventricle," *Circulation* 58, no. 3 Pt2 (Sep 1978): I133–I146.

18. William S. Pierce et al., "Ventricular-Assist Pumping in Patients with Cardiogenic Shock after Cardiac Operations," *NEJM* 305, no. 27 (1981): 1606–10; William S. Pierce, "Artificial Hearts and Blood Pumps in the Treatment of Profound Heart Failure, *Circulation* 68, no. 4 (1983): 883–88.

19. William S. Pierce and John L. Myers, "Left Ventricular Assist Pumps and the Artificial Heart," *J Cardiov Med* 6, no. 7 (1981): 667.

20. Peer M. Portner, "Economics of Devices," *Ann Thorac Surg* 71 (2001): S199.

21. See Victor Poirier, "The Quest for the Permanent LVAD: We Must Continue, We Must Push Forward," *Trans ASAIO* 36 (1990): 787; J. T. Watson, "The Present and Future of Cardiac Assist Devices," *Art Org* 9 (1985): 138–43.

22. "Company Developing 'Family' of Devices for Heart Patients," *American Medical News* (7 Jan 1983), Worcester Polytechnic Institute, Gordon Library, MS 66 Robert J. Harvey Collection, box 10, folder 9.

23. "Growth Markets: Biomaterials," *In Vivo* 5 (1982): 41, Worcester Polytechnic Institute, Gordon Library, MS 66 Robert J. Harvey Collection, box 10, folder 9.

24. Ibid.; Michael Shanley, "Of Miracle Berries, Second Skins and Plastic Hearts: The Rise and Fall and Rise of Dr Robert J Harvey '70 PhD," *Worcester Polytechnic Institute Journal* (Aug 1985): 21–22.

25. See Jeffrey L. Covell, "Thoratec Corporation," in *International Directory of Company Histories,* ed. Jay P. Pederson (Detroit: St. James Press, 2011), 122:447, 448.

26. Statistics taken from "New Heart, New Hopes," *Nursing Mirror* (21 Jun 1979): 24; American Heart Association, "Heart Disease and Stroke Statistics—2010 Update," *Circulation* 121, no. 7 (23 Feb 2010): e46–e215. See also "First Year of Cardiac Transplantation," *BMJ* (11 Jan 1969): 66; Thomas Thompson, "A New and Disquieting Look at Transplant: The Year They Changed Hearts," *Life,* 17 Sep 1971, 56–70.

27. J. Donald Hill, "Use of a Prosthetic Ventricle as a Bridge to Cardiac Transplantation for Postinfarction Cardiogenic Shock," *NEJM* 314, no. 10 (6 Mar 1986): 626–28.

28. D. J. Farrar et al., "Heterotopic Prosthetic Ventricles as a Bridge-to-Cardiac Transplantation: A Multicenter Study in 29 Patients," *NEJM* 318 (1988): 333–40; D. G. Pennington et al., "Use of the Pierce-Donachy Ventricular Assist Device in Patients with Cardiogenic Shock after Cardiac Operations," *Ann Thorac Surg* 47 (1989): 130–35; D. G. Pennington et al., "Eight Years' Experience with Bridging to Cardiac Transplantation," *JTCS* 107 (1994): 472–80; Demetrios Mavroidis, Benjamin C. Sun, and Walter E. Pae Jr., "Bridge to Transplantation: The Penn State Experience," *Ann Thorac Surg* 68, no. 2 (Aug 1999): 684–87.

29. See Lawrence R. McBride et al., "Clinical Experience with 111 Thoratec Ventricular Assist Devices," *Ann Thorac Surg* 67 (1999): 1233–39; Areo Saffarzadeh and Pramod Bonde, "Options for Temporary Mechanical Circulatory Support," *Journal of Thoracic Disease* 7, no. 12 (December 2015): 2102–11.

30. T. B. Icenogle et al., "Thromboembolic Complications of the Symbion AVAD System," *Art Org* 13, no. 6 (Dec 1989): 532–38; S. Lick et al., "Long-term Bridge to Transplantation with the Symbion Acute Ventricular Assist Device System," *Ann Thorac Surg* 52, no. 2 (Aug 1991): 308–9.

31. Portner, "Economics of Devices," S200.

32. P. M. Portner et al., "An Intrathoracic Solenoid Drive System for Chronic Left Ventricular Bypass," *Trans ASAIO* 22 (1976): 297–314.

33. P. M. Portner et al., "Evolution of the Solenoid-Actuated Left Ventricular Assist System: Integration with a Pusher-Plate Pump for Intra-Abdominal Implantation in the Calf," *Art Org* 2, no. 4 (1978): 402–12; P. M. Portner et al., "An Implantable Permanent Left Ventricular Assist System for Man," *Trans ASAIO* 24 (1978): 98–103.

34. Portner, "Economics of Devices," S200.

35. Oyer et al., "Development of Left Ventricular Assist System," 23.

36. Portner, "Implantable Permanent Left Ventricular System," 99–103; Oyer et al., "Development of Left Ventricular Assist System," 17–25.

37. V. A. Starnes et al., "Isolated Left Ventricular Assist as Bridge to Cardiac Transplantation," *JTCS* 96, no. 1 (Jul 1988): 62–71; P. M. Portner et al., "Implantable Electrical Left Ventricular Assist System: Bridge to Transplantation and the Future," *Ann Thorac Surg* 47, no. 1 (1989): 142–50.

38. Stanford University Medical Center Press Release, 18 Feb 1987, SU, Special Collections and University Archives, Norman Shumway Project (V0222), 2005-246, box 6, vol. 2.

39. Nicholas T Kouchoukos et al., *Kirklin/Barratt-Boyes Cardiac Surgery,* 4th ed. (Philadelphia: Elsevier Saunders, 2013), 880.

40. Starnes et al., "Isolated Left Ventricular Assist," 62–71; P. M. Portner et al., "Improved Outcomes with an Implantable Left Ventricular Assist System: A Multicenter Study," *Ann Thorac Surg* 71, no. 1 (2001): 205–9.

41. "10 Bay Area Leaders to Watch [D Keith Grossman, Thoratec Corp]," *Wall Street Journal Sunday Times,* 29 Dec 2002, section G, p. 1, Worcester Polytechnic Institute, Gordon Library, MS 66 Robert J. Harvey Collection, box 11, folder 11.

42. Starnes et al., "Isolated Left Ventricular Assist," 69.

43. Norman E. Shumway, Lecture to Community Hospital of Monterey Peninsula, 28 Jan 1978, SU, Special Collections and University Archives, Norman Shumway Project (V0222), box 6, vol. 3; Stanford Medical Center Press Release, 18 Feb 1987, SU; Stanford Medical Forum, 18 Nov 1992, SU, Special Collections and University Archives, Norman Shumway Project (V0222), box 6, vol. 3; Norman Shumway interview, 16 Oct 1997, William

S. Stoney Collection, Vanderbilt University Medical Center, Eskind Biomedical Library Special Collections, Collection no. 241, box 01A, folder 31.

44. Michael G. McGee et al., "Extended Clinical Support with an Implantable Left Ventricular Assist Device," *Trans ASAIO* 35 (1989): 614–16.

45. Quote taken from Mark S. Slaughter, "Bud Frazier's 1,000th Implantation of a Ventricular Assist Device," *THI Journal* 41, no. 2 (2014): 110. See also Eric A. Rose, "Bud Frazier Has Pioneered Mechanical Circulatory Support," *THI Journal* 41, no. 2 (2014): 109; O. H. Frazier, "Mechanical Circulatory Assist Device Development at the Texas Heart Institute: A Personal Perspective," *JTCS* 147, no. 6 (Jun 2014): 1738–44.

46. J. C. Norman et al., "Intracorporeal (Abdominal) Left Ventricular Assist Devices or Partial Artificial Hearts: A Five-Year Clinical Experience," *Arch Surg* 116 (1981): 1441–45, cited in Frazier, "Mechanical Circulatory Assist Device," 1738.

47. In 1983 Thermo formed Thermedics Inc. as a public company to continue developing VADs, and in 1989 Thermedics became Thermo Cardiosystems Inc. HeartMate: More Than a Medical Marvel [company literature], NLM, HMD, John Watson Papers, Accession 2003-054, box 27; Portner, "Economics of Devices," S200.

48. Victor Poirier stated that the reason for developing two different power sources was cost; electric systems were much costlier than the simpler pneumatic systems. Poirier interview, 2 Feb 2012, NLM; Jonathan B. Welch, "Heart, Soul and Cash at Thermo Cardiosystems, Inc.," unpublished case study, 2001, Smithsonian Institution, NMAH, Division of Medicine and Science, Artificial Heart vertical files.

49. Poirier, "Quest for the Permanent LVAD," 788; V. L. Poirier et al., "An Ambulatory, Intermediate Term Left Ventricular Assist System for Man," *Trans ASAIO* 35 (1989): 452–55.

50. W. F. Bernard et al., "A New Method of Temporary Left Ventricular Bypass," *JTCS* 70 (1975): 880; J. C. Norman et al., "An Intracorporeal (Abdominal) Left Ventricular Assist Device," *Arch Surg* 112 (1977): 1142; McGee et al., "Extended Clinical Support," 614–16.

51. Frazier, "Mechanical Circulatory Assist Device," 1739; O. H. Frazier, Project Bionics Pioneer Interview, 18 Jul 2013, NLM, HMD.

52. I thank Dr. Robert Bartlett for explaining FDA involvement in the commercialization stage of new devices and translational biomedical device research. Personal communication, 12 Aug 2012.

53. Robin Roberts Bostic and Tina Ommaya Ivovic, "Reimbursement and Funding Framework for Medical Circulatory Support," in *Mechanical Circulatory Support: A Companion to Braunwald's Heart Disease,* ed. Robert L. Kormos and Leslie W. Miller (Philadelphia: Saunders, 2012), 324.

54. Aaron V. Kaplan et al., "Medical Device Development: From Prototype to Regulatory Approval," *Circulation* 109 (2004): 3068–72; Carl Heneghan and Mathew Thompson, "Rethinking Medical Device Regulation," *Journal of the Royal Society of Medicine* 105 (2012): 186; Richard S. Stack and Robert A. Harrington, "Biomedical Innovation: A Risky Business at Risk," *Social Translational Medicine* 3, no. 96 (Aug 2011): 1–4; Christa Altenstetter, "EU and Member State Medical Devices Regulation," *International Journal of Technology Assessment in Health Care* 19, no. 1 (2003): 228–48.

55. See Health Canada, "Safe Medical Devices in Canada," at www.hc-sc.gc.ca, accessed 12 Jun 2013.

56. J. L. Pennock et al., "Cardiac Transplantation in Perspective for the Future: Survival, Complications, Rehabilitation, and Cost," *JTCS* 83, no. 2 (Feb 1982): 168–77.

57. The First International Congress on Cyclosporine: May 16–19, 1983, Houston, Texas, *Transplantation Proceedings* 15, suppl. 1–2 (1983): 2207–3187; Daniel J. Goldstein, Mehmet C. Oz, and Eric A. Rose, "Implantable Left Ventricular Assist Devices," *NEJM* 339, no. 21 (19 Nov 1998): 1522.

58. Lyle Joyce et al., "Mechanical Circulatory Support—A Historical Review," *ASAIO J* 50, no. 6 (Mar–Apr 2004): xi.

59. "Company Developing 'Family' of Devices," Worcester Polytechnic Institute, Gordon Library; "Half a Heart: Thoratec's Artificial Heart Parts," *Fortune,* 27 Dec 1982; Harold M. Schmeck Jr., "Artificial Heart Research Now Seeks a Portable and 'Forgettable' Device," *NYT,* 6 Dec 1982; "Pushing Back Medical Frontiers," *Venture,* Jun 1982, 42–44.

60. Portner, "Economics of Devices," S199.

61. Pierce, "Artificial Hearts and Blood Pumps," 883–88; Adrian Kantrowitz, "Early Mechanical Left Ventricular Assistance," *ASAIO J* (1993): 834–39; S. Westaby et al., "First Permanent Implant of the Jarvik 2000 Heart," *Lancet* 356, no. 9233 (9 Sep 2000): 900–903.

62. Portner, "Economics of Devices," S201.

63. See Laura E. Bothwell and Scott H. Podolsky, "The Emergence of the Randomized, Clinical Trial," *NEJM* 375, no. 6 (11 Aug 2016): 501–4; Laura E. Bothwell et al., "Assessing the Gold Standard—Lessons from the History of RCTs," *NEJM* 374, no. 22 (2 Jun 2016): 2175–81.

64. Harry M. Marks, *The Progress of Experiment: Science and Therapeutic Reform in the United States, 1900–1990* (New York: Cambridge University Press, 1997); Susan Lederer, *Subjected to Science: Human Experimentation in America before the Second World War* (Baltimore: Johns Hopkins University Press, 1995); Kenneth Stanley, "Design of Randomized Controlled Trials," *Circulation* 115 (6 Mar 2007): 1164–69; David S. Jones, "Visions of a Cure: Visualization, Clinical Trials, and Controversies in Cardiac Therapeutics, 1968–1998," *Isis* 91 (2000): 504–41; Marcia Meldrum, "Departures from the Design: The Randomized Clinical Trial in Historical Context, 1946–1970" (PhD diss., State University of New York at Stony Brook, 1994); Scott H. Podolsky, "Antibiotics and the Social History of the Controlled Clinical Trial, 1950–1970," *Journal of the History of Medicine and Allied Sciences* 65, no. 3 (Jul 2010): 327–67.

65. As Christopher Crenner states, the case series "proved both practical and influential and remains, with subsequent refinements, a mainstay of the surgical scientific literature." Christopher Crenner, "Placebos and the Progress of Surgery," in *Technological Change in Modern Surgery: Historical Perspectives on Innovation,* ed. Thomas Schlich and Christopher Crenner (Rochester, NY: University of Rochester Press, 2017), 157.

66. See R. S. McLeod, "Issues in Surgical Randomized Clinical Trials," *World Journal of Surgery* 23 (1999): 1210–14; N. S. Abraham, "Will the Dilemma of Evidence-Based Surgery Ever Be Resolved?," *Australian and New Zealand Journal of Surgery* 76 (2006): 855–60. Possible solutions to surgical RCT challenges are discussed in Lynne Warner Stevenson and Robert L. Kormos, "Mechanical Cardiac Support 2000: Current Applications and Future Trial Design," *J Am Coll Cardio* 37, no. 1 (2001): 340–70; Forough Farrokhyar et al., "Randomized Clinical Trials of Surgical Interventions," *Ann Surg* 251, no. 3 (March 2010): 409–16; Jeffrey S. Barkun et al., "Evaluation and Stages of Surgical Innovations," *Lancet* 374 (26 Sep 2009): 1089–96; Patrick L. Ergina et al., "Challenges in Evaluating Surgical Innovation," *Lancet* 374 (26 Sep 2009): 1097–1104; Nuh N. Rahbari et al., "Development and Perspectives of Randomized Clinical Trials in Surgery," *AJS* 194, suppl. (Oct 2007): S148–S152.

67. David S. Jones, *Broken Hearts: The Tangled History of Cardiac Care* (Baltimore: Johns Hopkins University Press, 2013).

68. Jones, "Visions of a Cure," 523, 529; see also John H. Alexander and Eric D. Peterson, "Translating Trials to Clinical Practice in Cardiac Surgery," *Nature Reviews* 10 (Jun 2013): 306–7.

69. Stevenson and Kormos, "Mechanical Cardiac Support 2000," 343; Eric A. Rose et al., "The REMATCH Trial: Rationale, Design and End Points," *Ann Thorac Surg* 67 (1999): 724.

70. O. H. Frazier et al., "Improved Mortality and Rehabilitation of Transplant Candidates Treated with a Long-Term Implantable Left Ventricular Assist System," *Ann Surg* 222, no. 3 (Sep 1995): 327–38.

71. Frazier, "Mechanical Circulatory Assist Device," 1739; O. H. Frazier, "First Use of an Untethered, Vented Electric Left Ventricular Assist Device for Long-Term Support," *Circulation* 89 (1994): 2908–14.

72. Frazier et al., "Improved Mortality and Rehabilitation," 334–35; O. H. Frazier et al., "Multicenter Clinical Evaluation of the Heart Mate 1000 IP Left Ventricular Assist Device, *Ann Thorac Surg* 53 (1992): 1080–90.

73. Portner et al., "Implantable Electrical Left Ventricular Assist System," 142–50; Pennington et al., "Eight Years' Experience," 472–81.

74. Frazier et al., "Improved Mortality and Rehabilitation," 333; David J. Farrar and J. Donald Hill, "Univentricular and Biventricular Thoratec VAD Support as a Bridge to Transplantation," *Ann Thorac Surg* 55 (1993): 279; M. M. Levinson et al., "Thromboembolic Complications of the Jarvik-7 Total Artificial Heart: Case Report," *Art Org* 10 (1986): 236; Portner, "Permanent Mechanical Circulatory Assistance," 545–46.

75. Frazier et al., "Improved Mortality and Rehabilitation," 334–35. See also Frazer et al., "Multicenter Clinical Evaluation," 1080–90.

76. Frazier et al., "Improved Mortality and Rehabilitation," 337.

77. Application submitted by Thermo Cardiosystems Inc. on 3/30/1992 and approved 9/30/1994, US FDA Premarket Approval (PMA) database for the HeartMate LVAD, www.accessdata.fda.gov.

78. D. Glenn Pennington et al., "Eleven Years' Experience with the Pierce-Donachy Ventricular Assist Device," *JHLT* 13 (1994): 803–10; Pennington et al., "Eight Years' Experience," 472–81; R. C. Robbins et al., "Bridge to Transplant with the Novacor Left Ventricular Assist System," *Ann Thorac Surg* 68 (1999): 695–97; D. R. Wheeldon et al., "The Novacor Electrical Implantable Left Ventricular Assist System," *Perfusion* 15 (2000): 355–61.

79. Mark S. Slaughter et al., "Results of a Multicenter Clinical Trial with the Thoratec Implantable Ventricular Assist Device," *JTCS* 133, no. 6 (Jun 2007): 1578.

80. Application submitted by Thoratec Corporation Inc. on 11/24/1987 and approved 12/20/1995, US FDA Premarket Approval database for the Thoratec PVAD, www.accessdata.fda.gov.

81. The Thoratec IVAD was an implantable version of the paracorporeal PVAD. It worked in the same manner, but the IVAD pump was smaller in size and weight and was positioned in the patient's chest cavity. The FDA awarded premarket approval for the IVAD in 2004. Thoratec Company website, www.thoratec.com, accessed 19 Jul 2012; US FDA Premarket Approval database for the Thoratec IVAD, www.accessdata.fda.gov.

82. D. Loisance et al., "Bridge to Transplantation with the Wearable Novacor Left Ventricular Assist System: Operative Technique," *European Journal of Cardiothoracic Surgery* 9 (1995): 95–98; H. O. Vetter et al., "Experience with the Novacor Left Ventricular Assist System as a Bridge to Transplantation, Including the New Wearable System," *JTCS* 109 (1995): 74–80.

83. Vetter et al., "Experience with the Novacor," 74–80; Application submitted by Novacor Inc. on 04/24/1998 and approved 9/29/1998, US FDA Premarket Approval database for the Novacor LVAS, www.accessdata.fda.gov.

84. Pierce, "Prolonged Mechanical Support," 1133–1146; Portner et al., "Implantable Permanent Left Ventricular System," 99–103; Victor Poirier, "The LVAD: A Case Study," *Bridge* 27, no. 4 (Winter 1997): 14–20.

85. Portner, "Economics of Devices," S199.

86. John T. Watson, "Food and Drug Administration Guidance Sections: A New Paradigm for Medical Devices," *ASAIO J* 40, no. 2 (Apr–Jun 1994): 138–44.

87. Quote by Poirier taken from David Stipp, "New Hope for the Heart," *Fortune* 133, no. 12 (24 Jun 1996): 108; see also Lawrence D. Maloney, "An Engineer for the Long Haul," *Design News* (10 Feb 1992): 66–76.

88. Portner, "Economics of Devices," S199.

89. Poirier, "LVAD," 19.

90. Portner, "Economics of Devices," S200. Details related to WorldHeart's product lines and acquisitions are also taken from "Company History" and "Milestones" pages on WorldHeart's company webpage, www.worldheart.com, accessed 25 Jan 2006.

91. The WorldHeart Corporation was founded in 1996 by Ottawa businessman Rod Bryden, who was dismissed in 2004 after failing to improve dismal company finances. See "Bryden Out at WorldHeart," *Ottawa Business Journal,* 28 Jul 2004. For information on the HeartSaver VAD, see Paul J. Hendry et al., "The HeartSaver Left Ventricular Assist Device: An Update," *Ann Thorac Surg* 71 (2001): S166–S170.

92. "WorldHeart Buys MedQuest Products," *San Francisco Business Times,* 31 Jan 2005.

93. "WorldHeart Will End Its Levacor(R) VAD Program and Will Focus on Developing Its Next-Generation MiFlow(TM) Miniature Ventricular Assist Device," WorldHeart Press Release, 29 Jul 2011, at www.worldheart.com.

94. This pattern of device company mergers and acquisitions was not unique to the Novacor LVAS. In 1982 Richard Wampler cofounded the Nimbus Corporation to develop the Hemopump; the firm was acquired in 1996 by Thermo Cardiosystems Inc., which in turn was acquired in 2001 by the Thoratec Corporation, which now owned this technology and applied aspects of it to its new HeartMate II pump. See Portner, "Economics of Devices," S200; Watson, "Present and Future," 138–43.

95. Alan S. Go et al., "Heart Disease and Stroke Statistics—2013 Update: A Report from the American Heart Association," *Circulation* 127 (2013): 143–52; J. Lopez-Sendon, "The Heart Failure Epidemic," *Medicographia* 33, no. 4 (2011): 363–69; "History Failure Fact Sheet," CDC, Division for Heart Disease and Stroke Prevention, www.cdc.gov, accessed 13 Jun 2013.

96. Covell, "Thoratec Corporation," 122:448.

97. Thoratec Laboratories Corporation, US Securities and Exchange Commission Form S-3, filed April 12, 2000, www.nasdaq.com.

98. By 2013 the Thoratec Corporation was selling four different mechanical circulatory support systems (CentriMag, PediVAS, Thoratec PVAD, and HeartMate II LVAD), to dominate the LVAD global market with a reported 50 percent share of the European market and a 75 percent share of the American market. Contributing to Thoratec's market dominance was its acquisition of competing technology, notably the HeartMate technology from Thermo Cardiosystems Inc. in 2001 for $572 million and the DuraHeart II ventricular assist system from Terumo Corporation in 2013 for $13 million. See "A Merger of 2 Medical Device

Makers," *NYT,* 4 Oct 2000, C10; "Heart Pump Wars Intensify as Thoratec Buys DuraHeart II," 2 Jul 2013, www.epvantage.com; Thoratec Corporation company website, www.thoratec .com.

99. Thoratec Commercial Literature available at www.thoratec.com, accessed 11 Jun 2013.

100. Bostic and Ivovic, "Reimbursement and Funding Framework," 324.

101. See National Coverage Determination for Artificial Hearts and Related Devices (20.9), Centers for Medicare and Medicaid Services, available online at www.cms.gov, accessed 5 Jun 2016.

102. See "The Increasing Use of Ventricular Assist Devices Will Drive Cardiac Assist Device Market Growth in Europe," 11 Aug 2015, at https://decisionresourcesgroup.com.

Chapter 6 · Securing a Place

Epigraph: Susan Page, "Taciturn Cheney Can't Stop Talking about Heart Device," *USA Today,* 31 Aug 2011.

1. See Dick Cheney and Jonathan Reiner, *Heart: An American Medical Odyssey* (New York: Scribner, 2013).

2. Ibid., 270–71.

3. "Cheney Recuperating from Heart Surgery," *Wash Post,* 14 Jul 2010; David Brown, "Pumps like Cheney's Can Extend Lives of Patients with Congestive Heart Failure," *Wash Post,* 16 Jul 2010.

4. Lawrence K. Altman, "Cheney File Traces Heart Care Milestones," *NYT,* 24 Apr 2012.

5. "Dick Cheney Speaks about Heart Troubles," *CNN: The Situation Room with Wolf Blitzer,* 6 Sep 2011; "Dick Cheney on 'Today': I May Need a Heart Transplant," *NBC Nightly News with Jamie Gangel,* 18 Jan 2011.

6. Page, "Taciturn Cheney."

7. Lawrence K. Altman and Denise Gray, "For Cheney, Pros and Cons in New Heart," *NYT,* 26 Mar 2012.

8. Cheney and Reiner, *Heart,* 273, 300.

9. Ibid., 278.

10. Ibid., 305.

11. Ibid., 303.

12. There were jokes made about Cheney not having a heart before his transplant and about Cheney acquiring new and quite different personality traits as a result of his donor heart, among other jabs. For example, see Ann Oldenburg, "Joan Rivers, Others Joke about Dick Cheney Heart Transplant," *USA Today,* 25 Mar 2012; Michael Posner, "Dick Cheney's Amazing Change of Heart," *Toronto Globe and Mail,* 1 Nov 2013.

13. See M. V. Badiwala, "Left Ventricular Device as Destination Therapy: Are We There Yet?," *Current Opinion in Cardiology* 24, no. 2 (Mar 2009): 184–89; M. G. McGee et al., "Extended Support with a Left Ventricular Assist Device as a Bridge to Heart Transplantation," *Trans ASAIO* 37, no. 3 (Jul–Sep 1991): M425–M426; K. R. Kanter et al., "Bridging to Cardiac Transplantation with Pulsatile Ventricular Assist Devices," *Ann Thorac Surg* 46, no. 2 (Aug 1988): 134–40.

14. Christopher Crenner, "Placebos and the Progress of Surgery," in *Technological Change in Modern Surgery: Historical Perspectives on Innovation,* ed. Thomas Schlich and Christopher Crenner (Rochester, NY: University of Rochester Press, 2017), 136, 177.

15. Ursula Maria Schmidt-Ott et al., "Challenges in Conducting Implantable Device Trials: Left Ventricular Assist Devices in Destination Therapy," in *Clinical Evaluation of*

Medical Devices: Principles and Case Studies, ed. K. M. Becker and J. Whyte, 2nd ed. (Totowa, NJ: Humana Press, 2006): 202–3.

16. "HeartMate VE LVAS," US FDA PMA Database, www.accessdata.fda.gov, accessed 29 Oct 2014; Eric A. Rose et al., "The REMATCH Trial: Rationale, Design and End Points," *Ann Thorac Surg* 67 (1999): 725.

17. Schmidt-Ott et al., "Challenges in Conducting Trials," 202–3.

18. The cost of the REMATCH trial was approximately $25 million. The Thoratec Corporation, as a partial sponsor, contributed $3.6 million plus all necessary LVADs and related equipment (approximately $60,000 each). US Securities and Exchange Commission Form 10-K, submitted by the Thoratec Corporation for the fiscal year ended December 29, 2001, at www.sec.gov; Schmidt-Ott et al., "Challenges in Conducting Trials," 205; Eric A. Rose et al., "Long-Term Use of a Left Ventricular Assist Device for End-Stage Heart Failure," *NEJM* 345, no. 20 (Nov 2001): 1436.

19. Rose et al., "Long-Term Use," 1435–43.

20. See R. D. Dowling et al., "HeartMate VE LVAS Design Enhancements and Its Impact on Device Reliability," *European Journal of Cardio-Thoracic Surgery* 25, no. 6 (2004): 958–63.

21. Ibid.

22. Rose et al., "Long-Term Use," 1438–39.

23. Ibid., 1440–41.

24. According to David Jones, heart surgeons and neurologists collaborated to document how cardiac surgery caused neurological and psychiatric complications in patients; however, in the 1990s, inattention to these issues was common. While neurological dysfunction was noted by artificial heart specialists, there was more concern expressed for infections, bleeding, and thromboembolic complications presenting in artificial heart recipients. See David S. Jones, *Broken Hearts: The Tangled History of Cardiac Care* (Baltimore: Johns Hopkins University Press, 2013).

25. Schmidt-Ott et al., "Challenges in Conducting Trials," 212.

26. J. W. Long et al., "Long-Term Destination Therapy with the HeartMate XVE Left Ventricular Assist Device: Improved Outcomes since the REMATCH Study," *Congestive Heart Failure* 11, no. 3 (May–Jun 2005): 133–38.

27. Rose et al., "Long-Term Use," 1442.

28. Schmidt-Ott et al., "Challenges in Conducting Trials," 211.

29. Rose et al., "Long-Term Use," 1435–43.

30. At this time, the one-year survival rate of cardiac transplant patients was more than 80 percent and the 10-year survival rate was nearly 50 percent. Taken from Rose et al., "Long-Term Use," 1442.

31. "The [REMATCH] trial was analogous to randomizing Titanic patients to a lifeboat or the sea," stated Stephen Westaby at the American Association for Thoracic Surgery meeting in Boston, Massachusetts, May 4–7, 2003. Soon J. Park et al., "Left Ventricular Assist Devices as Destination Therapy: A New Look at Survival," *JTCS* 129, no. 1 (Jan 2005): 16; Stephen Westaby, "Ventricular Assist Devices as Destination Therapy," *Surgical Clinics of North America* 84, no. 1 (Feb 2004): 91–123.

32. Robert O. Bonow et al., eds., *Braunwald's Heart Disease,* 9th ed. (Philadelphia: Elsevier/ Saunders, 2012), 619; Robert L. Kormos and Leslie W. Miller, eds., *Mechanical Circulatory Support: A Companion to Braunwald's Heart Disease* (Philadelphia: Elsevier/Saunders, 2012), 272.

33. Lynne Warner Stevenson, "Left Ventricular Assist Devices as Destination Therapy for End-Stage Heart Failure," *Current Treatment Options in Cardiovascular Medicine* 6 (2004): 471.

34. Ibid.; Lynne Warner Stevenson, "Ventricular Assist Devices for Durable Support," *Circulation* 112 (2005): e111–e115.

35. Anju Nohria, Eldrin Lewis, and Lynne Warner Stevenson, "Medical Management of Advanced Heart Failure," *JAMA* 287, no. 5 (6 Feb 2002): 638; Stevenson, "Left Ventricular Assist Devices," 471.

36. Larry A. Allen et al., "Decision Making in Advanced Heart Failure: A Scientific Statement from the American Heart Association," *Circulation* 125 (2012): 1928–52.

37. Mehmet C. Oz et al., "Left Ventricular Assist Devices as Permanent Heart Failure Therapy: The Price of Progress," *Ann Surg* 238, no. 4 (Oct 2003): 275–76.

38. Ibid., 276; Walter P. Dembitsky et al., "Left Ventricular Assist Device Performance with Long-Term Circulatory Support: Lessons from the REMATCH Trial," *Ann Thorac Surg* 78 (2004): 2128.

39. Oz et al., "Left Ventricular Assist Devices," 276.

40. Long et al., "Long-Term Destination Therapy," 138.

41. See Dembitsky et al., "Left Ventricular Assist Device Performance," 2129.

42. Barry M. Massie, "Comment—LVADs as Long-term Cardiac Replacement: Success but on What Terms and at What Cost?," *Journal of Cardiac Failure* 8, no. 2 (Apr 2002): 61.

43. Stevenson, "Left Ventricular Assist Devices," 471.

44. Massie, "Comment—LVADs," 61.

45. Mariell Jessup, "Mechanical Cardiac-Support Devices—Dreams and Devilish Details," *NEJM* 345, no. 20 (15 Nov 2001): 1490–93.

46. Alan J. Moskowitz, Eric A. Rose, and Annetine C. Geligns, "The Cost of Long-Term LVAD Implantation," *Ann Thorac Surg* 71 (2001): S198.

47. Oz et al., "Left Ventricular Assist Devices," 275, 278; Schmidt-Ott et al., "Challenges in Conducting Trials," 208; Rose et al., "Long-Term Use," 1442, table 6.

48. See A. el-Banaysy et al., "Preliminary Experience with the LionHeart Left Ventricular Assist Device in Patients with End-Stage Heart Failure," *Ann Thorac Surg* 75 (2003): 1469–75; W. E. Pae et al., "Does Total Implantability Reduce Infection with the Use of a Left Ventricular Assist Device? The LionHeart Experience in Europe," *JHLT* 26 (2007): 219–29; Katherine Lietz and Leslie W. Miller, "Will Left-Ventricular Assist Device Therapy Replace Transplantation in the Foreseeable Future?," *Current Opinion in Cardiology* 20 (2005): 133.

49. Joseph G. Rogers et al., "Chronic Mechanical Circulatory Support for Inotrope-Dependent Heart Failure Patients Who Are Not Transplant Candidates: Results of the INTrEPID Trial," *J Am Coll Cardio* 50, no. 8 (Aug 2007): 741–47.

50. Joseph G. Rogers and Francis D. Pagani, "Results of Clinical Trials to Date," in Kormos and Miller, *Mechanical Circulatory Support,* 287.

51. Lynne Warner Stevenson and Gregory Cooper, "On the Fledgling Field of Mechanical Support," *J Am Coll Cardio* 50, no. 8 (Aug 2007): 748–51. See also D. Checker, "Heart Failure: Issues and Guidelines—An Expert Interview with Lynne Warner Stevenson, MD," *Medscape Cardiology* 7, no. 2 (2003), www.medscape.org/viewarticle/462498.

52. Steve Stiles, "REMATCH: The Sickest Gain the Most from LVAD Destination Therapy," *Medscape* (16 Aug 2004), www.medscape.com/viewarticle/783205.

53. P. M. Portner, "Permanent Mechanical Circulatory Assistance," in *Heart and Lung Transplantation,* ed. W. A. Baumgartner et al., 2nd ed. (Philadelphia: W. B. Saunders, 2002), 544; J. Jassawalla et al., "Next Generation Novacor LVAS: A Miniaturized Pulsatile Pump," *ASAIO J* 45 (2000): 157; Rogers and Pagani, "Results of Clinical Trials," 287.

54. WorldHeart Corporation chose to focus its efforts on the next-generation Levacor VAD, technology rights to which it had acquired from MedQuest Products Inc. in 2005. On July 29, 2011, it announced the termination of its efforts to commercialize the Levacor VAD technology, stating that it felt the device was no longer commercially competitive. In 2012 the WorldHeart Corporation was acquired by Heart Ware International Inc. See US Securities and Exchange Commission, Form 10-K submitted by the World Heart Corporation for the fiscal year ended 31 Dec 2011, at www.sec.gov; "HeartWare Completes Acquisition of World-Heart Corporation," 2 Aug 2012, www.prnewswire.com.

55. Gideon Gil, "The Artificial Heart Juggernaut," *Hastings Center Report* 19, no. 2 (Mar–Apr 1989): 29–30.

56. Stevenson and Cooper, "Fledgling Field of Mechanical Support," 750.

57. James K. Kirklin et al., "Long-Term Mechanical Circulatory Support (Destination Therapy): On Track to Compete with Heart Transplantation?," *JTCS* 144, no. 3 (Sep 2012): 593–94; Sharon A. Hunt, "Mechanical Circulatory Support: New Data, Old Problems," *Circulation* 116 (2007): 462.

58. See Eugene Braunwald, ed., *Heart Disease: A Textbook of Cardiovascular Medicine*, 1st, 2nd, 3rd eds. (Philadelphia: W. B. Saunders, 1980, 1984, 1988).

59. Lyle Joyce et al., "Mechanical Circulatory Support—A Historical Review," *ASAIO J* 50, no. 6 (Mar–Apr 2004): xi.

60. Adrian Kantrowitz, "Origins of Intraaortic Balloon Pumping," *Ann Thorac Surg* 50, no. 4 (Oct 1990): 672–74.

61. D. Glenn Pennington and Marc T. Swartz, "Assisted Circulation and Mechanical Hearts," in *Heart Disease: A Textbook of Cardiovascular Medicine,* ed. Eugene Braunwald, 4th ed. (Philadelphia: W. B. Saunders, 1992), 538–40.

62. Richard K. Wampler et al., "In vivo Evaluation of a Peripheral Vascular Access Axial Flow Blood Pump," *ASAIO Transactions* 34 (1988): 450–54; Michael S. Sweeney, "The Hemopump in 1997: A Clinical, Political, and Marketing Evolution," *Ann Thorac Surg* 68 (1999): 761–63.

63. Kenneth C. Butler, John C. Moise, and Richard K. Wampler, "The Hemopump—A New Cardiac Prosthesis Device," *IEEE Transactions on Biomedical Engineering,* 37, no. 2 (Feb 1990): 193.

64. Robert Baldwin et al., "Management of Patients Supported on the Hemopump Cardiac Assist System," *THI Journal* 19, no. 2 (1992): 81–86.

65. Marco Caccom et al., "Current State of Ventricular Assist Devices," *Current Heart Failure Report* 8 (2011): 92.

66. I. Mandelbaum and W. H. Burns, "Pulsatile and Nonpulsatile Blood Flow," *JAMA* 191 (22 Feb 1965): 657–60; H. Wilkens et al., "The Physiological Importance of Pulsatile Blood Flow," *NEJM* 267, no. 9 (30 Aug 1962): 443–46.

67. Wilkens et al., "Physiologic Importance," 443–46; Mandelbaum and Burns, "Pulsatile and Nonpulsatile Blood Flow," 657–60.

68. I thank Dr. Robert Bartlett for drawing my attention to Bernstein's work on pulsatile blood flow. See E. F. Bernstein et al., "A Compact, Low Hemolysis, Non-Thrombogenic System for Non-Thoracotomy Prolonged Left Ventricular Bypass," *Trans ASAIO* 20B (1974): 643.

69. See Tohid Pirbodaghi et al., "Physiologic and Hematologic Concerns of Rotary Blood Pumps: What Needs to Be Improved? *Heart Failure Review* 19 (2014): 259–66.

70. O. H. Frazier, "Mechanical Circulatory Assist Device Development at the Texas Heart Institute: A Personal Perspective," *JTCS* 147, no. 6 (Jun 2014): 1740; O. H. Frazier,

Project Bionics Pioneer Interview, 18 Jul 2013, NLM, HMD; O. H. Frazier and Billy Cohn, "If You Have an Artificial Heart, Does That Make You Heartless?," lecture delivered at TED-MED 2012, an annual TED (Technology, Entertain, Design) conference focusing on health and medicine, Washington, DC, 11–13 Apr 2012; O. H. Frazier et al., "First Human Use of the Hemopump, a Catheter-Mounted Ventricular Assist Device," *Ann Thorac Surg* 49, no. 2 (Feb 1990): 299–304.

71. Caccom et al., "Current State of Ventricular Assist Devices," 92.

72. Richard K. Wampler, Project Bionics Pioneer Interview, 9 Jun 2011, NLM, HMD; Frazier, "Mechanical Circulatory Assist Device," 1741.

73. Jennifer Kerr, "Look for New Blood," *Sacramento Business Journal,* 10 Aug 2003; Bartley P. Griffith et al., "HeartMate II Left Ventricular Assist System: From Concept to First Clinical Use," *Ann Thorac Surg* 71 (2001): S116; Jeffrey L. Covell, "Thoratec Corporation," in *International Directory of Company Histories,* ed. Jay P. Pederson (Detroit: St. James Press, 2011), 122:448. After acquiring Thermo Cardiosystems Inc. in 2001, Thoratec Laboratories Corporation officially shortened its company name to Thoratec Corporation.

74. Griffith et al., "HeartMate II," S117–S119; HeartMate II, Smithsonian Institution, NMAH, Accession no. 2013.0017.

75. Ranjit John, "Current Axial-Flow Devices—the HeartMate II and Jarvik 2000 Left Ventricular Assist Devices," *Seminars in Thoracic and Cardiovascular Surgery* 20 (2008): 265.

76. Griffith et al., "HeartMate II," S116–S120.

77. Professional profile of Dr. Jacob Lavee at http://en.trustmed.co.il, accessed 6 Jun 2016.

78. Judy Siegel-Itzkovich, "Israeli Surgeons Implant First Permanent Artificial Ventricle," *British Medical Journal* 321 (12 Aug 2000): 399.

79. Griffith et al., "HeartMate II," S117; Timothy R. Maher et al., "HeartMate Left Ventricular Assist Devices: A Multigeneration of Implanted Blood Pumps," *Art Org* 25, no. 5 (2001): 424–25.

80. John, "Current Axial-Flow Devices," 268.

81. O. H. Frazier et al., "Initial Clinical Experience with the HeartMate II Axial Flow Left Ventricular Assist Device," *THI Journal* 34, no. 3 (2007): 281.

82. John, "Current Axial-Flow Devices," 268–69; Griffith et al., "HeartMate II," S118.

83. Frazier et al., "Initial Clinical Experience," 275–81; O. H. Frazier et al., "First Clinical Use of the Redesigned HeartMate II Left Ventricular Assist System in the United States," *THI Journal* 31, no. 2 (2004): 157–59.

84. L. W. Miller et al., "Use of a Continuous-Flow Device in Patients Awaiting Heart Transplantation," *NEJM* 357 (2007): 885–96.

85. F. D. Pagani et al., "Extended Mechanical Circulatory Support with a Continuous-Flow Rotary Left Ventricular Assist Device," *J Am Coll Cardio* 54 (2009): 312–21.

86. Mark S. Slaughter et al., "Advanced Heart Failure Treated with Continuous-Flow Left Ventricular Assist Device," *NEJM* 361, no. 23 (3 Dec 2009): 2241–51.

87. FDA Approval Order from Donna-Bea Tillman, director, Center for Devices and Radiological Health, FDA, to Donald A. Middlebrook, vice president, Regulatory Affairs and Quality Assurance, Thoratec Corporation, 21 Apr 2008, www.accessdata.fda.gov.

88. Research Support Provided to the University of Utah for Artificial Heart Research as of January 1986, 23 Jan 1986, NLM, HMD, John Watson Papers, Accession 2003-054, box 5.

89. T. B. Icenogle et al., "Thromboembolic Complications of the Symbion AVAD System," *Art Org* 13, no. 6 (Dec 1989): 532–38.

90. W. J. Kolff to Robert Levy (director, NLHBI), 29 Aug 1980, UU, MS 654 Willem J. Kolff Collection, box 175, folder 6.

91. "Withdrawal Asked in Bid for Symbion," *NYT,* 16 Apr 1987; "Symbion Board Ousts Jarvik," *NYT,* 27 Apr 1987.

92. Formed in 1988, the Manhattan company Jarvik Research Inc. was renamed Jarvik Heart Inc. in 1997 in anticipation of device clinical trials. www.jarvikheart.com.

93. O. H. Frazier et al., "Research and Development of an Implantable, Axial-Flow Left Ventricular Assist Device: The Jarvik 2000 Heart," *Ann Thorac Surg* 71 (2001): S125–S132; Jarvik 2000 FlowMaker, Smithsonian Institution, NMAH, Accession no. 2006.0234.

94. R. Jarvik, "Belt Worn Control System and Battery for the Percutaneous Model of the Jarvik 2000 Heart," *Art Org* 23 (1999): 487–89.

95. R. Jarvik et al., "LVAD Power Delivery: A Percutaneous Approach to Avoid Infection," *Ann Thorac Surg* 65 (1998): 470–73; S. Westaby et al., "Postauricular Percutaneous Power Delivery for Permanent Mechanical Circulatory Support," *JTCS* 123, no. 5 (May 2002): 977–83.

96. Frazier et al., "Research and Development," S125–S132.

97. A. K. Mahmood et al., "Critical Review of Current Left Ventricular Assist Devices," *Perfusion* 15 (2000): 401–2.

98. O. H. Frazier et al., "Initial Experience with the Jarvik 2000 Left Ventricular Assist System as a Bridge to Transplantation: Report of 4 Cases," *JHLT* 20 (2001): 201; S. Westaby et al., "First Permanent Implant of the Jarvik 2000 Heart," *Lancet* 356 (2000): 900–903.

99. Frazier et al., "Research and Development," S130; O. H. Frazier et al., "Initial Experience with Nonthoracic, Extraperitoneal, Off-Pump Insertion of the Jarvik 2000 Heart in Patients with Previous Media Sternotomy," *JHLT* 25 (2006): 499–503.

100. Westaby et al., "First Permanent Implant," 900–903; Westaby et al., "Postauricular Percutaneous Power Delivery," 977–83; Stephen Westaby et al., "Circulatory Support for Long-Term Treatment of Heart Failure: Experience with an Intraventricular Continuous Flow Pump," *Circulation* 105 (2002): 2588–91.

101. Stephen Westaby et al., "Six Years of Continuous Mechanical Circulatory Support," *NEJM* 355, no. 3 (20 Jul 2006): 325–27.

102. American Society for Artificial Internal Organs 48th Annual Conference, New York, 13–15 June 2002, attended by author; "The First Lifetime-Use Patient," www.jarvikheart.com, accessed 7 Jun 2013.

103. Lois Rogers, "The Human Dynamo," *Sunday Times Magazine,* 25 Mar 2001.

104. "Obituary: Peter Houghton," *Guardian* (London), 18 Dec 2007; P. Houghton, "Living with the Jarvik 2000: A Five-Plus Year Experience," *Art Org* 30, no. 5 (2006): 322–23; Stephen Westaby, *Open Heart: A Cardiac Surgeon's Stories of Life and Death on the Operating Table* (New York: Basic Books, 2017): 153–71; Stephen Westaby, "The Peter Houghton Legacy," *Artificial Organs* 32, 5 (2008): 363–65.

105. O. H. Frazier et al., "Initial Clinical Experience with the Jarvik 2000 Implantable Axial-Flow Left Ventricular Assist System," *Circulation* 105 (2002): 2855.

106. Frazier et al., "Research and Development," S130.

107. O. H. Frazier et al., "Use of the Jarvik 2000 Left Ventricular System as a Bridge to Heart Transplantation or as Destination Therapy for Patients with Chronic Heart Failure," *Ann Surg* 237 (2003): 631–37; S. Westaby et al., "The Jarvik 2000 Heart: Clinical Validation of the Intraventricular Position," *European Journal of Cardiovascular Surgery* 22 (2002): 228–32.

108. See "Jarvik 2000 Heart as a Bridge to Cardiac Transplantation—Pivotal Trial, completed May 2012, and Evaluation of the Jarvik 2000 Left Ventricular Assist System with Post-Auricular Connector—Destination Therapy Study," currently recruiting participants, https://clinicaltrials.gov, accessed 9 Nov 2016.

109. The MicroMed DeBakey Noon VAD was first implanted in a human in November 1998 in Berlin, Germany as a bridge-to-transplantation. The 56-year-old male patient survived one month before bleeding to death after a percutaneous tracheostomy. After more European implant cases, the pump was improved and evolved into the HeartAssist 5 VAD. Arvind Bhimaraj and Matthias Loebe, "An Interview with Dr George P. Noon," *Methodist DeBakey Cardiovascular Journal* 11, no. 1 (Jan 2015): 45–47; George P. Noon et al., "Clinical Experience with the MicroMed DeBakey Ventricular Assist Device," *Ann Thorac Surg* 71, no. 3, Suppl 1 (Mar 2001): S133–S138; George P. Noon and Matthias Loebe, "Current Status of the MicroMed DeBakey Noon Ventricular Assist Device," *THI Journal* 37, no. 6 (2010): 652–53; G. P. Noon et al., "Development and Clinical Application of the MicroMed DeBakey," *Current Opinion in Cardiology* 15 (2000): 166–71.

110. G. M. Wieselthaler et al., "First Experiences with Outpatient Care of Patients with Implanted Axial Flow Pumps," *Art Org* 25, no. 5 (2001): 331–35; D. L. S. Morales et al., "Lessons Learned from the First Application of the DeBakey VAD® Child: An Intracorporeal Ventricular Assist Device for Children," *JHLT* 24, no. 3 (March 2005): 331–37.

111. In 2013 MicroMed Inc. filed for bankruptcy, and within months, former members of the company founded ReliantHeart Inc., through which they acquired the HeartAssist pump technology. Like its predecessor, Reliant Heart Inc. is a stand-alone LVAD company and is based in Houston. As of 2017, the HeartAssist 5 VAD has CE Mark approval for use in Europe and FDA IDE approval for clinical trial use in the United States. See Jess Davis, "MicroMed Investors Say Execs Lied about Heart Pump Patents," 19 Dec 2013, www.law360 .com; "MicroMed Technology, Inc. Files for Chapter 11 Bankruptcy Protection in Delaware," 13 Jun 2013, http://chapter11cases.com; Gopal Chopra, "Details on ReliantHeart's Impressive LVAD Technology Cache," 15 Jul 2016, http://reliantheart.com.

112. Patients' stories and testimonials about living with an LVAD can be found online on various websites, including those of the device industries, medical centers, and the LVAD community. For example, see www.heartware.com; http://heartmateii.com; www.mylvad.com/.

113. "EMS Learn How to Treat LVAD Patients with No Pulse," http://mervsheppard .blogspot.ca, accessed 6 Jun 2016.

114. See Nader Moazami, "Patients with a Ventricular Assist Device Need Special Considerations," *Journal of Emergency Medical Services* (31 Jan 2012), www.jems.com/articles /print/volume-37/issue-2/patient-care/patients-ventricular-assist-device-need.html.

115. John, "Current Axial-Flow Devices," 265.

116. P. S. Joy et al., "Risk Factors and Outcomes of Gastrointestinal Bleeding in Left Ventricular Assist Device Recipients," *AJC* 117, no. 2 (15 Jan 2016): 240–44; S. Amer et al., "Gastrointestinal Bleeding with Continuous-Flow Left Ventricular Assist Devices," *Clinical Journal of Gastroenterology* 8, no. 2 (Apr 2015): 63–67; J. A. Morgan et al., "Gastrointestinal Bleeding with the HeartMate II Left Ventricular Assist Device," *JHLT* 31, no. 7 (Jul 2012): 715–18.

117. A. Guha et al., "Gastrointestinal Bleeding after Continuous-Flow Left Ventricular Device Implantation: Review of Pathophysiology and Management," *Methodist DeBakey Cardiovascular Journal* 11, no. 1 (Jan–Mar 2015): 24–27; J. Suarez et al., "Mechanisms of Bleeding and Approach to Patients with Axial-Flow Left Ventricular Assist Devices," *Circulation Heart Failure* 4, no. 6 (Nov 2011): 779–84.

118. John, "Current Axial-Flow Devices," 267.

119. Westaby et al., "First Permanent Implant," 902–3.

120. James B. Young and Lynne Warner Stevenson, "INTERMACS (Interagency Registry for Mechanically Assisted Circulatory Support) as a Tool to Track and Advance Clinical Practice," in Kormos and Miller, *Mechanical Circulatory Support*, 313–14.

121. The IMACS website became live in January 2013. See www.ishlt.org.

122. H. Hideo et al., "Third-Generation Blood Pumps with Mechanical Noncontact Magnetic Bearings," *Art Org* 30, no. 5 (May 2006): 324–38; J. J. Lee et al., "Development of Magnetic Bearing System for a New Third-Generation Blood Pump," *Art Org* 35, no. 11 (Nov 2011): 1082–94.

123. See Francis D. Pagani, "Continuous-Flow Rotary Left Ventricular Assist Devices with '3rd Generation' Design," *Seminar in Thoracic and Cardiovascular Surgery* 20 (2008): 255–63; J. Timothy Baldwin and John T. Watson, "Historical Aspects of Mechanical Circulatory Support," in Kormos and Miller, *Mechanical Circulatory Support*, 7–10; Victor Poirier, Project Bionics Pioneer Interview, 2 Feb 2012, NLM, HMD; N. Moazami et al., "Lessons Learned from the First Fully Magnetically Levitated Centrifugal LVAD Trial in the United States: The DuraHeart Trial," *Ann Thorac Surg* 97, no. 6 (Jun 2014); T. Sakaguchi et al., "Dura-Heart Magnetically Levitated Left Ventricular Assist Device: Osaka University Experience," *Circulation* 77, no. 7 (2013): 1736–41.

124. FDA Approval Order from Bram D. Zuckerman, director, Division of Cardiovascular Devices, Office of Device Evaluation, Center for Devices and Radiological Health, FDA, to Maritza Celaya, sr. director, Regulatory Affairs, HeartWare Inc., 20 Nov 2012, www.accessdata.fda.gov.

125. See Frazier, "Mechanical Circulatory Assist Device," 1742.

126. M. S. Slaughter et al., "HeartWare Miniature Axial-Flow Ventricular Assist Device: Design and Initial Feasibility Test," *THI Journal* 36 (2009): 12–16; G. M. Wieselthaler et al., "Initial Clinical Experience with a Novel Left Ventricular Assist Device with a Magnetically Levitated Rotor in a Multi-Institutional Trial," *JHLT* 29 (2010): 1218–25.

127. Sara Shumway, "VADs and Dad" lecture, 2011, at http://ctsurgery.stanford.edu.

128. K. D. Aaronson et al; "Use of an Intrapericardial, Continuous-Flow, Centrifugal Pump in Patients Awaiting Heart Transplantation," *Circulation* 125 (2012): 3191–3200; Veli K. Topkara et al., "HeartWare and HeartMate II Left Ventricular Assist Devices as Bridge to Transplantation: A Comparative Analysis," *Ann Thorac Surg* 97, no. 2 (Feb 2014): 506–12; Spencer D. Lalonde et al., "Clinical Differences between Continuous Flow Ventricular Assist Devices: A Comparison between Heart Mate II and Heart Ware HVAD," *Journal of Cardiac Surgery* 28, no. 5 (Sep 2013): 604–10; J. T. Magruder et al., "Survival after Orthotopic Heart Transplantation in Patients Undergoing Bridge to Transplantation with the HeartWare HVAD versus the HeartMate II," *Ann Thorac Surg* (17 Oct 2016): pii: S0003-4975(16)31128-6, doi: 10.1016/j.athoracsur.2016.08.060 (epub ahead of print).

129. Julie M. Donnelly, "HeartWare Warns of Heart Device Defect," *Boston Business Journal,* 8 Feb 2013, www.bizjournals.com.

130. HeartWare International Inc. Equity Research, 10 Jun 2010, p. 9, Worcester Polytechnic Institute, Gordon Library, MS 66 Robert J. Harvey Collection, box 11, folder 16, Wells Fargo Securities LLC; Covell, "Thoratec Corporation," 449.

131. Poirier interview, 2 Feb 2012, NLM; D. J. Farrar et al., "Design Features, Developmental Status, and Experimental Results with the HeartMate III Centrifugal Left Ventricular Assist System with a Magnetically Levitated Rotor," *ASAIO J* 53, no. 3 (May–Jun 2007): 310–15;

"MOMENTUM 3 IDE Clinical Study Protocol," ClinicalTrials.gov database, https://clinicaltrials.gov, accessed 4 Nov 2016.

132. Frazier, "Mechanical Circulatory Assist Device," 1742.

133. Muriel R. Gillick, "The Technological Imperative and the Battle for Hearts in America," *Perspectives in Biology and Medicine* 50, no. 2 (Spring 2007): 283.

134. Circulatory System Devices Panel Meeting Summary, 4–5 Mar 2002, US FDA, www.fda.gov.

135. National Coverage Determination for Artificial Hearts and Related Devices (20.9), Centers for Medicare and Medicaid Services, www.cms.gov/, accessed 21 Jun 2013.

136. Hunt, "Mechanical Circulatory Support," 461.

137. Rose et al., "Long-Term Use," 1438. See also Massie, "Comment—LVADs," 61.

138. Gillick, "Technological Imperative," 286.

139. See Shelley McKellar, "Disruptive Potential: The 'Landmark' REMATCH Trial, Left Ventricular Assist Device (LVAD) Technology and the Surgical Treatment of Heart Failure in the United States," in Schlich and Crenner, *Technological Change in Modern Surgery*, 129–55.

140. Kirklin et al., "Long-Term Mechanical Support (Destination Therapy)," 593.

141. See Dembitsky et al., "Left Ventricular Assist Device Performance," 2127; F. Pagani et al., "Improved Device Durability with Continuous Flow LVADs," *J Am Coll Cardio* 54 (2009): 312–21; Leslie W. Miller, "Left Ventricular Assist Devices Are Underutilized," *Circulation* 123 (2011): 1552–58.

142. NHLBI Working Group, *Next Generation Ventricular Assist Devices for Destination Therapy* (2004), www.nhlbi.nih.gov, accessed 19 Sep 2014.

143. See Miller et al., "Use of a Continuous-Flow Device," 885–96; Minutes of the FDA Circulatory System Devices Advisory Panel Meeting, 30 Nov 2007, www.fda.gov; FDA Approval Order from Donna-Bea Tillman, director, Center for Devices and Radiological Health, FDA, to Donald A. Middlebrook, vice president, Regulatory Affairs and Quality Assurance, Thoratec Corporation, 21 Apr 2008, www.accessdata.fda.gov.

144. See Slaughter et al., "Advanced Heart Failure," 2241–51; FDA Approval Order from Donna-Bea Tillman, director, Center for Devices and Radiological Health, FDA, to Donald A. Middlebrook, vice president, Regulatory Affairs and Quality Assurance, Thoratec Corporation, 20 Jan 2010, www.accessdata.fda.gov.

145. Kirklin et al., "Long-Term Mechanical Support (Destination Therapy)," 593.

146. US Securities and Exchange Commission Form 10-K, submitted by the Thoratec Corporation for the fiscal year ended 28 Dec 2013, www.sec.gov.

147. In 2015 St. Jude Medical Inc. acquired the Thoratec Corp for $3.4 billion. In 2016 Medtronic PLC purchased HeartWare International Inc. for a reported $1.1 billion. In early 2017, Abbott Laboratories completed its acquisition of St Jude Medical Inc. for a reported $25 billion to compete with rivals Medtronic PLC and Boston Scientific Corporation. See "St Jude Medical Completes Acquisition of Thoratec," 8 Oct 2015, http://media.sjm.com; Jof Enriquez, "Medtronic Buys Heart Failure Device Developer HeartWare for $1.1 Billion," *Med Device Online,* 28 Jun 2016; Marie Thibault, "What's Next for the LVAD Market?," *Medical Device and Diagnostic Industry Blog,* 27 Jun 2016, www.mddionline.com; "Abbott Completes the Acquisition of St. Jude Medical," 4 Jan 2017, http://abbott.mediaroom.com/press-releases.

148. The HeartWare ventricular assist system offers the Lavare Cycle, a controlled variation in speed that creates a pulse, which can be enabled or disabled by the clinician via the device's monitor. This provides pulsatile hemodynamics but also increased risk of thrombo-

embolism; the manufacturers strongly recommend that if thrombus is suspected within the device, the Lavare Cycle should be turned off until the thrombus is resolved. "HeartWare Ventricular Assist System: Instructions for Use (7.3.3 Lavare Cycle)," www.salute.gov.it, accessed 28 Jun 2016.

149. See Kevin G. Soucy et al., "Rotary Pumps and Diminished Pulsatility: Do We Need a Pulse?," *ASAIO J* 59 (2013): 355–66; Leslie Miller, "We Always Need a Pulse, Or Do We?," *Journal of Cardiovascular Translational Research* 5, no. 3 (Jun 2012): 296–301.

150. Frazier interview, 18 Jul 2013, NLM. See also John V. Pickstone, *Ways of Knowing: A New History of Science, Technology and Medicine* (Chicago: University of Chicago Press, 2000).

151. See Jennifer L. Hall and Guillermo Torre-Amione, "Cellular, Molecular, Genomic, and Functional Changes That Occur in the Failing Heart in Response to Mechanical Circulatory Support," in Kormos and Miller, *Mechanical Circulatory Support*, 265–67.

152. Slaughter et al., "Advanced Heart Failure," 2241–51.

153. James K. Kirklin, "Terminal Heart Failure: Who Should Be Transplanted and Who Should Have Mechanical Circulatory Support?," *Current Opinion in Organ Transplantation* 19, no. 5 (Oct 2014), 486–93.

154. See Stephen Westaby, "Cardiac Transplant or Rotary Blood Pump: Contemporary Evidence," *JTCS* 145, no. 1 (Jan 2013): 24–31; J. Garbade et al., "Heart Transplantation and Left Ventricular Assist Device Therapy: Two Comparable Options in End-Stage Heart Failure?," *Clinical Cardiology* (17 Apr 2013): 1–5; Markus J. Wilhelm, F. Ruschitzka, and V. Falk, "Destination Therapy—Time for a Paradigm Change in Heart Failure Therapy," *Swiss Medical Weekly* 143 (25 March 2013): 1–13; Robert Jarvik, "Transplant or VAD?," *Cardiology Clinics* 29, no. 4 (Nov 2011): 585–95; Michael Yamakawa et al., "Destination Therapy: The New Gold Standard Treatment for Heart Failure Patients with Left Ventricular Assist Devices," *General Thoracic and Cardiovascular Surgery* 61 (2013): 111–17; Daniel P. Mulloy et al., "Orthotopic Heart Transplant versus Left Ventricular Assist Device: A National Comparison of Cost and Survival," *JTCS* 145 (2013): 566–74.

155. Wilhelm, Ruschitzka, and Falk, "Destination Therapy," 1–13.

156. James C. Fang, "Rise of the Machines—Left Ventricular Assist Devices as Permanent Therapy for Advanced Heart Failure," *NEJM* 361, no. 23 (3 Dec 2009): 2282–85.

157. Tara Hrobowski and David E. Lanfear, "Ventricular Assist Devices: Is Destination Therapy a Viable Alternative in the Non-Transplant Candidate?," *Current Heart Failure Report* 10 (2013): 101–7. For similar articles, see Valluvan Jeevanandam, "Are We Ready to Implant Left Ventricular Assist Devices in 'Less Sick' Patients?," *Seminars in Thoracic and Cardiovascular Surgery* 24, no. 1 (2012): 8–10; Nader Moazami and David Feldman, "Rethinking the Terminology of Mechanical Circulatory Support," *JTCS* 144, no. 1 (Jul 2012): 2–3; Ana C. Alba and Diego H. Delgado, "The Future Is Here: Ventricular Assist Devices for the Failing Heart," *Expert Review of Cardiovascular Therapy* 7, no. 9 (2009): 1067–77; Thomas Krabatsch et al., "Ventricular Assist Devices for All?," *European Journal of Cardio-Thoracic Surgery* 42 (2012): 918–19; James K. Kirklin, "Long-Term Mechanical Circulatory Support: Could It Really Have a Public Health Impact?," *European Journal of Cardio-Thoracic Surgery* (2013): 1–3.

158. Patient Stories, Thoratec Corporation website, www.thoratec.com, accessed 14 Jun 2013.

159. Such patient issues and the need for palliative care for patients with advanced heart failure are discussed in the medical literature. See S. M. Dunlay et al., "Dying with a Left

Ventricular Assist Device as Destination Therapy," *Circulation Heart Failure* 9, no. 10 (Oct 2016), e003096, https://doi.org/10.1161/CIRCHEARTFAILURE.116.003096; Justin A. K. Phan et al., "Death on an LVAD—Two Sides of a Coin," *Heart, Lung and Circulation* 22, no. 11 (Nov 2013): 952–54; Belinda Linden, "Experiences of the Relatives of Patients with a LVAD," *British Journal of Cardiac Nursing* (27 Sep 2013); Jessie Casida, "The Lived Experience of Spouses of Patients with a Left Ventricular Assist Device before Heart Transplantation," *American Journal of Critical Care* 14, no. 2 (March 2005): 145–51; Keith M. Swetz et al., "Palliative Care and End-of-Life Issues in Patients Treated with Left Ventricular Assist Devices as Destination Therapy," *Current Heart Failure Reports* 8 (2011): 212–18; Lorelei A. Lingard et al., "Understanding Palliative Care on the Heart Failure Care Team: An Innovative Research Methodology," *Journal of Pain and Symptom Management* 45, no. 4 (May 2013): 901–11.

160. Quote taken from Dr. O. H. Frazier, 2012 Chancellor's Council Meeting and Symposium, University of Texas, 16 May 2012; see also Frazier and Cohn, "If You Have an Artificial Heart"; Dan Baum, "No Pulse: How Doctors Reinvented the Human Heart," *Popular Science* 280, no. 3 (Mar 2012).

Chapter 7 · *Artificial Hearts for the Twenty-First-Century*
Epigraph: Anita Hamilton, "Best Inventions of 2001: Abiocor Artificial Heart," *Time*, 19 Nov 2001.

1. Marvin J. Slepian, "The SynCardia Temporary Total Artificial Heart—Evolving Clinical Role and Future Status," *US Cardiol* 8, no. 1 (2011): 39–46; Jack Copeland, "Mechanical Circulatory Support in Heart Failure," *US Cardiol* 8, no. 1 (2011): 47–51.

2. Antonio Regalado, "CPR for the Artificial Heart," *Technology Review*, 1 May 1999.

3. Hamilton, "Best Inventions of 2001."

4. "How Technology Will Heal Your Heart," *Newsweek*, 25 Jun 2001.

5. T. Sloane Guy, "Evolution and Current Status of the Total Artificial Heart: The Search Continues," *ASAIO J* 44 (1998): 30; P. M. Portner, "Permanent Mechanical Circulatory Assistance," in *Heart and Lung Transplantation*, ed. W. A. Baumgartner et al., 2nd ed. (Philadelphia: W. B. Saunders, 2002), 534–35.

6. John T. Watson, "Prospects for Implantable Circulatory Support," in *Heart Replacement—Artificial Heart 6*, ed. T. Akutsu and H. Koyanagi (Tokyo: Springer-Verlage Tokyo, 1998), reprint, NLM, HMD, John Watson Papers, Accession 2003-054, box 25; A. J. Snyder et al., "In vivo Testing of a Completely Implanted Total Artificial Heart System," *ASAIO J* 39 (1993): M177–M184.

7. At Pennsylvania State University College of Medicine, William S. Pierce and his research team developed both VADs and TAHs. Initially, Penn State researchers collaborated with Sarns Inc., a manufacturer of heart-lung machines, which had been formed by Dick Sarns in 1960. During the 1970s, Pierce's team worked on pneumatically powered VADs (notably the Pierce-Donachy pump) and TAHs for temporary, bridge use in patients; by the later 1970s, they began developing electrically powered, self-contained device prototypes (notably the Penn State TAH) for longer-term implantation. In 1981 Sarns sold the company's product line to 3M; in 1999 3M sold its cardiovascular business to the Japanese medical device maker Terumo, who decided not to support work on the total artificial heart. Abiomed Inc. then purchased the Penn State TAH technology, attracted by its seam-free fabrication (to prevent stagnation of blood, reducing risk of blood clotting) and its ability to adjust automatically to changing patient blood flow requirements (unlike other TAHs, such as the

Jarvik heart, which required manual adjustment). "Penn State Artificial Heart Researchers to Work with Abiomed Inc.," 21 Sep 2000, PSU, Special Collections Library, PSUA 435, Milton S. Hershey Medical Center Records, The Penn State Ventricular Assist Device and Artificial Heart, box 10, folder PS Heart Media Packet; William J. Weiss et al., "The Development and Testing of the Penn State Artificial Heart and Ventricular Assist Device," *Cardiovascular Pathology* 5, no. 5 (Sep–Oct 1996): 288.

8. O. H. Frazier et al., "The Total Artificial Heart: Where We Stand," *Cardiology* 101 (2004): 117–21; Robert D. Dowling et al., "Initial Experience with the AbioCor Implantable Replacement Heart System," *JTCS* 127, no. 1 (Jan 2004): 131–41; Robert D. Dowling et al., "The AbioCor Implantable Replacement Heart," *Ann Thorac Surg* 75, no. 6, suppl. (2003): S93–S99.

9. Dowling et al., "Initial Experience with AbioCor System," 134.

10. Frazier et al., "Total Artificial Heart," 120–21.

11. "A Space Age Vision Advances in the Clinic," *Science* 295 (8 Feb 2002): 1000; Michael D. Lemonick, "Reviving Artificial Hearts," *Time,* 3 Jul 2001.

12. Dowling et al., "Initial Experience with AbioCor System," 141.

13. Dick Kaukas, "Implant Patient Conscious, Able to Breathe on His Own: Doctors Describe 'Flawless' Surgery," *Louisville (KY) Courier-Journal,* 5 Jul 2001; William Claiborne, "Patient with Artificial Heart Doing Well, Louisville Surgeons Say," *Wash Post,* 5 Jul 2001.

14. Lawrence K. Altman, "Manufacturer of Artificial Heart Forbids Doctors to Talk about Patient's Condition," *NYT,* 13 Jul 2001; Lawrence K. Altman, "Artificial Heart Maker Restricts News of Patient's Condition," *NYT,* 12 Jul 2001.

15. Dick Kaukas, "Artificial Heart's Maker Defends 'Quiet Period,'" *Louisville (KY) Courier-Journal,* 14 Jul 2001.

16. Jewish Hospital Press Release, 11 Jul 2001, www.heartpioneers.com.

17. Renée C. Fox and Judith P. Swazey, "'He Knows That Machine Is His Mortality': Old and New Social and Cultural Patterns in the Clinical Trial of the AbioCor Artificial Heart," *Perspectives in Biology and Medicine* 47, no. 1 (Winter 2004): 86.

18. E. Haavi Morreim, "High Profile Research and the Media: The Case of the AbioCor Artificial Heart," *Hastings Center Report* 34, no. 1 (Jan–Feb 2004): 11–24. For more on the Independent Patient Advocacy Council, a patient's assistance program conceived by Abiomed CEO David Lederman, see E. Haavi Morreim et al., "Innovation in Human Research Protection: The AbioCor Artificial Heart Trial," *American Journal of Bioethics* 6, no. 5 (2006): W6–W16.

19. Anne Lederman Flamm, "Medical Research and Media Circus," *Hastings Center Report* 34, no. 1 (Jan–Feb 2004): 3.

20. Andrew Wolfson, "'It Feels Great!' Tools Tells Reporters," *Louisville (KY) Courier-Journal,* 22 Aug 2001; Dick Kaukas, "Patient Grateful for Artificial Heart," *Louisville (KY) Courier-Journal,* 22 Aug 2001; Dick Kaukas, "Pioneer Heart Patient Identified," *Louisville (KY) Courier-Journal,* 21 Aug 2001.

21. Darla Carter, "Heart Patient Takes Field Trips, Tries Fast Food," *Louisville (KY) Courier-Journal,* 26 Sep 2001; Dick Kaukas, "Artificial Heart Patient Doing Better Than Expected," *Louisville (KY) Courier-Journal,* 17 Jul 2001; "Tools for Living," *Dateline NBC,* aired 2 Nov 2001.

22. Dowling et al., "Initial Experience with AbioCor System," 136; AbioCor Total Artificial Heart (that had been implanted in Robert Tools), Smithsonian Institution, NMAH, Accession no. 2003.0166.

23. Gideon Gil, "Heart Implant Patient Suffers Major Stroke," *Louisville (KY) Courier-Journal,* 15 Nov 2001; Gideon Gil, "Heart Patient Has 'Major Setback,'" *Louisville (KY) Courier-Journal,* 14 Nov 2001.

24. Guy Gugliottia, "Artificial Heart Pioneer Dies after Five Months," *Wash Post,* 1 Dec 2001; Gideon Gil, "First Heart Implant Patient Dies," *Louisville (KY) Courier-Journal,* 1 Dec 2001.

25. Dowling et al., "Initial Experience with AbioCor System," 136; Lawrence K. Altman, "Artificial Heart Is Implanted in a Second Gravely Ill Man," *NYT,* 14 Sep 2001.

26. Abiomed Inc. Press Release, "AbioCor Patient Achieves One-Year Milestone Today," 13 Sep 2002; images at www.heartpioneers.com, accessed 2 Aug 2013.

27. Abiomed Inc. Press Release, "Abiocor Patient Celebrates One Year," 10 Sep 2002.

28. Frazier et al., "Total Artificial Heart," 120.

29. Dowling et al., "Initial Experience with AbioCor System," 137; Frazier et al., "Total Artificial Heart," 120.

30. Debbie Goldberg, "Heart Patient Hears 'Miraculous' New Beat," *Wash Post,* 7 Dec 2001.

31. Guy Gugliotta, "Smiling to the Beat of a Normal Life," *Wash Post,* 4 Feb 2002; Goldberg, "Heart Patient Hears New Beat."

32. Gideon Gil, "AbioCor to Be Altered Slightly," *Louisville (KY) Courier-Journal,* 24 Jan 2002; "The Implantable Artificial Heart Project," Jewish Hospital—University of Louisville Health Sciences Center—Abiomed Inc., www.heartpioneers.com, accessed 2 Aug 2013.

33. "World's Third Recipient of AbioCor Artificial Heart Is Born Risk Taker, Continues Steady Recovery," News Release, Texas Heart Institute, 16 Jan 2002.

34. Dowling et al., "Initial Experience with AbioCor System," 137.

35. Sheryl Gay Stolberg, "Artificial Heart, Artificial Life," *NYT,* 10 Oct 2002.

36. Untitled News Service story bulletin, *Wash Post,* 17 Oct 2002.

37. Louis Samuels et al., "Use of the AbioCor Replacement Heart as Destination Therapy for End-Stage Heart Failure with Irreversible Pulmonary Hypertension," *JTCS* 128, no. 4 (Oct 2004): 643–45; Frazier et al., "Total Artificial Heart," 120; Abiomed Inc. Press Release, 26 Aug 2002; Hahnemann University Hospital Press Release, 26 Aug 2002.

38. Stacey Buring, "Widow Sues Artificial-Heart Maker," *Philadelphia Inquirer,* 17 Oct 2002; Sheryl Gay Stolberg, "Widow Sues over Artificial Heart," *NYT,* 17 Oct 2002; Debbie Goldberg, "Recipient's Wife Says She and Her Husband Were Misinformed and Misled on Risks, Benefits," *Wash Post,* 30 Nov 2002, A03.

39. The settlement amount was low owing to James Quinn's imminent death before the AbioCor TAH implant. I thank my Western University colleague Rande Kostal, lawyer and law historian, for reviewing the details of the Quinn case record with me. See Stacey Burling, "Widow of Man Who Received Artificial Heart Settles Lawsuit," *Philadelphia Inquirer,* 14 Jun 2003; Philadelphia Courts Civil Docket, Case 021001524 Quinn vs. Abiomed Inc. et al.

40. Frazier et al., "Total Artificial Heart," 117–21; David M. Lederman, Robert T. V. Kung, and Douglas S. McNair, "Therapeutic Potential of Implantable Replacement Hearts," *American Journal of Cardiovascular Drugs* 2, no. 5 (2002): 297–301; "Penn State Artificial Heart Researchers to Work with Abiomed, Inc.," Penn State News Release, 21 Sep 2000; US Securities and Exchange Commission Form 8-K, 21 Sep 21, 2000.

41. J. T. Juretich et al., "Development Progress on a Second General Total Artificial Heart," *ASAIO J* 52, no. 2 (Mar–Apr 2006): 48; Zakir Rangwala, Dalia Banks, and Jack Copeland, "The Total Artificial Heart: Is it an Appropriate Replacement for Existing Biven-

tricular Assist Devices?," *Journal of Cardiothoracic and Vascular Anesthesia* 28, no. 3 (Jun 2014): 837.

42. Corbin E. Goerlich, O. H. Frazier, and William E. Cohn, "Previous Challenges and Current Progress—the Use of Total Artificial Hearts in Patients with End-Stage Heart Failure," *Expert Review of Cardiovascular Therapy* 14, no. 10 (2016): 1095–98.

43. Dennis Hevesi, "David Lederman, Pioneer of Artificial Heart, Dies at 68," *NYT,* 28 Aug 2012.

44. Don B. Olsen, "ASAIO Presidential Address: Artificial Organs of the Future," *ASAIO J* (1992): M134.

45. CardioWest Total Artificial Heart, Smithsonian Institution, NMAH, Accession no. 2003.0337.

46. David Joyce, Lyle Joyce, and Matthias Loebe, *Mechanical Circulatory Support* (New York: McGraw-Hill, 2012), 174–78.

47. Jack Copeland et al., "Cardiac Replacement with a Total Artificial Heart as a Bridge to Transplantation," *NEJM* 351, no. 9 (26 Aug 2004): 866.

48. A. Platis and D. F. Larson, "CardioWest Temporary Total Artificial Heart," *Perfusion* 24, no. 5 (2009): 343; Copeland, "Cardiac Replacement," 859–66.

49. Jack G. Copeland et al., "Experience with More Than 100 Total Artificial Heart Implants," *JTCS* 143, no. 3 (Mar 2012): 727–34; Slepian, "SynCardia Temporary Total Artificial Heart," 39–46; Francisco A. Arabia, "Update on the Total Artificial Heart," *Journal of Cardiac Surgery* 16 (2001): 222–27.

50. Bram D. Zuckerman, FDA, to Sharon Rockwell, SynCardia Systems, 15 Oct 2004, US FDA Approval Letter, www.accessdata.fda.gov.

51. M. J. Slepian et al., "Translatable Performance with the Total Artificial Heart: The U.S. Postmarket Study," *JHLT* 31, no. 4S (Apr 2012): 88–89.

52. David Wichner, "SynCardia a Heartbeat from Leadership Role," *Tucson Arizona Daily Star,* 27 Jan 2013.

53. Jack G. Copeland, "SynCardia Total Artificial Heart: Update and Future," *THI Journal* 40, no. 5 (2013): 587–88; SynCardia Total Artificial Heart System, Smithsonian Institution, NMAH, Nonaccession no. 2015.3106.

54. Helen Laidlaw, "SynCardia's Freedom Driver—the Heart in a Bag," www.howitworks daily.com, accessed 3 Jul 2013.

55. See Intermacs Quarterly Statistical Report 2016 Q2, www.uab.edu/medicine /intermacs/, accessed 31 Oct 2016; Kristen E. Johnson et al., "Use of Total Artificial Hearts: Summary of World Experience, 1969–1991," *ASAIO J* 38, no. 3 (Jul–Sep 1992): M488.

56. Johnson lived for more than 19 months with her implanted SynCardia TAH before dying on August 24, 2013, during a cardiac transplant operation. See SynCardia Systems Press Release, "Cedars-Sinai Implants 1st Total Artificial Heart to Bridge Mother of Three to Second Heart Transplant," 20 May 2012, www.syncardia.com.

57. At Tucson's University of Arizona Medical Center, Shepherd received a heart transplant after being supported with a SynCardia TAH for 15 months, from June 20, 2013, to September 15, 2014. See "Arizona's 'Tin Man' Gets a Donor Heart after 15 Months on the SynCardia Total Artificial Heart," 8 Oct 2014; "Man's Real-Life Experiences with the SynCardia Total Artificial Heart Detailed on Social Media Site," 8 May 2014, both at www .syncardia.com.

58. "Florida Teen, 16, Youngest SynCardia Total Artificial Heart Patient Discharged on the Freedom Portable Driver," 27 May 2014, www.syncardia.com.

59. While most studies have focused on the LVAD patient, there is much crossover with the TAH patient. See C. H. Zambroski et al., "Edgar Allan Poe, 'The Pit and the Pendulum,' and Ventricular Assist Devices," *Critical Care Nursing* 29, no. 6 (2009): 29–39; L. S. Savage et al., "Life with a Left Ventricular Assist Device: The Patient's Perspective," *American Journal of Critical Care* 8, no. 5 (1999): 340–43; E. Chapman et al., "Psychosocial Issues for Patients with Ventricular Assist Devices: A Qualitative Pilot Study," *American Journal of Critical Care* 16, no. 1 (2007): 72–81; C. Hallas et al., "A Qualitative Study of the Psychosocial Experience of Patients during and after Mechanical Cardiac Support," *Journal of Cardiovascular Nursing* 24, no. 1 (2009): 31–39.

60. Highlights from Randy Shepherd's "Ask Me Anything" (AMA) on Reddit, www .syncardia.com, accessed 29 June 2014.

61. Laura S. Savage et al., "Living with a Total Artificial Heart: Patients' Perspectives," *Journal of Cardiovascular Nursing* 29, no. 1 (Jan–Feb 2014): E3.

62. Ibid.

63. I thank members of the Cedars-Sinai Centre for Health Care Ethics and Mechanical Circulatory Support service for their candid responses to my questions during my visit as the 2014 Leon Morgenstern, M.D., Lecturer in History, Ethics and Medicine.

64. Within a matter of minutes, if the TAH does not resume pumping, blood stops moving and pools in various organs, and the patient dies unpleasantly. Randy Shepherd's quote is from "Ask Me Anything" (AMA) on Reddit, www.syncardia.com, accessed 29 June 2014.

65. "Top Surgeon Says He'd Still Use Jarvik Heart," *Salt Lake Tribune,* 12 Jan 1990; statement by Jack Copeland, no date, Smithsonian Institution, NMAH, Division of Medicine and Science, Accession File 87.0474.

66. In 1990, as part of the Safe Medical Devices Act passed in the United States, a designation of Humanitarian Use Device (HUD) provided an alternative pathway for getting market approval for medical devices that may help people with rare diseases or conditions. The act grants HUD status to a "medical device intended to benefit patients in the treatment or diagnosis of a disease or condition that affects or is manifested in fewer than 4,000 individuals in the United States per year." See www.fda.gov, accessed 6 Jun 2016.

67. S. Spiliopoulos, R. Koerfer, and G. Tenderich, "A First Step beyond Traditional Boundaries: Destination Therapy with the SynCardia Total Artificial Heart," *Interactive CardioVascular and Thoracic Surgery* 18 (2014) 855–56.

68. David Wichner, "Artificial Heart Maker SynCardia Wins Bankruptcy Sale OK," *Tucson Arizona Daily Star,* 16 Sep 2016; Press Release, "SynCardia Systems Acquired by Versa Capital Management, LLC," 20 Sep 2016, www.syncardia.com.

69. According to one account, SynCardia approached more than 120 potential buyers, but all declined. See Donald L Swanson, "Total Artificial Heart: How Bankruptcy Provides a Valuable Service—And a Proactive Suggestion," *Mediatbankry Blog,* mediatbankry.com, accessed 4 Nov 2016.

70. Because of the patient's narrow chest cavity, the SynCardia TAH was not an option. See O. H. Frazier and W. E. Cohn, "Continuous-Flow Total Heart Replacement Device Implanted in a 55-year-old Man with End-Stage Heart Failure and Severe Amyloidosis," *THI Journal* 39, no. 4 (2012): 542–46; M. Loebe et al., "Initial Clinical Experience of Total Cardiac Replacement with Dual HeartMate-II Axial Flow Pumps for Severe Biventricular Heart Failure," *Methodist DeBakey Cardiovascular Journal* 7, no. 1 (Jan–Mar 2011): 40–44.

71. O. H. Frazier, "Mechanical Circulatory Assist Device Development at the Texas Heart Institute: A Personal Perspective," *JTCS* 147, no. 6 (Jun 2014): 1742–43; O. H. Frazier,

Project Bionics Pioneer Interview, 18 Jul 2013, NLM, HMD; W. E. Cohn et al., "Ninety-Day Survival of a Calf Implanted with a Continuous-Flow Total Artificial Heart," *ASAIO J* 60 (2014): 15–8.

72. H. Fumoto et al., "In vivo Acute Performance of the Cleveland Clinic Self-Regulation, Continuous-Flow Total Artificial Heart," *JHLT* 29 (2010): 21–26; M. Kobayashi et al., "Progress on the Design and Development of the Continuous-Flow Total Artificial Heart," *Art Org* 36, no. 8 (Aug 2012): 705–13; J. H. Karimov et al., "Human Fitting Studies of Cleveland Clinic Continuous-Flow Total Artificial Heart," *ASAIO J* 61 (2015): 424–28. See also the SmartHeart TAH and SmartHeart LVAD product pages on the Cleveland Heart Inc. company website, www.clevelandheart.com, accessed 3 Jul 2014.

73. Bioengineer-physician Len Golding joined the Cleveland Clinic in 1976 and worked on nonpulsatile pumps in Yukihiko Nosé's research group. One of the early papers representing this research is L. R. Golding et al., "Chronic Nonpulsatile Blood Flow in an Alive, Awake Animal 34-Day Survival," *Trans ASAIO* 26 (1980): 251–55.

74. Frazier interview, 18 Jul 2013, NLM.

75. Leslie Miller, "We Always Need a Pulse, or Do We?," *Journal of Cardiovascular Translational Research* 5, no. 3 (Jun 2012): 296–301; O. H. Frazier and Billy Cohn, "If You Have an Artificial Heart, Does That Make You Heartless?," lecture delivered at TEDMED 2012, an annual TED (Technology, Entertain, Design) conference focusing on health and medicine, Washington, DC, 11–13 Apr 2012.

76. University of Texas Medical Branch Health Center, "Cardiovascular Care at UTMB: It's About Getting Your Life Back" (advertisement in United Airlines Inflight Magazine), *Hemispheres,* Oct 2013.

77. Cheney and Reiner, *Heart,* 263.

78. Ibid., 247.

79. Piotr Ponikowski et al., "Heart Failure: Preventing Disease and Death Worldwide," *ESC Heart Failure* 1, no. 1 (Sep 2014): 4–25.

80. José Lopez-Sendon, "The Heart Failure Epidemic," *Medicographia* 33, no. 4 (2011): 363–69.

81. James K. Kirklin et al., "First Annual IMACS Report: A Global International Society for Heart and Lung Transplantation Registry for Mechanical Circulatory Support," *JHLT* 35, no. 4 (2016): 407–12.

82. Abraham J. Nunes et al., "A Systematic Review of the Cost-Effectiveness of Long-Term Mechanical Circulatory Support," *Value in Health* 19 (2016): 494–504.

83. Health Quality Ontario, "Left Ventricular Assist Devices for Destination Therapy: A Health Technology Assessment," *Ontario Health Technology Assessment Series* 16, no. 3 (Feb 2016): 1–60. Available at www.hqontario.ca/evidence/publications-andohtac-recommendations/ontario-health-technology-assessment-series/hta-lvad.

84. Patrycja Ganslmeier and Christof Schmid, "Chronic Mechanical Circulatory Support for Patients with End-Stage Heart Failure as a Definitive Treatment Option," *European Cardiology Review* 6, no. 4 (2010): 22–25; Copeland, "Mechanical Circulatory Support," 47–51.

85. Jason A. Cook et al., "The Total Artificial Heart," *Journal of Thoracic Disease* 7, no. 12 (Dec 2015): 2172–80.

86. "Exhibit 5: Implants per Year by Device Type," p. 10, INTERMACS Quarterly Report—2015 Q4, www.uab.edu/medicine/intermacs, accessed 22 Jun 2016.

87. As stated by O. H. Frazier, "the importance of this partnership cannot be underestimated." Frazier, "Mechanical Circulatory Assist Device," 1741; Richard K. Wampler, Project

Bionics Pioneer Interview, 9 Jun 2011, NLM, HMD; Victor Poirier, Project Bionics Pioneer Interview, 2 Feb 2012, NLM, HMD.

88. Renée C Fox and Judith P. Swazey, *Spare Parts: Organ Replacement in American Society* (Oxford: Oxford University Press, 1992), 208, 210; Thomas A. Preston, "The Case against the Artificial Heart," *Utah Holiday* (Jun 1983): 39–49; Thomas A. Preston, "The Artificial Heart," in *Worse Than the Disease: Pitfalls of Medical Progress,* ed. Diana B. Dutton (New York: Cambridge University Press, 1988), 91–126; Barton J. Bernstein, "The Misguided Quest for the Artificial Heart," *Technology Review* (Nov–Dec 1984): 13–19, 62–63; Barton J. Bernstein, "The Pursuit of the Artificial Heart," *Medical Heritage* 2 (1986): 80–100.

89. Robert H. Bartlett, "Extracorporeal Life Support: Gibbon Fulfilled," *J Am Coll Surg* 218, no. 3 (Mar 2014): 326.

90. Poirier interview, 2 Feb 2012, NLM.

91. I thank Renée Fox for our discussion regarding such ethos and values today, given the hospice care and end-of-life discussions in medical and lay communities. The "haunting" of treatment decision making by physicians and surgeons, as articulated in medical memoirs, was suggested to me by Dr. Fox, with reference to Henry Marsh, *Do No Harm: Stories of Life, Death, and Brain Surgery* (London: Weidenfeld & Nicholson, 2014). Personal communication with author, 16 Jun 2016.

92. For more on the shifting emphasis between cure and comfort, see Jacalyn Duffin, "Palliative Care: The Oldest Profession?," *Canadian Bulletin of Medical History* 31, no. 2 (Winter 2014): 205–28.

Abbott Laboratories, 237, 330n147

AbioCor TAH, 5, 27, 178, 241–51, 334n39; assessment of, 250–51; cost of, 245; design of, 244; implantation of, 241, 244–51; media coverage of, 245–46; photograph of, 244

ABIOMED BVS 5000, 184

Abiomed Inc., 172, 178; circulatory support systems developed by, 243–44; and TAH research and development, 243–51, 332–33n7; and VAD research, 184, 185

Acute Ventricular Assist Device (AVAD), 311n197

advance directives, 155

Aerojet-General, 98

Akers, William, 40

Akutsu III TAH, 6, 156; design of, 136; implanted in a human patient, 135–38; media interest in, 137–38

Akutsu, Tetsuzo, 112; as pioneer in artificial heart research and development, 33–34, 50, 54, 86, 136, 138

Altman, Lawrence K., 145, 151, 166, 246

American College of Cardiology, 74

American Heart Association, 39

American Society for Artificial Internal Organs (ASAIO), 31–32, 85

Anderson, Rudolph, 71

Anderson, Suzanne, 82

Andreopoulos, Spyros, 95–96

Andros Inc., 190, 207

angiocardiograms, 15

angioplasty, 13–14

Annas, George, 96, 165, 166, 170

antirejection drugs, 90–91

Arkon Scientific Labs, 190, 207

Artificial Heart Assessment Panel (NHLI), 112–13, 116, 117, 118

artificial heart implantation: costs associated with, 147, 245; at for-profit institutions, 148–49; media coverage of, 144–46, 151–52, 154–55; "success" of, as assessed by physicians and researchers, 48–49, 51–54, 56, 86, 146–47, 266. See also AbioCor TAH; artificial hearts; Burcham, Jack; Christerson, Tom; Clark, Barney; Haydon, Murray; Jarvik-7 artificial heart; Meuffels, Willebror-

dus; Schroeder, William; Stenberg, Leif; SynCardia TAH; Tools, Robert

Artificial Heart Program (NHI), 10, 22–23, 26, 31, 42, 54, 56, 93, 158–59; congressional hearings relating to, 169–70; early years of, 57–59; establishment of, 42–48, 97; evaluation of, 168–69; Myocardial Infarction Branch of, 47; name changes for, 276n60

artificial heart research: academic-industry partnerships involved in, 26, 57, 158, 175, 178, 182, 184, 185, 189, 200, 220, 242–43, 264; advocates for, 170–71; animal testing relating to, 33–34, 35, 36, 38, 40, 42, 53, 54, 75, 84, 104, 107, 116–17, 128, 129–31, 132–33, 136, 156, 159, 160, 187, 195, 196, 206, 218, 224, 225–26, 229–30, 237, 243; at Baylor College of Medicine, 38–41, 52, 54, 74–75; diverse approaches to, 30–31, 32–37, 54–59, 177–79; and expectations for the future, 258–62, 264–65; government funding for, 22–23, 26, 39–40, 41–45, 47–48, 54, 57, 74–75, 80, 86, 97, 121, 126, 158–59, 171–72, 178, 242–43, 276n60; oversight of, 170; at University of Utah Medical Center, 24, 25, 26, 103, 124–31, 242. See also Cooley, Denton; DeBakey, Michael; Jarvik-7 artificial heart; Kantrowitz, Adrian; Kolff, Willem; Pierce, William S.; Poirier, Victor

artificial hearts: American leadership in, 10–11; bioethical issues associated with, 9–10, 25, 111–15, 124, 163, 164–71, 174, 176, 246, 265; as bridge-to-recovery devices, 92; as bridge-to-transplant devices, 27–28, 61, 77, 87, 89, 92, 135–36, 155–58, 161–62, 310–11n197; clinical trials for, 197; congressional hearings relating to, 169–70; commercialization of, 159–62, 175, 176, 266; as compared with heart transplantation, 23–24, 86–88; as complementary to heart transplantation, 91–92; complications associated with, 143, 144, 152, 153–54, 158, 172–73, 247–48, 250, 261; controversial history of, 1–2, 28, 85–86; Cooley-DeBakey feud relating to, 80–86; cost-effectiveness of, 167; critics of, 162–63, 175; costs associated with, 147, 254–55, 260–61;

artificial hearts (*continued*)

debate surrounding, 7–10, 21–22, 24, 25–26, 86–91, 262–66; design of, 76–77; early experimentation with, 29–31, 32–37, 74–76; early expectations of, 14–15, 21, 31, 47–48, 124; efficacy of, 33–34, 86–87; as engineering challenge, 19–21, 23, 24–25, 26, 29, 31, 33–36, 39–40, 46–47, 57, 58; FDA's role in, 119–20, 135, 169, 172, 174; as first used on a human patient, 76–80; government regulation of, 27, 110–11, 119–20, 197; growing acceptance of, 27; illustrations and photographs of, 3, 4, 34, 77, 88, 93, 103, 127, 131, 139; media coverage of, 22, 24, 25, 61, 79–80, 86, 168, 175–76, 241, 245–46, 248–49, 263; Medicare reimbursement for, 253; nuclear-powered, 24–25, 95–101, 115; obstacles to, 90; patient eligibility for, 134–41, 261; power sources for, 120, 178, 254–55; phases of development for, 197–99; public sentiment toward, 5, 154–55, 173–74; and readiness for implantation in a human, 131–35, 197–98; regulatory process required for, 132–35, 197–98; risks associated with, 24–25, 86, 119–120; socioeconomic issues associated with, 46; stakeholders involved in, 174–75; and transplant surgery, 18, 23–24; types of, 3–4; well-known recipients of, 5. *See also* artificial heart research; assist pumps; atomic hearts; Jarvik-7 artificial heart; Karp case; left ventricular assist devices; total artificial hearts; ventricular assist devices

artificial heart valves, 136, 143 bileaflet, 19; development of, 18–19, 20–21; materials used for, 18–19

artificial kidneys, 32, 126

assist pumps, 56; clinical successes with, 48–54; complications associated with, 39; DeBakey's use of, 48–49, 63; as developed by DeBakey, 38–40; research relating to, 74–75. *See also* intraaortic balloon pump; left ventricular assist devices; mechanical auxiliary ventricle; ventricular assist devices

Atomic Energy Commission (AEC), 24; atomic heart design developed by, 101–4, 106–7; and atomic heart research, 97–101; as critic of the NHLI atomic heart design, 107; and phasing out of atomic heart research, 116, 117–18

atomic hearts: ambivalence about risks versus benefits of, 116–17, 119; competing approaches to development of, 24, 97–107, 120–21; and concerns about radiation exposure, 116–17; design proposals for, 98–99, 101–7; fictional account of, 95–96, 121; first animal implantation of, 104; illustrations of, 103, 104; phasing out of research on, 116–19; research and development relating to, 96–107; problems inherent in, 118–19; risks associated with, 111–15, 116–17, 121

atrial septal defect, 17

Avco-Everett Research Labs, 184, 185

AVCO LVAD, 184, 185

azathioprine, 91

Baby Fae, 151

Bailey, Charles P., 16

Bakken, Earl, 20

balloon pumps, 221–22. *See also* intraaortic balloon pump

Barnard, Christiaan: criticism of, 69, 284n50; first heart transplant performed by, 23, 60, 68–69, 70; medical background of, 67–68; as public figure, 68–69, 91

Bartlett, Robert, 10, 18, 173, 262, 263

batteries: as used in pacemakers, 20

Bavoleck, Cecilia, 17

Baxter Healthcare Corporation, 26, 182, 184, 204, 207

Bayh-Dole Act, 159

Baylor College of Medicine: as cardiovascular surgical center, 17, 62, 64; and collaboration with Rice University, 39–40, 52, 54, 74–75; heart research at, 37–42; and the Karp case, 76–85. *See also* Cooley, Denton; DeBakey, Michael

Beall, Arthur, 110

Beck, Ulrich, 111

BeneCor Heart Systems, 243

Berlin heart, 177, 314n280

Berlin Heart Pediatric VAD, 180

Bernard, William, 195

Bernstein, Barton, 46, 47, 96, 167

Bernstein, Eugene, 180, 223–24

Bigelow, Wilfred, 16

Billroth, Theodor, 15

bioengineering: as applied to artificial heart research, 2, 19–21, 23, 24–25, 26, 29, 31, 33–36 bioethical issues: associated with artificial hearts, 9–10, 25, 111–15, 163, 164–71, 174, 176, 246, 265; and the Barney Clark case, 164, 165–67; and medical innovation, 111–12, 163–69; and patient self-determination, 25, 165–66

Bivacor, 258

Bjork, Viking, 19

Bjork-Shiley valve, 19, 136, 143, 150

Blaiberg, Philip, 68

Blalock, Alfred, 15, 16, 63

Blitzer, Wolf, 239

blood oxygenator devices, 32

blue baby operations, 15, 16

body parts, replaceable, 4, 5, 6–7. *See also* artificial hearts; artificial heart valves; organ transplantation

Bonnell Inc., 160

"booster heart." *See* mechanical auxiliary ventricle

Borovetz, Harvey, 224

Bosso, John, 147

Boudia, Soraya, 97

Boyle, Joseph, 145, 148

Bricker, Eugene, 49, 278–79n105

bridge-to-recovery (BTR) devices, 30, 180

Brighton, John, 185

Brock, Russell, 15, 63

Brown, Harold, 84

Brown, Nik, 21

Bryden, Rod, 207

Büecherl, Emil S., 177, 314n280

Burcham, Jack, 154

Butler, Ken, 222, 224

Callahan, Daniel, 164

Campbell, Gordon, 311n197

Canada: approval system for medical devices in, 199

Caplan, Arthur, 96, 165

CardioWest TAH. *See* SynCardia TAH

CardioWest Technologies Inc., 177–78, 251–52, 315n282. *See also* SynCardia TAH

Carrel, Alexis, 14

Carroll, William C., 72

Centers for Medicare and Medicaid Services (CMS): and device reimbursement, 199, 209, 253, 260; and support for clinical trials, 215

centrifugal pumps, 221, 222

Ceraso, Louise, 51

Chaim Sheba Medical Center (Israel), 226

Cheney, Dick, 5, 239; complications experienced by, 212–13; HeartMate II LVAD implanted in, 27, 211–13, 214, 259–60; as heart transplant patient, 213, 322n12

Cheng, Kevin, 156

chimpanzee heart: implanted in a human, 66

Christerson, Tom, 245, 248–49

circulatory support systems. *See* mechanical circulatory support systems

Clark, Barney: assessment of, 146–47, 173; bioethical issues relating to case of, 164, 165–67, 263; complications experienced by, 143, 144; consent form presented to, 164, 165; death of, 144; media interest in, 144–46, 176; as recipient of the Jarvik-7 heart, 5, 25, 141–44

Clark, Una Loy, 141, 142, 143, 144, 147, 155

Clarke, Lee, 117

Cleveland Clinic: artificial heart research at 178, 243; Kolff's research at, 32–33

Cleveland Heart Inc., 258–59

clinical trials: as applied to surgical procedures, 201–2; required by the FDA, 110, 182, 189, 197, 198; for VADs, 181, 182, 184, 197, 198, 199–200, 202–5, 207, 208, 214–21, 235–38

Cole, Donald, 118

Columbia Presbyterian Medical Center, 215

Conformité Européene (CE): and approval for medical devices, 198–99; and the Jarvik 2000 Flowmaker, 231

continuous flow technology: as applied to the total artificial heart, 259

continuous-flow VADs, 213–14, 221, 222–27, 237–39; as compared with pulsatile blood flow, 223–24; problems associated with, 231–33. *See also* HeartMate II LVAD

Cooley, Denton, 10, 16, 17, 23, 54, 59, 120, 262, 289n162; and the AbioCor TAH, 249; and artificial heart research, 75–76, 86, 87, 88; artificial hearts implanted by, 76–80, 135–38, 165; censuring of, 81; and the Karp case, 76–86, 92–93, 286–87n102; as DeBakey's rival, 64–65; and feud with DeBakey, 24, 61, 62, 80–83, 92–94; heart transplants performed by, 72; as prominent heart surgeon, 60, 63–65, 196

Cooper, Theodore, 80, 99, 100, 101, 104, 108
Cooper Committee: and medical device
    legislation, 108–9, 110
Copeland, Jack, 10, 28, 120, 172, 257, 262,
    315n282; as advocate for artificial heart
    technology, 170, 177–78; artificial heart
    technology as used by, 155–57, 161, 169,
    251–52, 253; as heart transplant surgeon, 155
Crafoord, Clarence, 15, 16, 17
Creager, Angela, 96
Creighton, Thomas, 156
Crenner, Christopher, 201–2, 214
Cruz, Anatolio, 19
Cullen Cardiovascular Laboratories, 75, 136
cyclosporine, 90, 91, 189–90

Dacron graft: as used in heart surgery, 37,
    39, 62
Daggett, Ronald, 19
Dalkon Shield IUD, 109
Darvall, Denise, 68
Davies, Lawrence, 71
death: definition and determination of, 67, 91
DeBakey, Michael, 112; as Cooley's rival,
    64–65; criticism and censure of, 49,
    279n108; and feud with Cooley, 24, 61, 62,
    80–83, 92–94; heart transplants performed
    by, 72; and the Karp case, 80, 81–82, 83–85;
    left ventricular assist pump developed by,
    48–49, 186; as pioneer in artificial heart
    research and development, 7, 10, 16, 17, 22,
    23, 28, 30, 31, 37–43, 54, 63, 74–75, 86–87,
    94, 97, 262; as prominent heart surgeon, 60,
    62–63, 65, 70, 200; as public figure, 37, 39,
    40–42, 44–45, 48, 49, 54–55, 57, 61, 63–64;
    and VADs, 182, 199, 214, 232, 286n101
Dennis, Clarence, 117, 118
DeRudder, Marcel, 48
Desai, Shashank, 213
Deseret Research Inc., 159
DeVries, William, 25, 54, 120, 165, 172,
    307n131; as advocate for artificial heart
    research, 170; and the artificial heart
    program at Humana Hospital Audubon,
    147–53; and the artificial heart program at
    the University of Utah, 127, 130, 131–32,
    144–47; and the Jarvik-7 heart, 132, 133–34,
    135, 139–47, 149–54, 166, 169
DeWall bubble oxygenator, 17

dialysis, 32, 126
Dong, Eugene, 95–96
donor hearts: shortage of, 28, 75, 92, 123, 194,
    260, 260; viability of, 91. *See also* organ
    rejection
Donovan artificial heart, 126
Dowling, Robert, 245, 247, 248
Drummond, Michael, 5, 156–57, 161, 162
Duffy, Robert, 111
Dwan, John, 144

Edwards, Lowell, 19
Edwards Lifesciences LLC, 184, 207
Eichwald, Ernst, 305n76
Eisenhower, Dwight D., 11
electrocardiograph, 15
Elema Company, 20
Elmquist, Rune, 20
Energy Research and Development Adminis-
    tration (ERDA), 118
ethics. *See* bioethical issues
Europe: approval system for medical devices
    in, 198–99; VAD implant reimbursement
    in, 209. *See also* Conformité Européene
Evans, Barbara, 78
extracorporeal membrane oxygenation
    (ECMO), 18, 64, 180, 249, 272n62

FK-506, 91
Flamm, Anne Lederman, 246
Flannery, Ellen, 166
Fletcher, James, 125
Fogarty, John, 43
Food and Drug Administration (FDA): and
    bridge-to-transplant devices, 156; clinical
    trials required by, 110, 182, 189; and regulation
    of artificial hearts, 119–20, 135, 169, 172, 254;
    and regulation of medical devices, 107–10,
    197; and ventricular assist devices, 181, 182,
    184, 204–5
Foote, Susan, 109
Ford, Gerald, 110
Fouquet, Simone, 114
Fowler, Eugene, 99, 101
Fox, Renée, 8–9, 73, 74, 96, 166, 167, 246,
    338n91; and the Jarvik-7 heart, 131, 134, 135,
    148, 152–53, 171, 175; and the Karp case,
    82–83, 85
Framingham Heart Study, 11

Frazier, O. H., 10, 82, 86, 173, 223, 224, 237, 258, 259, 262; and the AbioCor TAH, 245, 249; and the HeartMate LVAD, 194–96, 203, 204, 214, 227; and the Jarvik 2000 Flowmaker, 230–31, 239
Fredrickson, Donald, 98
Frommer, Peter, 183
Fye, Bruce, 10, 13, 16, 71

Gaylin, Willard, 164
Geffen, Maxwell, 49
Gibbon, John, Jr., 16, 17, 30
Giddens, Anthony, 111
Gil, Gideon, 167, 176
Gillick, Muriel, 235, 236
Godden, Matthew, 5
Golden, Troy, 1
Golding, Len, 258–59
Gott, Vincent, 19
Gott-Daggett valve, 19
government regulation: of medical devices, 22, 107–11
Grant, Robert, 47
Gray, Laman, 245, 248
Greenberg, Daniel, 96
Griffith, Bartley P., 224
Grondin, Pierre, 74
Groote Schuur Hospital, 67, 68
Gross, Robert E., 15, 16, 18
guidelines for experimental procedures, 80–81
Gumbel, Bryant, 161

Hahnemann University Hospital, 249–50
Hall, C. William, 38, 74, 275n43
Hamilton, David, 6
Hansen, Bert, 123
Hansen, Lisa and Elisa, 145
Hardy, James, 66
Harken, Dwight, 16
Harmison, Lowell, 106, 107
Harrison, Bobby, 249
Harvey, Robert, 189, 200–201
Hastings, Frank W., 28, 37, 106, 277n76; as director of the Artificial Heart Program, 43–44, 97
Hastings Center, 112, 164, 165
Hatch, Orrin, 171–72
Haupt, Clive, 68

Haydon, Murray, 152–53
Health Canada, 199
Health Industry Manufacturers Association, 297n89
Heart and Vascular Center EKN Duisburg (Germany), 257
HeartAssist 5, 232
HeartAssist VAD, 232, 328n111
Heart Beat (Dong and Andreopoulos), 95–96, 121, 300–301n157
heart catheterization, 15
heart disease: causes of, 11, 13; diagnostic technologies as applied to, 15; as leading cause of death in the US, 11–13; prevention versus treatment of, 8, 162–63, 167; mortality rates from, 13; types of, 11–12
heart failure: artificial heart as treatment for, 2, 3–4, 10–11; classification system for, 12; prevalence of, 12–13, 207–8, 260, 266; prognosis for, 12; symptoms of, 12; VADs used to treat, 187–88; well-known patients suffering from, 5. *See also* artificial hearts; left ventricular assist devices, 259; ventricular assist devices
heart-lung machine: complications associated with, 18, 32, 310n180; importance of, 17–18; invention of, 16–17, 29
HeartMate LVAD, 184, 194–96, 321n98; clinical trial of, 203–5; design of, 195, 196; FDA approval for, 204; premarket approval for, 196
HeartMate II LVAD, 5, 224–28, 231, 234, 258, 321n94; as bridge-to-transplant device, 227, 236–37; Dick Cheney as recipient of, 27, 211–13; clinical trial of, 227; complications associated with, 227; design problems in, 226–27; as destination therapy, 227–28; implantation of, 226, 227; patient testimonials for, 238–39; photograph of, 225; power source for, 212, 225
HeartMate III, 234
HeartMate VE LVAD: as compared with drug therapy, 215–17; physicians' concerns regarding, 217–18
HeartMate XVE LVAD, 216, 236; compared with the Novacor LVAS, 220; as destination therapy, 235; FDA approval for, 235; photograph of, 225
HeartSaver VAD, 207

heart surgery: bypass, 13–14, 17; closed-heart, 64; history of, 13–16; hypothermia as used in, 16, 17, 64; mortality rates for, 17; neurological complications associated with, 310n180, 323n24; open-heart, 63, 64. *See also* Cooley, Denton; DeBakey, Michael
heart transplantation: animal research relating to, 66–67, 69; Dick Cheney as recipient of, 213; as compared with artificial hearts, 23–24, 86–88; as complementary to artificial hearts, 91–92; complications resulting from 71, 137; early experiences with, 18, 66–74, 155; early research and development relating to, 66–67; limitations of, 60; media coverage of, 24, 61, 68–69, 91; mortality rates for, 60, 72, 87, 200; obstacles to, 90; organ rejection as concern with, 18, 60, 67, 68, 71, 72, 73, 74; patient eligibility for, 216, 221; patient outcomes following, 68, 70–71, 72, 74, 87; prevalence of, 72–73, 74, 91, 200, 260; survival rate following, 260. *See also* Barnard, Christiaan; Cooley, Denton; DeBakey, Michael; Kantrowitz, Adrian; Shumway, Norman
heart valves: diseases of, 18. *See also* artificial heart valves
HeartWare International Inc., 207, 234, 325n54, 330n147
HeartWare VAD (HVAD), 234, 237, 330–31n148
Hellums, J. David, 75, 82
Hemopump, 222–23, 224, 321n94
Henderson, Nalexia, 256
Henry Ford Heart and Vascular Institute, 238
Hernandez, Nelva Lou, 72
Hill, Donald, 189, 190
Hill, Lister, 43
Hiller, Kirby W., 36
Hoff, Hebbel E., 80
Holter, John W., 37
Houghton, Peter, 5, 230
Hrobowski, Tara, 238
Hufnagel, Charles, 19
Humana Hospital Audubon: artificial heart program at, 147–53, 175
Humanitarian Use Device (HUD) status, 257, 336n66
Hume, David, 67
Hunt, Sharon, 235–36

hypertension, 11
hypothermia: as used in heart surgery, 16, 17, 64

Illich, Ivan, 163
Illinois Institute of Technology Research Institute, 296n63
immunosuppressant drugs, 90–91, 189–90
implantable cardiac defibrillator, 20
In My Time (Cheney), 211
Inova Fairfax Hospital and Vascular Institute, 211, 213
Institute for Biomedical Engineering (University of Utah), 102–3
institutional review boards (IRBs): for artificial heart implantation, 92; and the Jarvik-7 heart, 132–35
Interagency Registry for Mechanically Assisted Circulatory Support (INTERMACS), 233–34, 236, 261
International Society for Heart and Lung Transplantation Registry for Mechanically Assisted Circulatory Support (IMACS), 234
International Society for Heart and Lung Transplantation, 91
intraaortic balloon pump, 52–54, 136, 180, 187, 221–22
Investigation of Nontransplant-Eligible Patients Who Are Inotrope Dependent (INTrEPID) clinical trial, 219–20, 235
Investigational Device Exemption (IDE) applications: for the CardioWest temporary TAH, 178; for the Jarvik-7 heart, 135, 176; for the Pierce-Donachy VAD, 188
IUDs: problems with, 109

Jarvik, Robert, 10, 25, 26, 54, 126, 127, 128–29, 176; as advocate for artificial heart research, 170, 176; artificial heart developed by, 126, 129–30, 131, 148, 159; celebrity status of, 146; and dismissal from Symbion, 162; and friction with Kolff, 160–61; on the readiness of the Jarvik-7 heart, 132–33; and VADs, 214. *See also* Jarvik-7 artificial heart; Jarvik 2000 FlowMaker Pump
Jarvik Research Inc., 172, 228
Jarvik-7 artificial heart (Utah TAH), 8–9, 25, 126, 127, 168, 177–78, 204, 263; adapted as a VAD, 228; as bridge-to-transplantation

device, 155–62, 173, 190; commercialization of, 159–62, 176; complications associated with, 143, 144, 152, 153–54, 158, 172–73; costs associated with implantation of, 147; design of, 129; FDA concerns regarding, 135, 169, 172, 174; IRB concerns regarding, 134–35, 165; media interest in, 132, 140, 144–46; patient eligibility for, 139–41; phasing out of, 172; photographs of, 131, 139, 149; and readiness for use on human patients, 131–35; as a success, 146–47; as tested on animals, 130–31. *See also* Clark, Barney; DeVries, William; Haydon, Murray; Kolff, Willem; Olsen, Don B.; Schroeder, William; Stenberg, Leif; SynCardia TAH

Jarvik 7–70 artificial heart, 157–58

Jarvik 2000 FlowMaker Pump, 26, 172, 182, 228–31; design of, 228–29; implantation of, 230; Investigational Device Exemption status for, 231; photograph of, 229; power source for, 229; testing of, 229–30

Jassawalla, Jal, 207

Jeffrey, Kirk, 108, 114

Jessup, Mariell, 219

Jewish Hospital—University of Louisville: artificial heart implantation at, 245–49

Johnson, Lyndon B., 43, 44, 98

Johnson, Michelle, 255–56

Joint Committee on Atomic Energy (JCAE), 99, 100–101, 118

Jones, David, 13, 14, 202, 323n24

Jongbloed, Jacob, 16, 17

Jonsen, Albert R., 96, 166, 167, 170–71

Joyce, David, 200

Joyce, Lyle, 200

Jurgens, John, 78

Kantrowitz, Adrian: auxiliary ventricle developed by, 49–51, 280n13; heart transplants performed by, 69–70, 87, 284n60; intraaortic balloon pump developed by, 52–54, 180, 221–22; as pioneer in artificial heart research and development, 10, 22, 23, 28, 30–31, 42, 54–55, 56, 85, 86, 262

Kantrowitz, Arthur, 49–50

Kantrowitz, Jean, 56

Karolinska Hospital: artificial heart implanted at, 153–54

Karolinska Institute, 20

Karp, Haskell, 5; death of, 79; as heart transplant patient, 60–61, 76–80, 93, 137. *See also* Karp case

Karp, Shirley, 78, 83

Karp case: investigation of, 80–83, 286–87n102; malpractice suit relating to, 83–85

Kasperak, Mike, 70–71

Katz, Jay, 166

Kefauver-Harris drug amendments, 108

Kennedy, Edward, 171–72

Kennedy Institute of Ethics, 164

Keon, Wilbert, 310–11n197

Kessler, Tom, 130

kidney failure. *See* renal failure

kidney transplants, 67, 68

Kirklin, James, 221

Kirklin, John, 17

Knutti, Ralph, 23, 46

Kolff, Jack, 159

Kolff, Willem, 29, 93, 112, 138, 262, 305n76; and artificial heart research at the University of Utah, 124–32, 148; and atomic heart research and development, 102–3, 116, 118, 121; and friction with Robert Jarvik, 160–61; and the Jarvik-7 heart, 141, 176; and marketing of the artificial heart, 158–61; as pioneer in artificial heart research and development, 7, 10, 22, 23, 24, 25, 26, 28, 30, 31, 32–36, 42, 43, 54–55, 74, 85, 94, 121; and VADs, 182

Kolff Associates Inc., 158–61

Kolff Medical, 160–61

Kormos, Robert, 224

Kralios artificial heart, 126

Kranich, Herb, 223

Kung, Robert, 243

Kusserow, Bert, 28, 36–37, 42

Kwan-Gett, Clifford, 126, 127–28, 159

Kwan-Gett artificial heart, 127; design of, 128

Lanfear, David, 238

Lavare Cycle, 330–31n148

Lasker, Mary, 47

Laurence, William, 14

Lavee, Jacob, 226

Leclair, Noella, 310–11n197

Lederberg, Joshua, 45

Lederer, Susan, 6–7, 65, 69, 284n50

Lederman, David, 184, 185, 243, 246, 251

left ventricular assist devices (LVADs), 3, 4, 27, 48–49; clinical trials of, 214–21, 235–38; as compared with drug therapy, 215–17; compared with optimal medical management, 219–20; complications associated with, 216–17, 221; as destination therapy, 214, 219, 236–37; limitations of, 236; mortality rate associated with, 220; as used in atomic heart design, 105; prevalence of, 261–62. *See also* HeartMate LVAD; Heartmate II LVAD; HeartMate VE LVAD; HeartMate XVE LVAD; Novacor LVAS; Thoratec PVAD system; ventricular assist devices

Lenfant, Claude, 162, 173, 178, 242; and the Artificial Heart Program, 168, 170–72

Lerner, Barron H., 96, 124, 164, 166

Levacor VAD, 325n54

Leviev Heart Center (Israel), 226

Levinson, Mark, 157

Levy, Robert I., 168

Lewis, John, 16

Life Extenders Corporation, 159

Lillehei, C. Walton, 16, 19, 67

Lillehei pump-oxygenator, 17

Lindbergh, Charles, 14

Liotta, Domingo: and artificial heart research and development, 37, 38, 54, 74, 75; and the Karp case, 75, 78, 79, 80, 81, 82–83, 92, 287n102

Loebe, Matthias, 218–19

Long, James, 1

Lott, Dale, 140

Love, Robert, 1

Lower, Richard: and heart transplantation, 66, 68, 88

L-VAD Technologies, 56

Lyman artificial heart, 126

MagLev technology, 207

Mann, Alfred, 114

Marks, Harry, 201

Massie, Barry, 219

McCabe, Selwyn, 28, 32

McCans, Walter, 49

McCollum, Leonard F., 80

McDonnell-Douglas, 98

McGowan Institute for Organ Engineering, 224–26

McIntosh, Charles, 169, 170

McKeown, Thomas, 163

McRae, Donald, 67

mechanical auxiliary ventricle ("booster heart"): clotting as problem with, 51; as developed by Kantrowitz, 49–52

mechanical circulatory support systems (MCSSs), 29, 54–55, 243–44; for short-term use, 199–200. *See also* artificial hearts; artificial heart valves; medical devices; pacemakers; total artificial hearts; ventricular assist devices

MedForte Research Foundation, 178, 251

media coverage: of hypertension research, 276n55; of the Jarvik-7 heart, 138, 144–46, 151–52; relating to artificial heart development and implantation, 22, 24, 25, 37, 39, 40–42, 48, 61, 79–80, 86, 168, 175–76, 241, 245–46, 248–49, 263; and the Meuffels case, 137–38

Medical College of Virginia (MCV), 67–68

Medical Device Amendments (1976), 97, 110, 119, 188–89, 197

medical device innovation: bioethical concerns relating to, 111–12, 163–69, 265; costs of, 206–7; federal oversight of, 119–20. *See also* artificial hearts; ventricular assist devices

medical devices: classification of, 108–9, 110, 120; commercialization and marketing of, 198; government regulation of, 22, 107–11, 119–20, 197, 198, 300n152; legislation affecting, 109, 110–11, 119–20; phases in development of, 197–99; proliferation of, 4, 5, 106–8, 109; reimbursement for, 199, 253; risks posed by, 108–9; safety concerns relating to, 109–10. *See also* artificial hearts; artificial kidneys; ventricular assist devices

medical ethics. *See* bioethical issues

Medicare. *See* Centers for Medicare and Medicaid Services

MedQuest Products Inc., 207, 325n54

Medtronic Inc., 20, 237, 330n147

Medtronic-Alcatel device, 113

Medtronic-Hall valve, 143, 150

Methodist Hospital (Houston), 37

Meuffels, Willebrordus, 6, 136–38

MicroMed DeBakey Noon VAD, 232, 328n109

MicroMed Inc., 232, 328n111

MiFlow VAD technology, 207
Model-7 ALVAD, 195
Moise, John, 222, 224
Montreal Heart Institute, 74
Morreim, E. Haavi, 246
Motion Control, 159
Mott, William, 98, 101, 105, 107, 111, 116, 118
Moulopoulos, Spyridon, 52
Murray, Gordon, 16
Mustard, William, 16

Nader, Ralph, 109
Nathoo, Ayesha, 68
National Advisory Heart Council, 43
National Aeronautics and Space Administration (NASA): and artificial heart research, 35, 36
National Council on Radiation Protection (NCRP), 113
National Heart Act, 11
National Heart and Lung Institute (NHLI), 101, 276–77n61; atomic heart design developed by, 104–7; and ethical issues relating to artificial hearts, 112, 167–71; and phasing out of atomic heart research, 117
National Heart Institute (NHI), 11, 23, 39–40, 42–47, 276–77n61; and atomic heart research, 97–101, 117. *See also* Artificial Heart Program
National Heart, Lung, and Blood Institute (NHLBI), 276–77n61; and review of the artificial heart program, 162, 167–71; and funding for artificial heart research, 172, 175, 178, 242–43; and funding for VAD research, 182–85, 215, 224
National Institutes of Health (NIH): and funding for artificial heart research, 7, 42–48, 57–58, 74, 86, 97, 158–59, 167–68, 171–72, 181, 276n60; and funding for VAD research, 26, 87, 121, 215; and the Karp case, 80–81, 93. *See also* Artificial Heart Program; National Heart Institute
Nelkin, Dorothy, 96, 175–76
Nellen, Maurice, 67
Nimbus Inc., 178, 222, 224, 321n94; and artificial heart research, 243
Noon, George, 200, 214, 262
Norman, John C., 24, 104, 112, 117, 262; and VAD development, 184, 194–95, 199

Norton, S. Harry, 36
Nosé, Yukihiko, 50, 54, 295n50
Novacor II LVAS, 207
Novacor LVAS, 90, 173, 184, 190–94, 261; clinical trial of, 219–20; compared with the HeartMate XVE LVAD, 220; complications associated with, 192–93; design of, 191–92; development of, 207; European clinical trials of, 205; FDA approval for, 204–5; premarket approval for, 196
Novacor Medical, 204–5, 207, 208
nuclear energy: as power source for artificial hearts, 95–101. *See also* atomic hearts
Nuclear Materials and Equipment Corporation (NUMEC), 113, 114
Nuclear Regulatory Commission, 118
Nuetfield, Debbie, 157

O'Bannon, William, 40, 75, 81–82
O'Brien, James, 192
Office of Management and Budget (OMB): role of in artificial heart research, 100
Olsen, Don B., 159; and artificial heart research at the University of Utah, 25, 129–30, 131, 132, 133; and CardioWest Technologies, 177–78, 251–52
organ rejection: drugs used to alleviate, 90–91; as problem with heart transplantation, 18, 60, 67, 68, 71, 72, 73, 74, 200
organ transplantation, 65–66. *See also* heart transplantation
Oxford Heart Centre, 230
Oyer, Philip, 90, 162, 192

pacemakers, 18; development of, 19–20, 21; manufacturer recalls involving, 109; lithium-powered, 115; plutonium-powered, 24–25, 97, 113–14; power sources for, 20, 113–14, 115; with transistor circuitry, 20
Page, Irvine H., 41, 49, 73, 276n55
Paget, Sir Stephen, 15
Parsonnet, Victor, 113, 114, 115
Penn State TAH, 177, 243, 332–33n7; photograph of, 242
Penn State University College of Medicine: and partnering with Thoratec, 189–90; VAD research at, 184, 185–90, 332n7
Penn State University Hershey Medical Center, 178, 187, 242–43

perfusionists, 17

perfusion pump: development of, 14

personhood, concept of, 7

Peterson, Chase, 144, 145

Philips of North America, 102–3, 105

Phillips, Steven J., 54

Phillips, Winfred, 185

Phoenix TAH, 156

Pierce, William S., 10, 37, 172–73, 177, 262; and VAD research and development, 184, 185–89, 206, 332n7

Pierce-Donachy pump, 184, 185–89; complications associated with, 188; design of, 186–87; shortcomings of, 190

plutonium-238, 295n46; as used in pacemakers, 97, 113–14; as power source for the atomic heart, 97, 102, 104, 105–6, 111, 112, 115; risks associated with, 112–14, 115

Poirier, Victor, 10, 106, 262, 264; and the HeartMate LVAD, 184, 195, 200, 206, 207, 224

Portner, Peer, 10, 162, 173, 201; and the Novacor LVAS, 184, 190–91, 193, 200, 206

Potter, William H., 37

prednisone, 91

PREMATCH clinical trial: for VADs, 214–15

Preston, Thomas, 43, 57, 167

Public Citizen Health Research Group, 170

quality of life: as issue for artificial heart patients, 6, 7, 46, 167. *See also* bioethical issues

Quinn, Irene, 250

Quinn, James, 6, 334n39

radiation: as concern regarding atomic hearts, 116–17, 298n104

radioisotope thermoelectric generator (RTG), 98. *See also* atomic hearts

randomized controlled trials (RCTs): as basis for evaluating new treatments, 201–2; of VADs, 201, 202, 214–21

Randomized Evaluation of Mechanical Assistance for the Treatment of Congestive Heart Failure (REMATCH) study, 27, 323n31; cost of, 323n18; and VADs, 213, 214–20, 235–38

Randomized Evaluation of Novacor LVAS in a Non-Transplant Population (RELIANT) trial, 220, 235

rapamycin, 91

Ray, Dixy Lee, 117

Reagan, Ronald, 151

Reiner, Jonathan, 211, 212, 213, 259–60

Reiser, Stanley, 166

ReliantHeart Inc., 328n111

Relman, Arnold, 145, 148

renal failure: mechanical devices for treatment of, 32

Rice University: and collaboration with Baylor College of Medicine, 39–40, 52, 54, 74–75

risks: associated with atomic hearts, 111–15; associated with science and technology, 96

Rizor, Joseph, 71

Rogers, Paul, 109

roller pumps, 221, 222

Rose, Eric, 215

Rosenberg, Gerson, 10, 177, 185, 242

Rothman, David, 179

Rush, Boyd, 66

Safe Medical Devices Act (1990), 119, 336n66

St. Jude Medical, 20, 330n147

St. Jude Medical bileaflet valve, 19

St. Luke's Hospital (Houston), 64–65, 75

Salisbury, Peter, 32, 42

Salter, James, 138

Samuels, Louis, 249

Sarns, Dick, 332n7

Sarns 3M, 178, 243, 332n7

Savant, Marilyn vos, 146

Schlich, Thomas, 6

Schrire, Velva, 67

Schroeder, William: complications experienced by, 152; as recipient of Jarvik-7 heart, 52, 149–52, 176;

Seaborg, Glenn, 98, 100–101

Searle Cardiopulmonary Systems, 189

Segal, Howard, 96

Semb, Bjarne, 153–54

Senning, Åke, 20

Shanks, Haskell, 53–54, 58

Shannon, James, 31, 42–43, 46–48, 57, 97, 278n97

Sharp, Lesley, 32, 36
Shepherd, Randy, 256, 257, 335n57
Shores, Kathleen, 1
Shumacker, Harris, 13
Shumakov, Valeriy I., 10
Shumway, Norman, 16, 155, 300–301n157; as
    advocate for heart transplantation, 88–91;
    heart transplants performed by, 70–71; on
    the Jarvik-7 heart, 161; as pioneer in heart
    transplantation research and development,
    66–67, 68–69, 74, 91; on VADs, 194
Sigerist, Henry E., 15
Slepian, Marvin, 240, 253, 315n282
SmartHeart Left Ventricular Assist Device,
    258–59
SmartHeart Total Artificial Heart, 258–59
Smith, Lee, 159
Smith, Richard G., 157, 253, 315n282
Smithsonian Institution: artificial hearts
    donated to, 77, 93, 162, 275n43, 279n110,
    289n162, 295n49, 302n17, 308n153, 311n209,
    333n22
Soviet Union: artificial heart research in, 10
Starr, Albert, 19
Starr-Edwards ball valve, 19
Starzl, Thomas, 67–68
Stenberg, Leif, 153–54
Stevenson, Lynne, 217–18, 219, 220
Stinson, Edward, 73
Stirling mechanical converter: as applied in
    atomic heart design, 102
Strait, George, 151
Strauss, Michael J., 58
Sutherland, Donald, 138
Swazey, Judith, 8–9, 73, 74, 96, 167, 246; and
    the Jarvik-7 heart, 131, 134, 135, 148, 152–53,
    161, 171, 175; and the Karp case, 82–83, 85
Symbion Inc., 146, 161–62, 172, 175, 176, 190,
    228, 251, 311n197
SynCardia Systems Inc., 253–58, 315n282;
    financial problems of, 258
SynCardia TAH (CardioWest TAH), 3, 27,
    241, 252–58, 261, 315n282, 335n57; clinical
    trial for, 252–53; as compared with the
    AbioCor TAH, 252, 257; costs associated
    with, 254–55; design of, 253–54; FDA
    approval for, 257; patient experiences with,
    255–57; photograph of, 255; power source
    for, 254–55

Taussig, Helen, 15, 284n60
Terumo Corporation, 321n98, 332n7
Texas Children's Hospital, 64, 65
Texas Heart Institute (THI), 17, 33, 65, 75,
    135–36, 178, 243; and the HeartMate II LVAD,
    224, 226, 227; VAD research at, 194–95
Thermedics Inc., 195, 196
Thermo Cardiosystems Inc., 321n94, 321n98;
    VADs developed by, 26, 26, 183, 184, 195, 224
Thermo Electron Engineering Corporation,
    97–98; and atomic heart design, 105–6; and
    VAD development, 184, 195, 196
Thomas, Everett, 72
Thompson, Thomas, 41, 65, 83
Thompson Ramo Wooldridge Inc. (TRW),
    101–2
Thoratec IVAD, 320n81
Thoratec Laboratories Corporation, 321n94,
    321n98, 330n147; revenues generated by,
    208; VADs developed by, 26, 182, 184,
    189–90, 215–19, 224–28, 237
Thoratec PVAD system (Pierce-Donachy
    pump), 184, 185–90, 193, 200–201, 204, 208,
    261; FDA approval for, 204–5; marketing of,
    208; premarket approval for, 196
Threshold (film), 138
Tools, Robert: complications experienced by,
    247–48; as recipient of the AbioCor TAH,
    5, 241, 245–48, 249
total artificial hearts (TAHs), 3, 4, 6, 24,
    25–26; as bridge-to-transplantation devices,
    27–28, 155–58, 161; as compared with VADs,
    181–82, 205–6, 209–10; DeBakey's research
    on, 54; early experimentation with, 33–34,
    54; obstacles to use of, 63; in the twenty-
    first century, 240–41. *See also* AbioCor
    TAH; artificial hearts; Jarvik-7 artificial
    heart; Penn State TAH; SynCardia TAH;
    Utah TAH
transplantation: of body parts, 4, 5, 6–7.
    See also heart transplantation
Trasoff, Nina, 157
Truman, Harry, 42

Unger, Felix, 177, 314n280
Unger artificial heart, 126, 177, 314n280
University of Arizona Medical Center:
    artificial heart research at, 155–58, 178,
    251, 253

University of Ottawa Heart Institute, 207, 310–11n197
University of Pittsburgh, 224
University of Utah Medical Center: animal research at, 129–30; artificial heart research at, 24, 25, 26, 103, 124–31, 172, 242; and collaborations with private industry, 159–60. *See also* Jarvik-7 artificial heart; Utah TAH
Utah TAH, 5, 25; media spotlight on, 123–24. *See also* Jarvik-7 artificial heart

VADs. *See* ventricular assist devices
Vascular International Inc., 159
Vasquez, Esperanza del Valle, 5, 52–53, 58, 63
ventricular assist devices (VADs), 3, 158, 311n197; academic-industry partnerships involved in development of, 183–85, 189, 215, 224, 232; applications of, 200–201, 259–60; and artificial hearts, 181–82; as bridge-to-recovery devices, 30, 180, 181, 192, 231; as bridge-to-transplant devices, 161–62, 172, 177, 181, 185, 190, 192, 200, 203, 209; clinical trials for, 181, 182, 184, 197, 198, 199–200, 202–5, 207, 208, 214–21, 235–38; commercialization of, 189, 193–94, 196–97, 203, 204–5, 207–10, 321n98; as compared with TAHs, 181–82, 205–6, 209–10; complications associated with, 188, 204, 216–17, 218, 233; continuous-flow, 213–14, 221, 222–27, 228–33, 237–39; costs of developing, 206–7; costs of, for patients, 219; data collection relating to, 233–34; as destination therapy, 214, 219; development of, 26–27, 30, 180–83, 206–9; FDA involvement in development and approval of, 181, 184, 200, 201, 203; government funding for research and development of, 171, 172, 178, 181, 182–85, 188, 195, 207, 215, 224; implantable, 190–94; as implanted in patients, 187–88, 190, 192–93, 194; infection management relating to, 217, 218; malfunctions of, 218–19; marketing of, 208, 236; Medicare reim-

bursement for, 209; national coverage determination for, 209; photographs of, 186, 193; power sources for, 190, 191, 206, 225; premarket approval for, 196–97; prevalence of, 261–62; randomized controlled trials of, 201, 202, 214–21, 235; second-generation, 210, 213–14, 232–33, 238; and TAH research, 240–41; temporary versus permanent use of, 221; third-generation, 234–35; venture capital for, 206–7. *See also* HeartMate LVAD; HeartMate VE LVAD; Hemopump; Jarvik 2000 Flowmaker Pump; Novacor LVAS; Thoratec PVAD system
Versa Capital Management LCC, 258
Vineberg, Arthur, 16
Vlaco, Duson, 72
Volkmer, Harold, 123

Walker, Rich, 5
Wampler, Richard, 10, 222, 223, 224, 228, 321n94
Wangensteen, Owen, 67
Warburg Pincus and Company, 162, 228
Washkansky, Louis, 68
Watson, John, 10, 206, 276n60; and the artificial heart program, 132, 143, 171, 183–84
Watson, Thomas, 17
wearable artificial kidney (WAK), 126
Weisse, Allen, 51
Westaby, Stephen, 217, 230, 233, 232n31
Westinghouse Electric, 98, 101–3, 295n50
White, Paul Dudley, 11, 13
White, Virginia Mae, 71
Wilson, Carole, 113
Wolfe, Sidney, 170
Woolley, F. Ross, 135, 166
WorldHeart Corporation, 184, 207, 220, 325n54
Wyngaarden, James B., 172

Zion, Libby, 174
Zoll, Paul, 19–20